# Sexually Transmitted Diseases

L.C. Parish F. Gschnait
Editors

# Sexually Transmitted Diseases

## A Guide for Clinicians

With 145 Illustrations

Springer-Verlag New York Berlin Heidelberg
London Paris Tokyo

Lawrence Charles Parish, M.D.
Clinical Professor of Dermatology and Director, Jefferson Center for International Dermatology, Jefferson Medical College, Thomas Jefferson University, Philadelphia, Pennsylvania 19107, USA
Visiting Professor of Dermatology, Yonsei University College of Medicine, Seoul, South Korea

Friedrich Gschnait, M.D.
Associate Professor of Dermatology and Venerology, University of Vienna, and Chief, Department of Dermatology, City Hospital Vienna-Lainz, 1130 Vienna, Austria

Library of Congress Cataloging-in-Publication Data
Sexually transmitted diseases; a guide for clinicians/ [edited by]
Lawrence Charles Parish and Friedrich Gschnait.
p. cm.
Includes bibliographies and index.
1. Sexually transmitted diseases—Handbooks, manuals, etc.
I. Parish, Lawrence Charles. II. Gschnait, F.
[DNLM: 1. Sexually Transmitted Diseases. WC 140 551763]
RC200.S496 1988
616.95' 1—dc19
DNLM/DLC 88-16004
Printed on acid-free paper.


Softcover reprint of the hardcover 1st edition 1989



Typeset by Publishers Service, Bozeman, Montana.

9 8 7 6 5 4 3 2 1

ISBN-13: 978-1-4612-8142-9 e-ISBN-13: 978-1-4612-3528-6
DOI: 10.1007/978-1-4612-3528-6

*To*
*Sheila and Irene*

# Introduction

In 1943, the introduction of penicillin therapy for the treatment of syphilis had great promise for the demise of venereal diseases, or so the optimists thought. Had not the same scenario been written nearly 40 years before, when 606 was to eradicate the newly identified treponeme? By the 1950s, academic institutions were deleting syphilology from the title of departments of dermatology, and the American Board of Dermatology and Syphilology adopted a more concise name [1].

Such haste! By the 1970s, public health authorities were reporting increases in the incidence of infectious syphilis. Gonorrhea was now not so easily treated, as resistant strains of *Neisseria gonococcus* were being recognized. Chancroid and lymphogranuloma venereum were going unrecognized, as physicians had assumed that they were nearly extinct or were simply weird tropical diseases.

Then came the autoimmune deficiency syndrome. Although we know the exact day and location when syphilis arrived in Florence [2], our knowledge of AIDS is less exact. In fact, we understand little more than the truism that AIDS is not simply a punishment for the promiscuous. Just as syphilis swept much of the civilized world, so this newly recognized viral epidemic is affecting both the heterosexual and the homosexual population, the sexually active, and even infants.

*Chlamydia trachomatis*, an organism whose recognition may have been limited in the older textbooks of venereal disease, is now known to cause 4 million infections a year in the United States. The cost of this sexually transmitted disease exceeds $1.4 billion annually [3]. Yet much of the population is unaware of this condition.

"*Syphilis in the Innocent*" [4] may have been a Victorian term, but congenital syphilis is again appearing. In Zambia, 20 to 30% of perinatal deaths are thought to be due to syphilis [5]. Even in developed countries, congenital syphilis is becoming a problem, particularly in children of teenage mothers who have had no prenatal care.

The facts are very evident. There is a crisis in contemporary society. Sexually transmitted diseases are increasing in number and in the damage and destruction they cause. No longer can observers be content to say: "Men persist in seeing themselves as erection machines" [6]. Sexually transmitted diseases can involve everyone, not just overtly sexually active people. This guide is designed to bring the practitioner up to date on the various aspects of conditions and diseases considered to be sexually transmitted.

## References

1. Crissey JT, Denenholz DA: Development of the modern forms and concepts of syphilis. *Clin Dermatol*, **2**(1):1–10, 1984.
2. Panconesi E, Mazzi M: The day syphilis came. *Int J Dermatol*, **23**:284–286, 1984.
3. Washington AE, Johnson RE, Sanders LL: *Chlamydia trachomatis* infections in the United States: What are they costing us? *JAMA*, **257**:2070–2074, 1987.
4. Bulkley LD: *Syphilis in the Innocent*. New York: Bailey and Fairchild, 1894.
5. Syphilis: Major perinatal killer. *Med World Trib*, **28**(16):2, 1987.
6. Renshaw DC: Management of impotence. I. Psychological considerations. *Clin Therap*, **9**:142–148, 1987.

*Acknowledgments*. We are very grateful to our teachers for the stimulation they provided in our studies of dermatology and sexually transmitted diseases. We particularly acknowledge the impetus given by Herman Beerman, M.D., Emeritus Professor of Dermatology, University of Pennsylvania School of Medicine, Philadelphia.

Our office staffs have been particularly helpful, and we would like to recognize the contributions of Mrs. Carmela Ciferni. Lastly, this book was conceived through the inspiration of Dr. Jerry Stone, late Senior Medical Editor of Springer-Verlag, New York.

Philadelphia, Pennsylvania — Lawrence Charles Parish
Vienna, Austria — Friedrich Gschnait

# Contents

# Contributors

FULVIO ALLEGRA, M.D.
Professore ordinario di Clinica Dermosifilopatica, Instituto di Clinica Dermosifilopatica, Universita di Parma, 43100 Parma, Italy

MOHAMED AMER, M.D.
Professor and Chairman of Dermatology and Venereology, University of Zagazig, Senior Consultant of Dermatology and Venereology, Zagazig University Medical Center, Zagazig, Egypt

HARRY L. ARNOLD, JR., M.D.
Clinical Professor of Dermatology, University of California School of Medicine; Attending Dermatologist, Children's Hospital of San Francisco, San Francisco, California 94118, USA

DANIEL S.F. CHENG, M.D., DIP., DERM. (London), DIP. VEN.
Associate Professor of Dermatology, China Medical College; Section Chief, Dermatology, China Medical College Hospital, Taichung, Taiwan, Republic of China

BLAISE L. CONGENI, M.D.
Associate Professor of Pediatrics, Northeastern Ohio University College of Medicine; Director, Infectious Disease Department, Children's Hospital, Akron, Ohio 44308, USA

JOHN THORNE CRISSEY, M.D.
Clinical Professor of Medicine (Dermatology), University of Southern California School of Medicine, Los Angeles, California 90330, USA

R.F.E. DE WIT, M.D.
Associate Professor of Dermatology and Venereology, University of Utrecht, Academische Ziekenhuis Utrecht, Utrecht 3511 GV, The Netherlands

PETER DUSCHET, M.D.
Staff Dermatologist, Hospital Vienna-Lainz, 1130 Vienna, Austria

JOSEPH EL-ON, PH.D.
Senior Lecturer in Microbiology and Immunology, Faculty of Health Sciences, Ben Gurion University of the Negev, Beer-Sheva, Israel

STEVEN D. EMMET, M.D.
Assistant Professor of Dermatology, University of California at San Diego School of Medicine, San Diego, California 92075, USA

BENJAMIN K. FISHER, M.D., F.R.C.P. (C.)
Associate Professor of Medicine (Dermatology), University of Toronto School of Medicine; Chief, Division of Dermatology, The Wellesley Hospital, Toronto, Ontario, M4Y 1J3, Canada

FRIEDRICH GSCHNAIT, M.D.
Associate Professor of Dermatology and Venereology, University of Vienna; Chief, Department of Dermatology, City Hospital Vienna-Lainz, Vienna, Austria

JERE D. GUIN, M.D.
Professor and Chairman of Dermatology, University of Arkansas for Medical Sciences; Chief of Dermatology, John L. McClellan Veterans Administration Hospital, Little Rock, Arkansas 72205, USA

MARIE LAGA, M.D.
Assistant in Microbiology, Institute of Tropical Medicine, 2000 Antwerp, Belgium

HILARY A. LAVERY, M.D., M.R.C.P. (UK)
Consultant Physician, Queen's University of Belfast; Consultant Physician, Department of Midwifery and Gynecology, Royal Victoria Hospital, Belfast, BT19 1UB, Northern Ireland

ANTON F.H. LUGER, M.D.
Hofrat, a.o. University Professor of Dermatology and Venereology, University of Vienna; Head, Ludwig Boltmann Institute for Dermato-venereological Seodiagnostics, 1130 Vienna, Austria

ANNE G. MATLOW, M.D., M.SC., F.R.C.P. (C.)
Assistant Professor of Medical Microbiology, University of Toronto School of Medicine; Consultant, Infectious Diseases, The Wellesley and Princess Margaret Hospitals, Toronto, Ontario M4Y 1J3, Canada

LOIS Y. MATSUOKA, M.D.
Associate Professor of Dermatology, Jefferson Medical College, Thomas Jefferson University, Philadelphia, Pennsylvania 19107, USA

LARRY E. MILLIKAN, M.D.
Professor and Chairman of Dermatology, Tulane University School of Medicine, New Orleans, Louisiana 70112, USA

TOMASZ F. MROCZKOWSKI, M.D.
Assistant Professor of Venereology, Medical Academy, Warsaw, Poland; Visiting Professor of Dermatology, Tulane University School of Medicine, New Orleans, Louisiana 70112, USA

MICHIHITO NIIMURA, M.D., PH.D.
Professor and Chairman of Dermatology, The Jikei University School of Medicine, Tokyo 105, Japan

LAWRENCE CHARLES PARISH, M.D.
Clinical Professor of Dermatology and Director, Jefferson Center for International Dermatology, Jefferson Medical College, Thomas Jefferson University, Philadelphia, Pennsylvania 19107 USA; Visiting Professor of Dermatology, Yonsei University College of Medicine, Seoul, South Korea

PETER PIOT, M.D.
Professor of Microbiology, Institute of Tropical Medicine, 2000 Antwerp, Belgium

ROBERT L. RIETSCHEL, M.D.
Associate Chairman of Dermatology, Ochsner Clinic; Clinical Associate Professor of Dermatology, Tulane University School of Medicine; Clinical Assistant Professor of Dermatology, Louisiana State University Medical School, New Orleans, Louisiana 70121, USA

BARBARA M. ROCK, M.D.
Senior Clinical and Research Fellow in Dermatology and Immunodermatology, Johns Hopkins School of Medicine, Baltimore, Maryland 21205, USA

ALLAN R. RONALD, M.D., F.R.C.P. (C.)
Distinguished Professor and Chairman of Internal Medicine, University of Manitoba; Physician-in-Chief of Internal Medicine, Health Sciences Centre, Winnipeg, Manitoba R3E 0Z3, Canada

VIRENDRA N. SEHGAL, M.B., B.S., M.D.
Professor and Head of Dermatology and Venereology, Maulana Azad Medical College and Associated Lok Nayak Jai Prakash Narain and Govind Ballabh Pant Hospitals, New Delhi; Member, Faculty of Medical Sciences, Academic Council and Board of Research Studies, Head of Group of Gynecology and Obstetrics, Dermatology and Venereology and Radiology, University of Delhi, Delhi 110 033, India

KEVIN J. SHANLEY, D.V.M.
Assistant Professor of Dermatology, University of Pennsylvania School of Veterinary Medicine, Philadelphia, Pennsylvania 19104, USA

ANGELIKA STARY, M.D.
Senior Physician for Dermatology and Venereology, Hospital Vienna-Lainz, 1130 Vienna, Austria; Head of Institute for Diagnosis of Infectious Venerologic-Dermatologic Diseases, 1210 Vienna, Austria.

DOWLING B. STOUGH, III, M.D.
Chief Resident in Dermatology, University of Arkansas for Medical Sciences, Little Rock, Arkansas 72205, USA

LEONARD C. WARNER, M.D.
Resident in Internal Medicine, Sunnybrook Medical Center, Toronto, Ontario, Canada

LOUIS WEINRAUCH, M.D.
Lecturer in Dermatology and Venereology, Hadassah Medical School, Hebrew University; 91120 Jerusalem, Israel

JOSEPH A. WITKOWSKI, M.D.
Clinical Professor of Dermatology, University of Pennsylvania School of Medicine; Philadelphia, Pennsylvania 19104, USA

REYNOLD C. WONG, M.D.
Clinical Instructor of Dermatology, University of California at Davis, School of Medicine, Davis, California 95616, USA

# What are Sexually Transmitted Diseases?

CHAPTER 1

# History

Lois Y. Matsuoka

Sexually transmitted (venereal) diseases have been associated with human beings for thousands of years. Anthropologic studies have found bone changes compatible with syphilis in skeletons of prehistoric North and South American and European humans [1,2]. Descriptions of venereal diseases can be found in the earliest written records, including Chinese (2697 B.C.), Biblical (approximately 3000 B.C.), Hindu (1000 B.C.), and Greek (460 B.C.) [1,3,4]. For example, Chinese scholars during the reign of Huang-ti (China, 2697 B.C.) provided a detailed description of a venereal disease that appears to be syphilis. They noted the appearance of a genital chancre followed by a skin eruption and delayed manifestations (oral lesions, destruction of nasal septum, etc.) [3].

## Ancient and Medieval Experience

The clinical recognition of syphilis was promptly followed by the institution of preventive measures to control the spread of the disease. In the first five books of Moses, the Bible prescribes strict legal penalties for illicit sexual behavior, and recommends careful hygiene and sexual quarantine for married couples [4].

Western civilization followed a similar pattern of awareness of sexually transmitted diseases. Hippocrates (Greece, 460 B.C.) mentioned genital lesions that followed sexual contact [5]. Celsus (Rome, 30 A.D.) distinguished between the dry, clean genital ulcer and the moist, purulent type [3]. Galen (Greece, born 131 A.D.) coined the word *gonorrhea* to describe the semen-like flow draining from the urethra. He also described "moist, ulcerating tubercles," which may be analogous to the mucous patches of secondary syphilis. Galen also characterized a chronic stage of disease with ulcerating and "serpiginous affection of the tibia" and deep-seated pain that he believed originated from direct involvement of bones and periosteum [3].

By the end of the 16th century, clinicians were fully aware of the consequences of syphilis. Fevri (Italy, 1538) gave descriptions of the oral, cutaneous, and joint involvements [6]. The neurologic involvement had been described in detail by Massa (Italy, 1532) [6,7] and the syphilitic etiology of aortic aneurysm of syphilis by Paré (France, 1510–1590) [6,7]. The contagiousness of syphilis was noted by Cataneus

(Italy, 1505) [6]. Treatment with mercury salts and arsenic was widespread and thought to be beneficial by Paracelsus (Switzerland, 1493–1541) [6]. The name *syphilis* was coined by the Italian pathologist Girolamo Fracastoro in 1530. He gave a clinical description of the disease affecting a shepherd named Syphilus in his poem, "Syphilis Sive Morbus Gallicus" [8].

## Early Research

An experiment performed by the Scottish physician John Hunter in 1767 represents a milestone in the understanding of venereal disease [9]. Hunter inoculated his own penis with a lancet dipped in pus obtained from a patient with a genital lesion and was able to document, for the first time, transmission of a venereal disease via a nonsexual route. The lesion that resulted is still known as the Hunterian chancre. As a marginal note, because the pus donor was simultaneously affected by gonorrhea and also incubating syphilis, Hunter concluded, mistakenly, that gonorrhea and syphilis were a single disease.

The first controlled study of venereal disease was performed by Ricord (France, 1838) and involved inoculations of 2,500 "normal" volunteers [6]. Ricord clearly defined gonorrhea and syphilis as distinct disease entities and delineated syphilis into three phases: primary, secondary, and late or tertiary [7].

The histopathology of syphilis was described in detail by Virchow (Germany, 1854). He noted infiltrative changes with typical histologic features in the organs and tissues of patients affected with syphilis. On the basis of his own observations and those of Ricord, Virchow developed a comprehensive understanding of the pathophysiology of syphilis by establishing the correlation between distribution of the infection through the blood and disease activity or apparent inactivity [6]. All this took place before the actual discovery of the causative organism.

The cause of gonorrhea and its unique characteristic as a separate venereal disease were established by Neisser (Germany, 1879). He discovered the gonococcus after isolation of the bacteria from purulent secretions of urethritis, cervicitis, and conjunctivitis [10]. Bumm (Germany, 1885) was able to maintain the gonococcus organism in pure cultures and to inoculate the infective organism in "normal volunteers," fulfilling all of Koch's postulates [10].

Schaudinn and Hoffmann (Germany, 1905) were finally able to see the mobile spirochete (*Treponema pallidum*) in fresh, unstained material, using a primitive type of darkfield microscope. Schaudinn and Hoffmann simply used an ordinary microscope and cut the source of light to a very low level [6,11]. The microorganism became easier to visualize with the development of the true darkfield microscope by Landsteiner (Germany, 1907) [6]. A complement fixation blood test for the diagnosis of syphilis was subsequently developed by Wassermann (Germany, 1906) [12]. The availability of serologic testing made it possible to diagnose syphilis at a latent stage, when no outward manifestations were evident [12]. Ehrlich and Hata discovered the arsphenamine Salvarsan (compound 606) (Germany, 1910). Salvarsan, the precursor of modern chemotherapy, represented a partially effective agent for the treatment of syphilis [12].

## Venereal Disease Control

A number of approaches to venereal disease control were attempted during World War I. The French and German governments licensed prostitutes and mandated treatment [13,14]. More significantly, the British developed modern epidemiologic techniques for the control of venereal disease such as case findings, compulsory reporting, and follow-up of contacts [13,14]. Similar measures were adapted by the Medical Corps of the United States Armed Forces, at a time when it was estimated that 7.5% of men on active duty were affected with venereal disease [10]. These principles of sexual hygiene were extended to the civilian population during the post-World War I period by the U.S. Public Health Service [13,14].

## Other Sexually Transmitted Diseases

A recent advance in the field of venereal disease has been the inclusion of conditions that were previously considered to be of a nonvenereal nature. Current evidence strongly indicates a sexual mechanism of transmission for *Chlamydia trachomatis, Entamoeba histolytica, Giardia lamblia,* and hepatitis A and B [15]. The latest addition to this list is the acquired immune deficiency syndrome (United States, 1981) [16]. This sexually transmitted disease has a highly unusual clinical presentation characterized by absence of local alterations at genital areas but profound and lethal involvement of the immune system [15,16]. Calling it GRID, the homosexual disease, or AIDS does not changes its etiology.

### References


1. Buret F: *Syphilis in Ancient and Prehistoric Times.* Philadelphia: FA Davis, 1891, pp. 34–35, 107–123.
2. Marshall CF, French EG: *Syphilis and Venereal Disease.* New York: Williams and Wood, 1921, pp. 4–6.
3. Lancereaux E: *A Treatise on Syphilis.* London: New Sydenham Society, 1868, pp. 8–13.
4. Leviticus 15,16.
5. Kelly EC: *Hippocrates: Theory and Practice of Medicine.* New York: Philosophical Library, 1964.
6. Goodman, H: *Notable Contributions to the Knowledge of Syphilis.* New York: Froben Press, 1944, pp.30,38–40,88–89,95,115–116.
7. Garrison FH: *An Introduction to the History of Medicine.* Philadelphia: WB Saunders, 1929, pp. 204–208,225,416.

8. Fracastoro G: *Fracastor Syphilis: Or the French Disease: A Poem in Latin Hexameters.* London: William Heineman, 1935.
9. Hunter J: Experiments made to ascertain the progress and effects of the venereal poison, 1786. Quoted in S. Rapport, H. Wright: *Great Adventures in Medicine.* New York: Dial Press, 1961, pp. 162–165.
10. Brown WJ, Donohue JF, Axnick NW, Blount JH, Elven NH, Jones D: *Syphilis and Other Venereal Disease.* Cambridge: Harvard Press, 1958, p. 83.
11. Dennie C: *A History of Syphilis.* Springfield, Ill.: Charles C Thomas, 1962, pp. 93–95.
12. Singer C, Underwood E: *A Short History of Medicine.* New York: Oxford Press, 1962, pp. 417–690.
13. Holmes KK, Mardh P, Sparling PF, et al: *Sexually Transmitted Disease.* New York: McGraw-Hill, 1984, pp. 30–35.
14. Brandt AM: *No Magic Bullet.* New York: Oxford University Press, 1987, pp. 7–161.
15. Oxtrow D, Sandholzer T, Felman Y: *Sexually Transmitted Disease in Homosexual Men: Diagnosis, Treatment and Research.* New York: Plenum Press, 1982, pp. 1–272.
16. U.S. Department of Health and Human Services: Morbidity and Mortality Weekly Report, June 5, 1981.

# CHAPTER 2

# Definition

Harry L. Arnold, Jr.

The world moves on, and as it moves it becomes less simple. Once it was sufficient to speak of "venereal disease," or "VD." But people read something into *venereal* (not originally there) that seemed to exclude conjugal sexual relations. That was not unintentional, or unreasonable; but no matter–it was a bit misleading. Thus, the term "sexually transmitted diseases"–STD– was born, probably about 1950, give or take a decade.

## Truly Sexually Transmitted Diseases

Strictly speaking, the term should be reserved for diseases transmitted most often by sexual intercourse, oftener than in other ways involving comparably intimate contact. Diseases caused by microbes requiring almost constant moisture and warmth, like *Treponema pallidum* and *Neisseria gonorrheae,* had no trouble being included: Syphilis and gonorrhea were in the category of venereal diseases and were "grandfathered" as sexually transmitted (note: not *transmissible* but *transmitted*) from the start. Chancroid, too, was a member of the group from the beginning, for good reason: Certainly it is very rarely acquired from other than sexual activity. Granuloma inguinale likewise: Its location and the site of its complications establish its right to be included in the group. Condyloma acuminatum–in a franker day "venereal wart"–is very unlikely to be transmitted otherwise than in sexual intimacy, and so deserves inclusion in this category. The same is true of trichomoniasis.

The other diseases often classified as sexually transmitted are not so secure in their classification. All of them are undoubtedly transmitted far more commonly by asexual contact; however, they are likely not to *fail* to be transmitted under conditions of intimacy, and by such reverse reasoning it seems proper to include them under the broad umbrella of sexually transmitted diseases. None of them, however–unlike those just mentioned–prompt the suspicion that they are transmitted sexually. Sometimes the site of the index lesion–on the genitalia in herpes "progenitalis," on the anterior pelvis or buttocks in molluscum contagiosum–can raise or lessen the suspicion of sexual transmission considerably.

## The Current Plague

Among the organisms responsible for sexually transmitted diseases, just one has no peer for its frightful pathogenic potential. It was originally called HTLV-III, because it was the third virus that preferentially infected T cells and modified their behavior; its predecessors were HTLV-I and HTLV-II. The initials stand for human T-cell lymphotropic virus no. 3. The virus causes AIDS—acquired immunodeficiency syndrome.

Its simultaneous discoverers in France named it LAV, for lymphadenopathy-associated virus, and it was also briefly known as ARV, or AIDS-related virus, but these names never were widely accepted. Since about 1984 it has been generally called HIV-1, for human immunodeficiency virus.

Although all of these designations are formed like acronyms, only one—AIDS—is actually an acronym, because it is the only one that can be, and is, pronounced like a word. The others are examples of "initialese," or as the famous etymologist John Dirckx calls them, "initialisms."

In retrospect, it would be unwieldy to have to speak of "certainly," "probably," and "possibly" sexually transmitted diseases, and as a practical matter, we can probably do no better than to speak and write of just "sexually transmitted diseases" and let the qualifying adjective remain implicit. It is a pragmatic solution.

# Diseases

CHAPTER 3

# Syphilis

John Thorne Crissey

Once the most feared and formidable of the sexually transmitted diseases, syphilis is much diminished now in the eyes of both the public and the medical profession. The worldwide drop in incidence, the virtual disappearance of the late, destructive forms of the disease, and the ease with which it can be treated with antibiotics have all contributed to this decline. Yet the situation is dangerous. The number of cases falls now in the troublesome zone—high enough to ensure that health care providers in urban settings will inevitably be confronted with examples in practice, but not high enough to maintain the index of suspicion necessary for routine recognition of the disease. In 1986, 27,098 new cases of primary and secondary syphilis were reported in the United States, up very slightly from 1985 (26,868). It was the second most common reportable disease, a distant second to gonorrhea, but more common than any single form of viral hepatitis [1].

## Definition

Syphilis is a chronic, contagious infection caused by *Treponoma pallidum.* It is usually contracted through sexual activities, is often self-limited, and is characterized in its course by an extraordinary variety of clinical manifestations [2–6].

## Clinical Findings

With respect to signs and symptoms, syphilis is an intermittent disease. After an incubation period of 9 to 90 days, a primary lesion appears. This is often followed by multiple generalized manifestations, referred to collectively as the secondary stage. Untreated, these manifestations heal spontaneously, sometimes reappear briefly, heal again, and are followed in a minority of cases by late or tertiary lesions entirely different from the early forms of the disease. Latent syphilis, that is, the period between healing of the secondary signs and the appearance (if any) of late manifestations, is now divided in the United States into early (1 year or less), and late (more than 1 year). In Europe the dividing time is often set at 2 years. It is

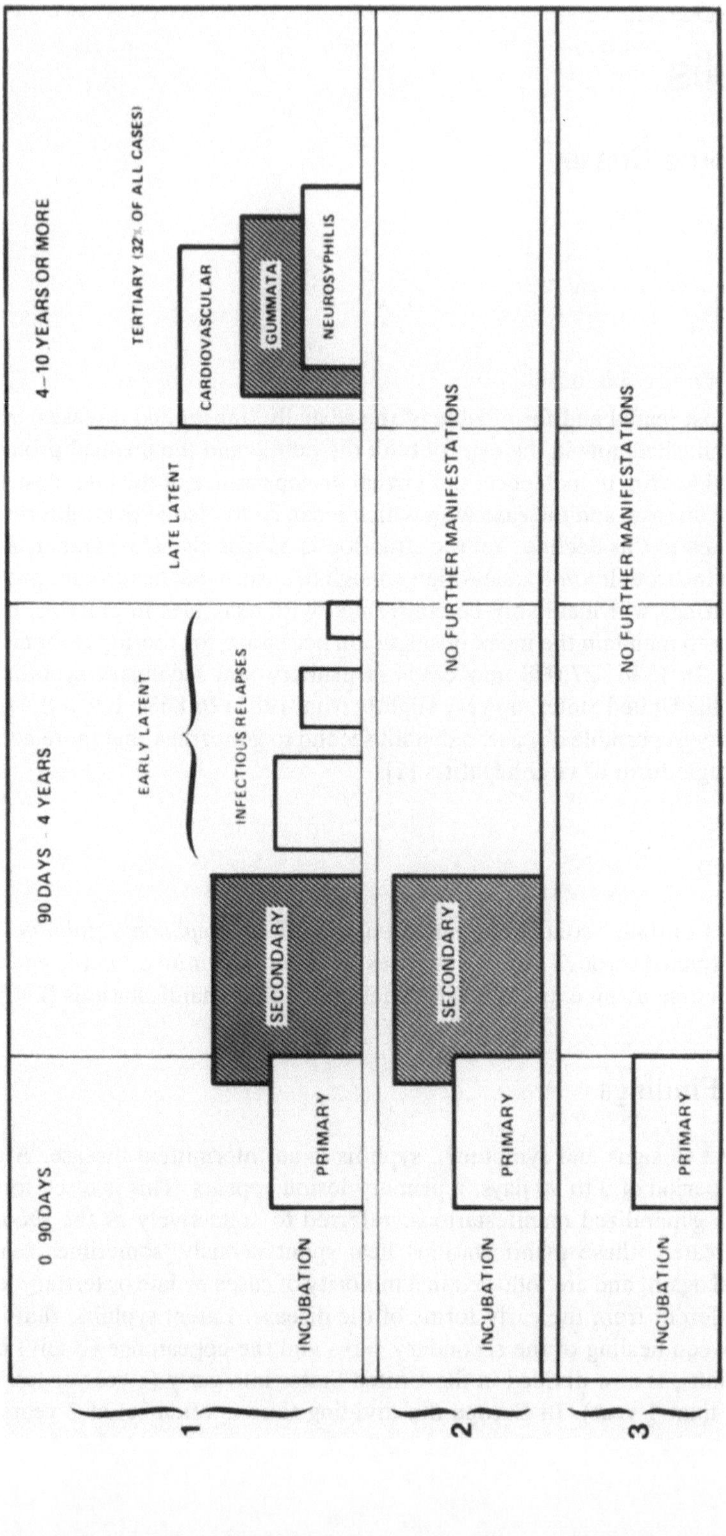


FIGURE 3.1. Common variations in the course of syphilis.

presumed that early latent cases are potentially infectious, while late latent cases are not. Common variations in the course of syphilis are shown diagrammatically in Figure 3.1.

## Primary Syphilis

The primary lesion, or chancre, begins as a reddish macule, often at a point of injury and usually on the genitalia. It is usually solitary. The coronal sulcus of the penis and the labia majora are the most common sites, but no area is exempt. Extragenital chancres occur most often on the lip and finger. Figures 3.2 through 3.4 show typical lesions.

In a day or two the initial macule becomes papular, firm or cartilaginous to the feel, and develops a central erosion. Fully developed chancres vary in size from a few millimeters to several centimeters. Borders are sharp and often delineated by a fine hemorrhagic line. The central erosion does not bleed easily, and unless complicated, the edges are not undermined, ragged, or necrotic. The base of the erosion is clean, the color of raw muscle, and is commonly covered with a faint grayish pellicle. Exudate, when present, is serous.

Chancres are seldom painful. The are indolent, persisting 3 to 8 weeks before healing spontaneously, and they leave either no trace or a faint atrophic scar. Regional lymphadenitis appears a week or so after the primary lesion in 70 to 80% of cases. The palpable nodes are firm and rubbery, not fixed to surrounding tissue, and not tender. Characteristics of the typical primary lesion are shown in Table 3.1.

Exceptions to the usual clinical findings are not uncommon. Chancres may be multiple, especially when they are superimposed, so to speak, on the lesions of herpes progenitalis or scabies. Induration may be lacking, so the lesion appears as a simple nondescript erosion. Edema at the site of the lesion may be massive, especially around chancres of the female genitalia. Primary syphilis in men can present as balanoposthitis, with moderate to severe swelling of the glans and foreskin.

Table 3.1. Characteristics of the typical primary lesion.

| |
|---|
| Tends to be single rather than multiple |
| Has relatively long incubation period (10 to 90 days) |
| Is relatively painless when uncomplicated |
| Is indurated |
| Features an eroded surface rather than ulceration |
| Is characterized by sharply defined border, limited by fine hemorrhagic line; border not undermined, ragged, or necrotic unless complicated |
| Has clean, raw-muscle-colored base, covered by faint grayish pellicle |
| Exudes serous rather than purulent material |
| Is indolent, persisting 3 to 8 weeks before healing |
| Is followed a week after appearance by development of painless, nontender, discrete, firm regional adenopathy |
| Heals with no trace or leaves thin atrophic scar |

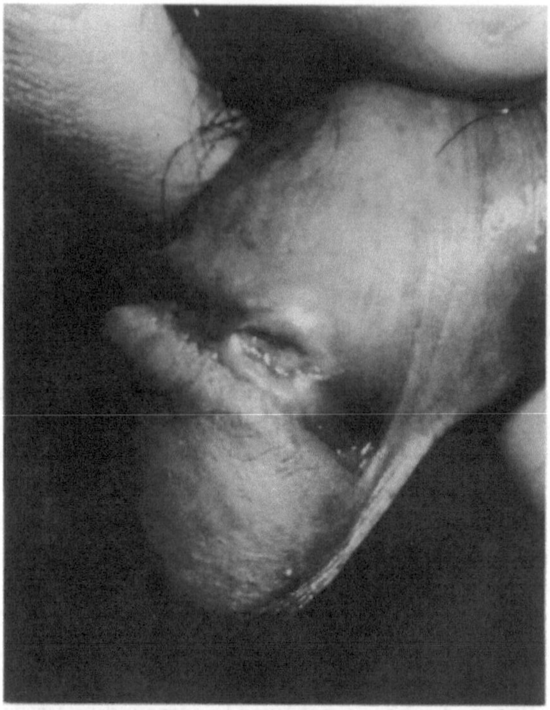
a

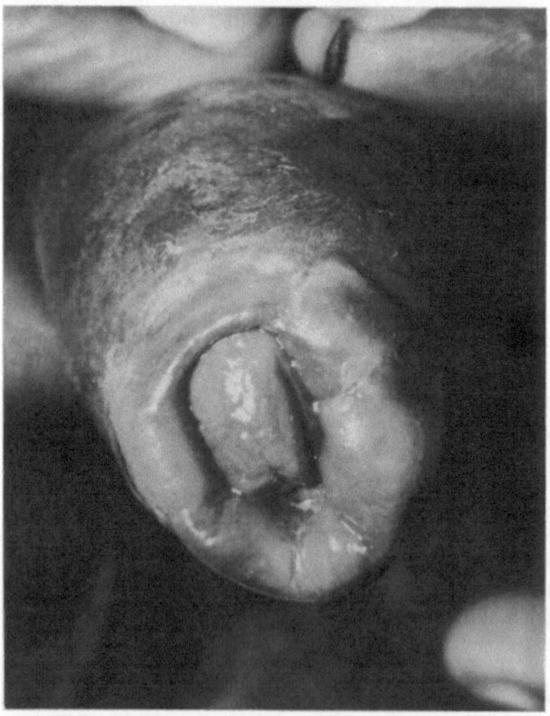
b

FIGURE 3.2. Primary syphilis. (a) Hunterian chancre, coronal sulcus. (b) Phimotic chancre.

FIGURE 3.3. Primary syphilis.
(a) Multiple chancres.
(b) Chancre, labium majorum.

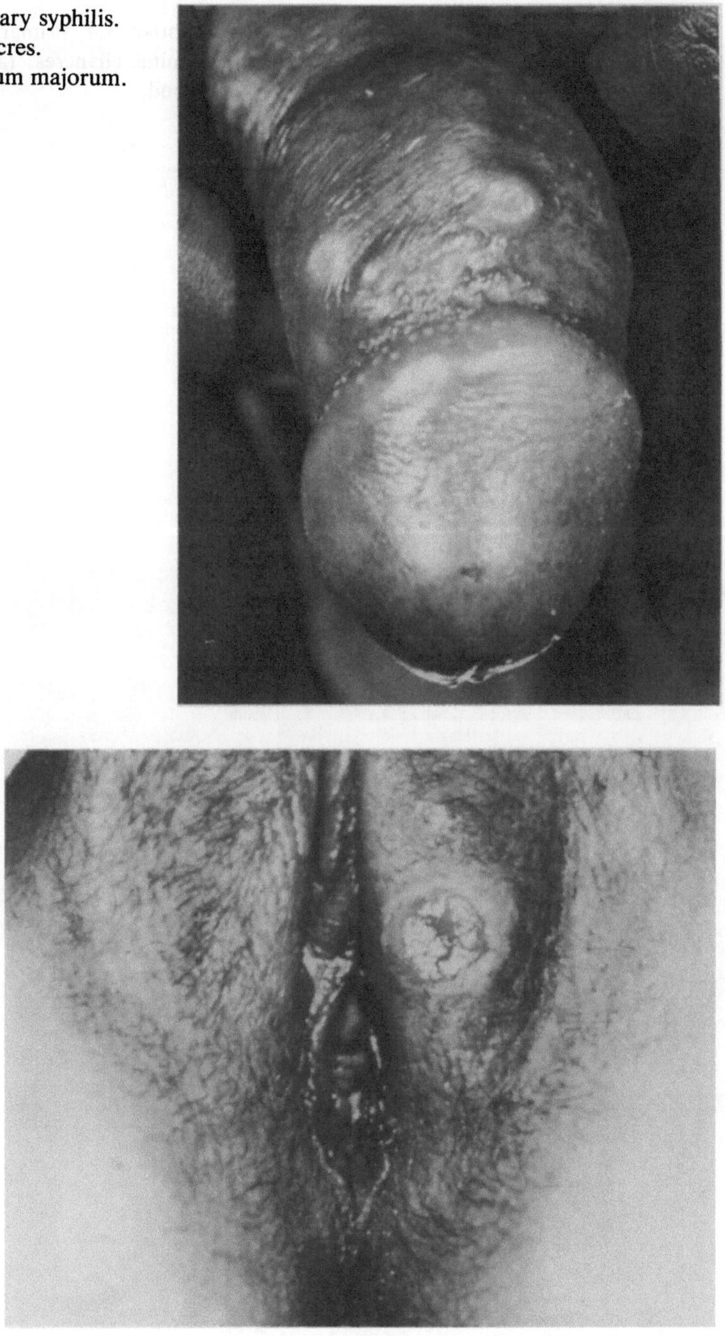

a

b

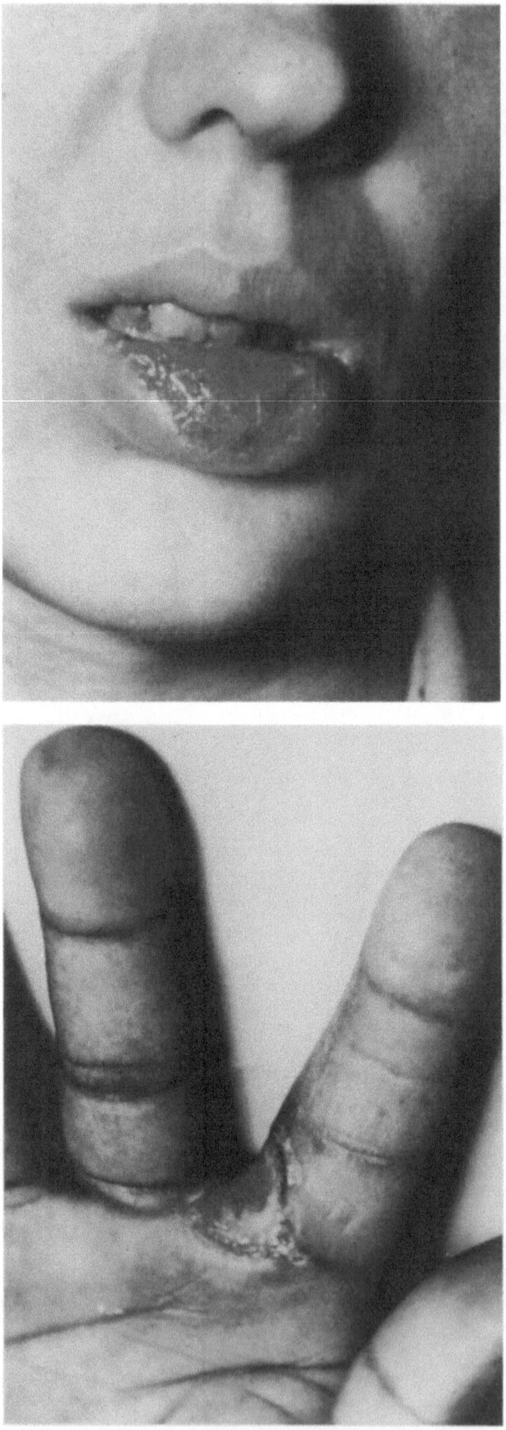

a

b

FIGURE 3.4. Primary syphilis, extragenital chancres. (a) Lower lip. (b) Hand.

## Secondary Syphilis

The line between primary and secondary stages is not sharp; in 15% of cases the chancre is still present when secondary signs appear. Typical lesions are shown in Figures 3.5 through 3.10. Signs and symptoms of secondary syphilis occur in perhaps half of the cases, and appear from 1 week to several months after the primary lesions, the average interval being 8 weeks.

Secondary syphilis often begins with a prodrome consisting of malaise, depression, low-grade fever, stiff neck, lacrimation, arthralgia, aching bones (especially at night), runny nose, and a distinct feeling that something is very wrong. In other instances, systemic symptoms are entirely absent. In decreasing order of frequency, organs and organ systems participating in the clinical picture of secondary syphilis are the skin and its appendages, throat and mouth, genitalia, central nervous system, eye, and viscera.

### Skin Lesions (Syphilids, Syphiloderms)

The integument is involved in more than 80% of cases. Many eruption varieties have been described, but fully 97% fall in one of four categories: macular, maculopapular, papular, and annular papular. Pustular syphilids occur, but unless complications are present, vesicles and bullae are never seen. The rashes of secondary syphilis are subacute. Unlike the exanthemata, they do not spring suddenly into existence, evolve rapidly, and vanish. Itching is not a prominent feature in most cases.

The macular syphilid, which makes up some 10% of cases, presents as discrete pink, oval spots 1 to 2 cm in diameter, faint and difficult to see. The spots are distributed on the flanks and over the shoulders, and to some extent on chest and back. Palms and soles are also involved, but except for the chin, which takes on a mottled appearance, the face and scalp are spared.

More common is the maculopapular syphilid that occurs in some 70% of the cases now seen in practice. Well illustrated in this form is the occurrence of the lesions of secondary syphilis in successive waves. Here lesions different in character from their predecessors, and usually more infiltrated, make their appearance before earlier lesions have healed. It is this phenomenon that results in the polymorphism seen in many syphilids. Previously macular lesions become thickened and assume darker copper-colored hues. Along with the trunk, the face is heavily involved, especially in the seborrheic areas and along the hairline (the corona veneris). Genital lesions are common. The highly distinctive discrete brownish or coppery macules and papules on palms and soles are a part of this picture; more than any other feature, this should alert the examiner to the possibility of syphilis. Papular forms on the palms and soles are often surrounded by a thin white ring or collar of scale, the "collarette of Biett," which, while not pathognomonic of syphilis, should certainly act as a clinical red flag.

Purely papular syphilids constitute some 4 to 12% of cases seen. The elementary lesion is an oval or circinate papule, 5 mm or so in diameter, reddish brown in color, and shiny. The lesions bear a striking resemblance to the papules of lichen planus. The polygonal shape of the latter, the violaceous color, and the absence of other

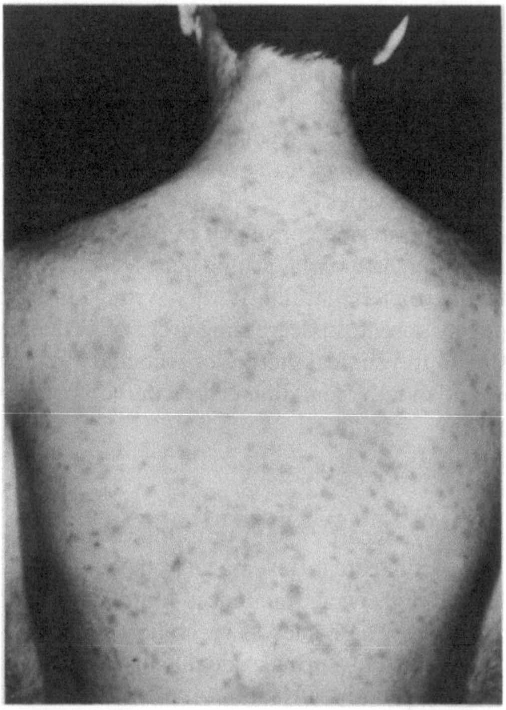
a

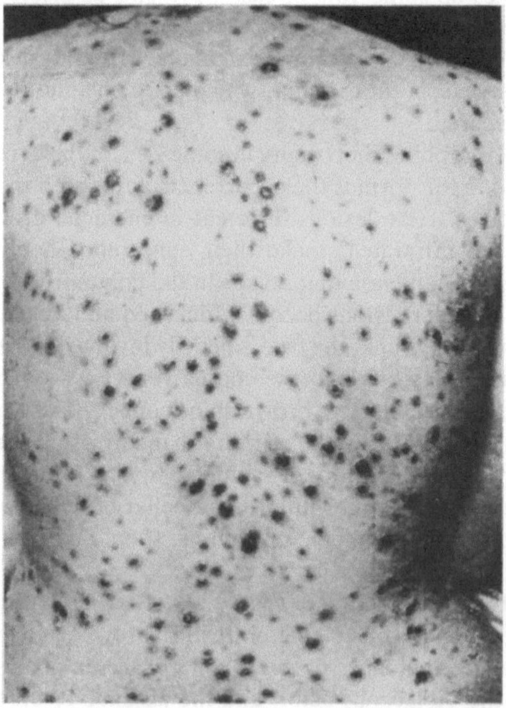
b

FIGURE 3.5. Secondary syphilis. (a) Maculopapular eruption on the neck and back. (b) Papulosquamous eruption on the back.

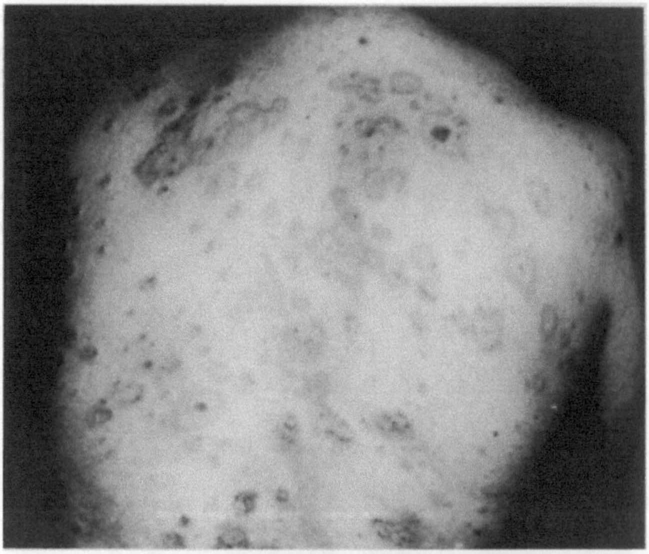

a

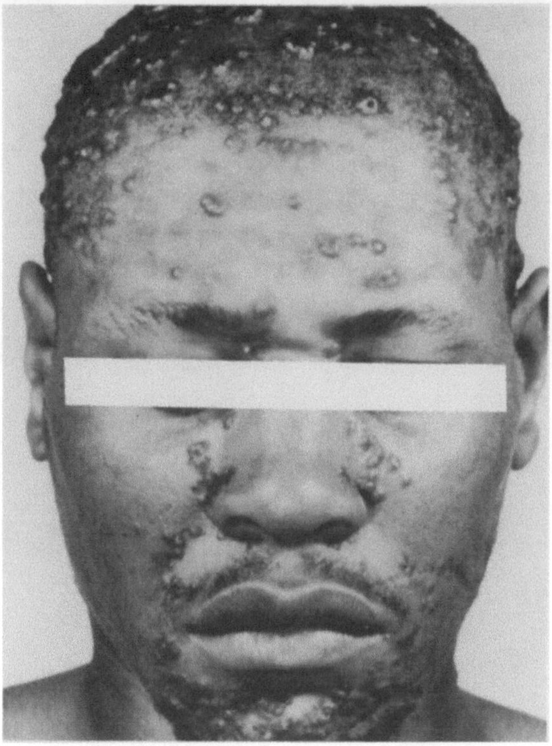

b

FIGURE 3.6. Secondary syphilis. (a) Annular papular eruption on the back. (b) Papular eruption with predilection for seborrheic areas. Note the corona veneris along the hairline.

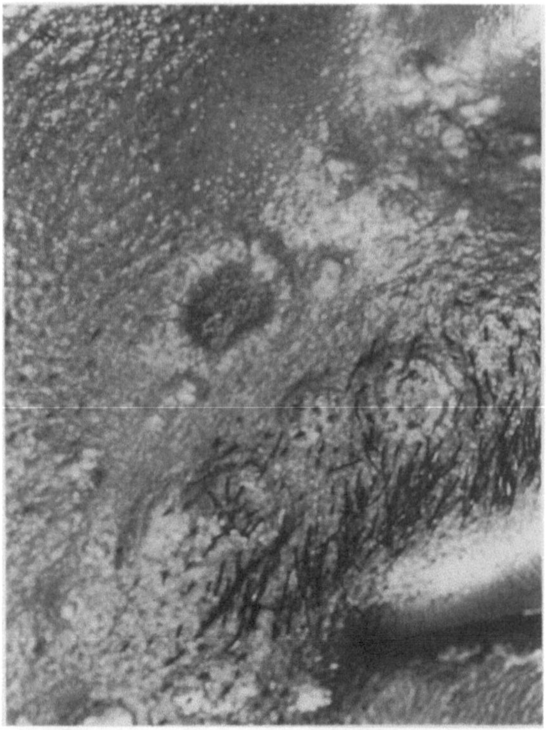

a

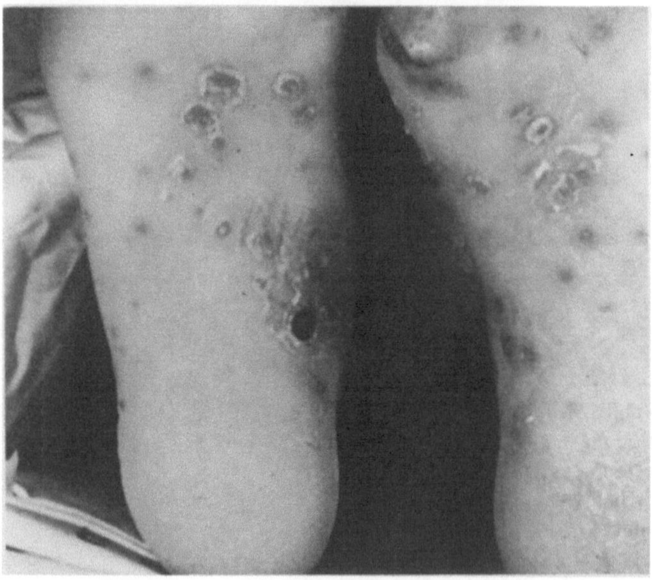

b

FIGURE 3.7. Secondary syphilis. (a) Annular papular eruption, upper lip and nasolabial fold. This is the "nickel and dime" syphilid. (b) Papular scaling eruption of the soles. The white rings of scales are examples of the "Collarette of Biett."

FIGURE 3.8. Secondary syphilis. (a) Distinctive coppery maculopapular eruption of the palms. (b) Mucous patches, lower lip.

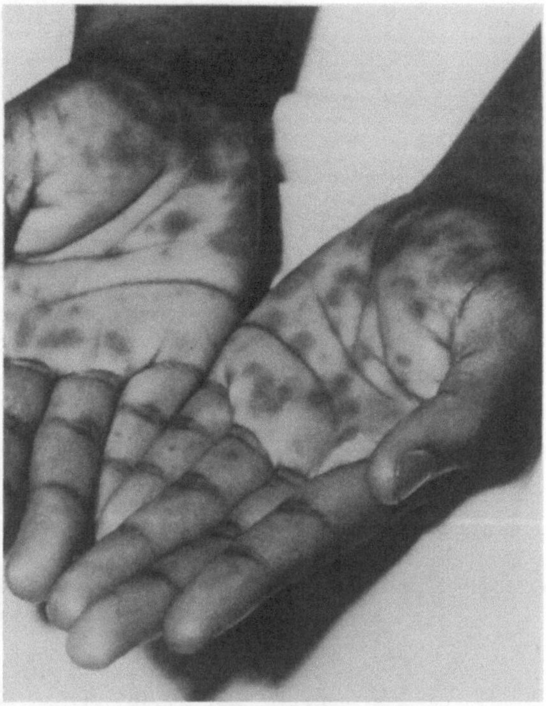

a

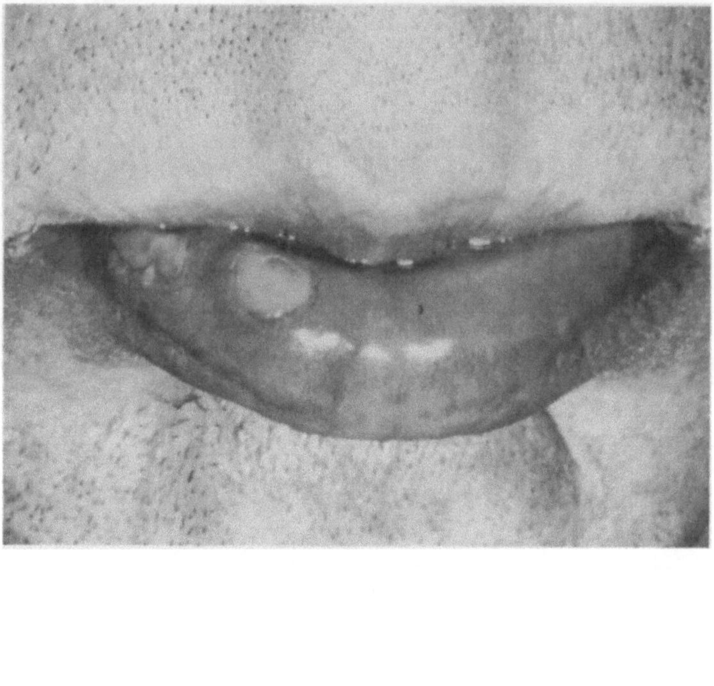

b

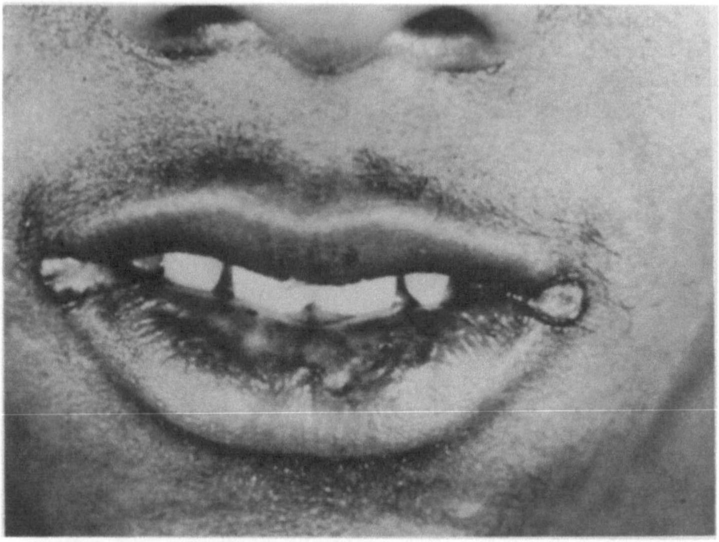

a

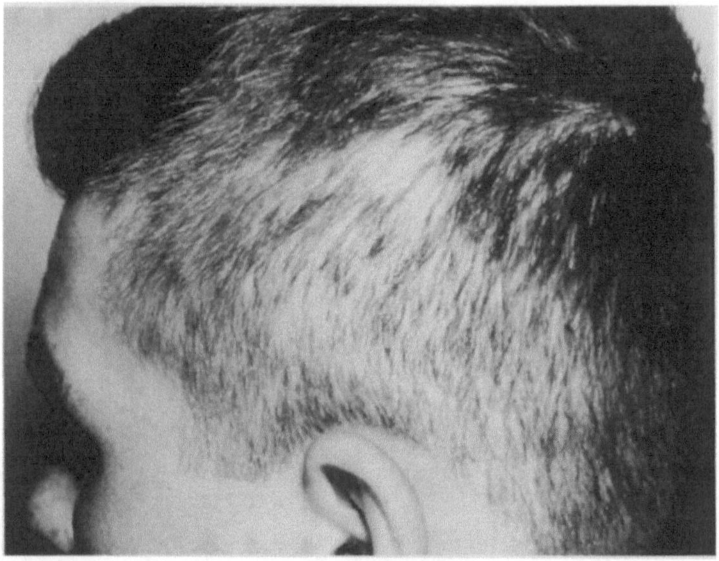

b

FIGURE 3.9. Secondary syphilis. (a) "Split papules" at the labial commissures. (b) "Moth eaten" alopecia.

FIGURE 3.10. Secondary syphilis. (a) Condylomata lata, posterior fourchette and perianal areas. (b) Condylomata lata, vulva.

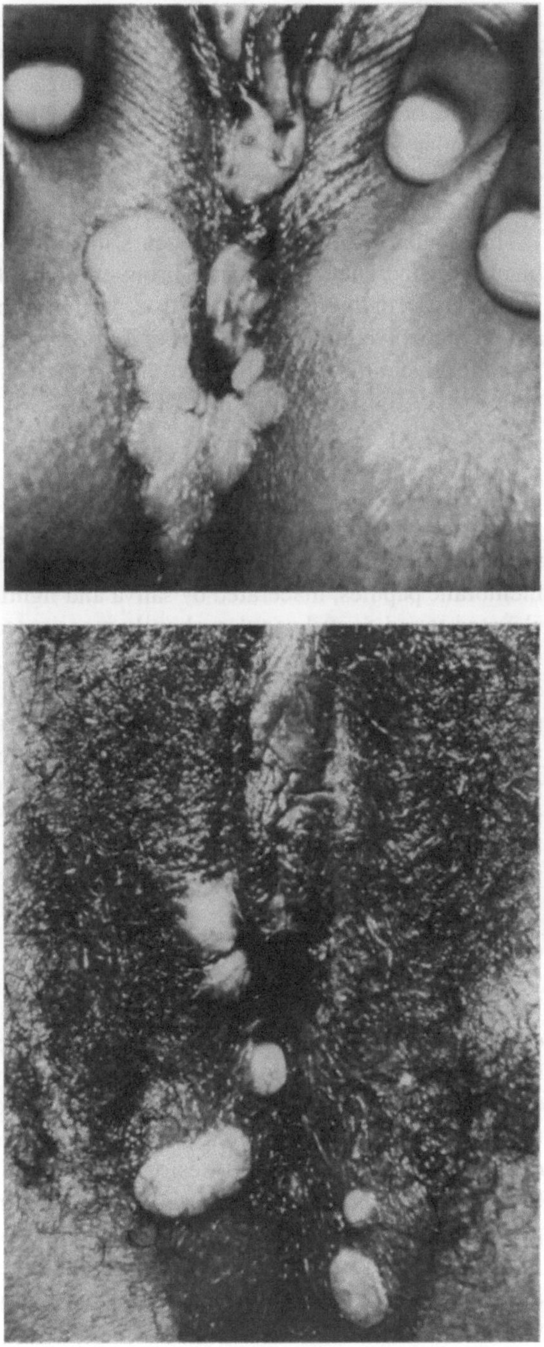

a

b

signs of secondary syphilis will usually allow the two diseases to be separated on clinical grounds alone. Scale is minimal on most lesions of the papular syphilid, but occasionally it is pronounced enough to suggest a diagnosis of guttate psoriasis. Again, the other signs of secondary syphilis will usually point to the correct diagnosis. Papular syphilids show the same distribution as the maculopapular variety. Older syphilitic papules on palms and soles can also take the form of small corns or punctate keratoses (clavi syphilitica).

The annular papular syphilid occurs in about 6% of cases and is largely seen in black patients. The lesions have a pronounced tendency to ring configurations. Anogenital areas, palms and soles, axillae, periumbilical areas, and particularly the face are often involved. In the latter case, in the United States the disease is often called "the nickel and dime syphilid", and in fact the lesions often do assume the approximate size of those coins.

### Mucous Membrane Lesions

A transient diffuse redness of the throat may occur—"syphilitic sore throat"—but more characteristic are the so-called mucous patches. They are essentially mucous membrane papules, macerated by saliva and lightly eroded. They appear as slightly elevated round or oval papules, sharply marginated, 5 to 12 mm in diameter, faintly inflammatory, and covered with a pearly or grayish membrane. No part of the mouth is exempt. Lesions on the tongue are particularly striking because of the loss of papillae. Lesions at the labial commissures may take the form of "split" or fissured papules, easily confused with ordinary pèrleche. Mucocutaneous lesions in the genitalia and anal areas may resemble mucous patches or nondescript-looking erosions, and sometimes raise up as the exuberant excrescences known as condylomata lata. These condylomata vary in morphology from slightly pedunculated, flat, papular lesions, smooth and buttonlike, to large cauliflowerlike vegetations.

### Other Signs of Secondary Syphilis

More or less generalized lymphadenopathy occurs in more than 85% of cases and is one of the most important clinical signs of the disease. Nodes are nontender, rubbery, and discrete. They occur, in descending order of frequency, in the inguinal areas, axillae, cervical triangles, epitrochlear regions, and femoral and supraclavicular areas. A nonscarring patchy or "moth-eaten" scalp alopecia occurs in some 7% of cases of secondary syphilis. Lesions occur throughout the scalp, but are most visible at the margins, where the hair is cut short. Hair loss within the patches is incomplete, and the borders are not so sharp as in alopecia areata.

Periostitis is occasionally seen, especially in the long bones, where it shows itself as slightly swollen areas 1 or 2 cm in diameter, doughy to the touch and exquisitely tender.

Acute glomerulonephritis, which usually presents as the nephrotic syndrome, can occur. Liver involvement, with nontender hepatomegaly, is sometimes seen.

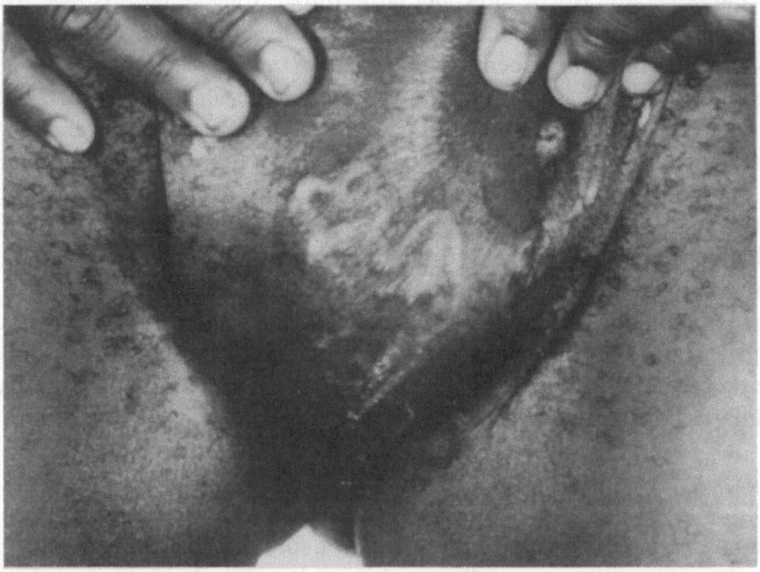

FIGURE 3.11. Relapsing syphilis. Annular lesions on the underside of the scrotum.

## Relapsing Syphilis

Some 20% or more of untreated cases of secondary syphilis that have healed without treatment will relapse within a year. Any manifestation of the secondary stage can reappear, but recurrence of mucous and mucocutaneous lesions is the usual story. Relapsing skin lesions show a marked predilection for the anogenital area and an increased tendency to assume annular forms (Fig. 3.11).

## Late Syphilis

It is convenient to discuss the manifestations of late syphilis under three headings: benign tertiary syphilis, cardiovascular syphilis, and neurosyphilis.

### Benign Tertiary Syphilis (BTS)

This designation includes all forms of symptomatic acquired syphilis occurring beyond the secondary or relapsing stages, with the exception of cardiovascular syphilis and neurosyphilis. BTS is sometimes also called late benign syphilis. The characteristic lesion is the granuloma called the gumma. Gummata occur in some 16% of cases of untreated syphilis. They appear as early as 2 years and as late as 35 years after the initial infection; the great majority appear in the 2- to 7-year range. All forms are now extremely rare.

Skin and bone are favorite sites, but nose, throat, tongue, larynx, eye, liver, and stomach may be involved. In the skin the lesions usually appear as firm pinkish or purplish nodules that spread centrifugally to form ring-shaped lesions with atrophic scars at the center and an indurated, hyperpigmented, ulcerated border. Eccentric spread and coalescence of several lesions can result in bizarre shapes and configurations. Cutaneous gummata can also present as a solitary dusky red nodule that breaks down to form a punched-out, clean, and more or less cylindrical ulcer, the floor of which is a tough, yellowish-white, chamois-like slough. Forehead, chin, neck, buttocks, and outer aspects of the thigh are the most common locations for cutaneous gummata, but no area can be considered immune.

Osseous gummata favor the long bones and the skull. These lesions usually present as painful, tender doughy swellings beneath the skin. Later the skin overlying the process can become livid. Gummata of the bones of the nose and face can result in gross disfigurement.

### Cardiovascular Syphilis

Once common, cardiovascular syphilis is now a rare disease. Some 10% of cases of untreated syphilis will show cardiovascular involvement. In most cases the disease appears from 5 to 15 years after the initial infection. In its simplest form, cardiovascular syphilis presents as an uncomplicated aortitis, usually involving the ascending aorta, producing neither signs nor symptoms and usually discovered postmortem. Aortitis may progress to the point where the weakened aortic wall dilates to form an aneurysm, again usually in the ascending portion. The danger of rupture in these cases is ever present and real. Coronary artery disease with stenosis and anginal symptoms is also sometimes seen in association with syphilitic aortitis. Syphilitic aortic valvular disease with valvular incompetence is another late complication and usually occurs in association with aortic aneurysm. Aortic regurgitation results, with volume overload, hypertrophy of the left ventricle, and eventually congestive heart failure.

### Neurosyphilis

Symptomatic involvement of the central nervous system develops in some 6 to 7% of cases of untreated syphilis. Neurosyphilis is seldom encountered now in practice, and has become more difficult than ever to diagnose because the disease, perhaps modified by subcurative doses of antibiotics administered for other diseases, seldom appears in its classic forms. But the diagnosis of neurosyphilis has never been easy; the disease can mimic other disturbances of the central nervous system in virtually every category. It is for this reason that examination of the cerebrospinal fluid is recommended as a part of the work-up in all cases of syphilis, especially beyond the primary stage. Neurological consultation is also recommended when either laboratory or clinical evidence of neurologic disease is encountered. The clinical varieties of neurosyphilis are outlined in Table 3.2.

TABLE 3.2. Classification of neurosyphilis.*

| Group | Type | Involvement |
|---|---|---|
| I | Asymptomatic | Abnormalities in cerebrospinal fluid with no signs or symptoms attributable to syphilis |
| II† | Meningeal and vascular | Diffuse: Increased intracranial pressure and cranial nerve palsies |
| | Cerebral meningeal | Focal (gummatous): Increased intracranial pressure; Focal cerebral symptoms and signs; slow in onset |
| | Cerebral vascular | Focal cerebral symptoms and signs, sudden in onset |
| | Spinal meningeal and vascular | Paresthesias, weakness, atrophy, and sensory loss in extremities and trunk |
| III | Parenchymatous | Neurons and axons degenerate |
| | | General paresis (paresis): Progressive mental deterioration, convulsions, coma, and death |
| | | Tabes dorsalis: Ataxia, areflexia, paresthesias, bladder and eye disturbances, impotence, and pain |
| | | Optic atrophy |

* Adapted from Merritt, Adams, and Solomon, pp. 5, 6;
† Overlap of groups II and III is not uncommon.

## Histopathology

Despite the extreme variability of the clinical signs and symptoms, the microscopic picture of syphilis is characterized by several relatively simple and constant features, the hallmarks of syphilis [2]:

1. Obliterative endarteritis, in which capillaries and arterioles exhibit swelling and proliferation of endothelial cells to produce partial or complete occlusion of the vessels.
2. Periarteritis, in which lymphocytes, monocytes, large numbers of plasma cells, and proliferating adventitial cells surround or "cuff" the dilated swollen vessels.

The basic changes may be found regardless of the anatomic site, stage of the disease, or appearance of the lesions. They are not always present, and cannot be called pathognomonic for syphilis. Nevertheless, they occur in the great majority of cases, and when noted, should always suggest the diagnosis.

## Natural History

Untreated, approximately one third of individuals with syphilis will develop some late manifestation of the disease. The 1955 study of Gjestland, in which 953 patients who had received no treatment in the early stages of syphilis were followed up, set the percentages as follows: benign tertiary lesions, 16.6%; cardiovascular syphilis,

9.7%; symptomatic neurosyphilis, 6.5%. Syphilis was judged to be the primary cause of death in 10.8% of the cases studied [7].

## Differential Diagnosis

Syphilis, "the great imitator," can resemble a host of diseases involving almost any organ or organ system. Darkfield, microscopic, or serologic tests provide the key to the proper diagnosis.

## Diagnosis and Management

The management of syphilis is, of course, intimately tied in with diagnostic considerations [2,8,9]. A diagnosis of syphilis should not be made on clinical grounds alone. Present-day diagnosis of primary, secondary, and tertiary syphilis depends on the interpretation of serologic laboratory tests performed on patients with suspicious lesions, while a diagnosis of latent syphilis depends entirely on evaluation of serologic tests with or without supporting evidence supplied by the history. Follow-up assessment of treatment results also depends on serologic testing.

It is useful to distinguish between those serologic tests employed in the diagnosis and control of syphilis that measure antibodies directed against *T. pallidum* itself (treponemal tests) and those that measure antibodies formed in response to products of tissue destruction (nontreponemal tests). Antibodies measured in the latter are sometimes called reagenic. In general, nontreponemal tests are suited to the tasks of screening for the disease and monitoring response to treatment, while treponemal tests are best suited to confirmation of diagnosis. Five tests are currently in widespread use in North America in the diagnosis and control of syphilis; three are nontreponemal—the VDRL, RPR, and ART tests—and two are treponemal—the FTA-ABS and MHA-TP tests. The approximate percentages of positive reactions in each procedure in the various stages of untreated syphilis are shown in Table 3.3.

### Primary Syphilis

Darkfield microscopic examination of serum from suspected lesions is the best approach. A positive darkfield examination makes the diagnosis, and treatment can be instituted on the spot, although a titered RPR or VDRL should also be drawn for treatment follow-up. When darkfield microscopy is unavailable or untrustworthy (as in mouth and anal lesions), serologic tests should be done, and should be repeated at weekly intervals for 3 weeks if negative. As shown in Table 3.3, the RPR is the test of choice under these circumstances. Positive nontreponemal tests should be confirmed by treponemal tests. The best of the latter in primary syphilis is clearly the FTA-ABS.

TABLE 3.3. Positive reactions (approximate percentages) in serologic tests in various stages of untreated syphilis.*

| Test | Stage | | |
|---|---|---|---|
| | Primary | Secondary | Latent and tertiary |
| VDRL | 70 | 100 | 70 |
| RPR (and ART) | 85 | 100 | 80 |
| FTA-ABS | 88 | 100 | 98 |
| MHA-TP | 65 | 100 | 95 |
| TPI | 50 | 95 | 95 |

*Adapted from Crissey and Denenholz [2].

Treatment of choice is benzathine penicillin G, 1.2 million IU injected into each buttock, a total of 2.4 million IU. European centers prefer to repeat the treatment 1 week later. Seroreversal to negativity should occur within 1 year. Patients allergic to penicillin can be treated with tetracycline HCL or erythromycin base or stearate, 500 mg by mouth four times per day for 15 days.

## LATENT SYPHILIS

In the United States, early latent syphilis is syphilis without signs or symptoms, present less than 1year. Beyond 1year the disease is considered to be in the late latent stage. The duration is determined by history. Diagnosis is made on the basis of a positive RPR or VDRL, confirmed by FTA-ABS.

Treatment of choice is benzathine penicillin G, 1.2 million IU injected into each buttock at weekly intervals for 3 weeks, a total of 7.2 million IU. Seronegativity is usually achieved in 2 years, but serofastness, with continuous low-level positive reactions, are common. Titers are important. A fourfold rise in titer in RPR or VDRL means relapse or reinfection; treatment should be repeated.

Patients with early latent syphilis who are allergic to penicillin can be treated with tetracycline hydrochloride or erythromycin base or stearate, 500 mg by mouth four times per day for 15 days. In late latent cases, these schedules should be continued for 30 days.

## SECONDARY AND RELAPSING SYPHILIS

Diagnosis is best made by darkfield microscopic examination of material from moist genital lesions. Positive cases can be treated immediately, but a titered RPR or VDRL should be drawn for treatment monitoring. When darkfield examination is negative or the technique is not available, the diagnosis is made by positive RPR or VDRL tests, confirmed by the FTA-ABS tests. It is well to mark the blood specimens "check for pro-zone reactions." High antibody concentrations present in secondary syphilis can interfere in some cases with nontreponemal test flocculations, giving false-negative results. This can be avoided in the laboratory by serum dilution.

Treatment of choice is benzathine penicillin G, 1.2 million IU injected intramuscularly into each buttock at weekly intervals for 2 weeks, a total of 4.8 million IU. Patients allergic to penicillin can be treated as in latent syphilis.

### Late Syphilis

Signs appropriate to the organ system involved, associated with a positive FTA-ABS test, serve to make the diagnosis. Nontreponemal tests are unreliable in late syphilis and may be negative even in the presence of active disease. There is a great deal of controversy on the significance of cerebrospinal fluid (CSF) findings in neurosyphilis; neurologic consultation is necessary. The clinical consequences of failure to treat neurosyphilis are so great that it is wise in questionable cases to treat in the spirit of the therapeutic trial. Continuous CSF monitoring of several years, with particular reference to cell counts and protein levels, is essential.

The preferred treatment for late forms of syphilis other than neurosyphilis is benzathine penicillin G, 1.2 million IU injected intramuscularly into each buttock at weekly intervals for 3 weeks, a total of 7.2 million IU. Patients allergic to penicillin can be treated as in latent syphilis, but for 30 days.

Benzathine penicillin alone is probably not effective in certain cases of neurosyphilis. The preferred combination and schedule are aqueous crystalline penicillin G, 2.4 million IU given intravenously each day (2 to 4 million IU every 4 hours), followed by benzathine penicillin G, 2.4 million IU injected intramuscularly every week for 3 weeks.

## Prognosis

Untreated, approximately 10% of patients can be expected to die of the disease. With adequate antibiotic treatment, cure rates in syphilis approach 100%. Tissue damage in cardiovascular syphilis and neurosyphilis is not reversible, and in some cases further deterioration occurs even after adequate treatment. Nevertheless, gratifying improvement can occur after treatment, even in neurosyphilis of long standing, and the lack of prospects for spectacular results should not be a contraindication to treatment.

### References

1. *MMWR* **35**:798–801, 1987.
2. Crissey JT, Denenholz DA: Syphilis. *Clin Dermatol* **2**(1):1–166, 1984.
3. Chapel TA: The variability of syphilitic chancres. *Sex Trans Dis* **5**:68–70, 1978.
4. Chapel TA: The signs and symptoms of secondary syphilis. *Sex Trans Dis* **7**:161–164, 1980.
5. Merritt HH, Adams RD, Solomon HC: *Neurosyphilis.* New York: Oxford University Press, 1946.

6. Merritt HH: *Textbook of Neurology.* 6th ed. Philadelphia: Lea & Febiger, 1979, p. 135.
7. Gjestland T: The Oslo study of untreated syphilis. *Acta Derm Venereol* (Stockh) 1955 **35,** Supple. 34.
8. Stratigos JD, Felman YM: Syphilis. In A Rook, LC Parish, and JM Beare (Eds.): *Practical Management of the Dermatologic Patient.* Philadelphia: JB Lippincott, 1986, pp. 192–197.
9. Fiumara N: Therapy guidelines for sexually transmitted diseases. *J Am Acad Dermatol* **9**:600, 1983.

CHAPTER 4

# Endemic Treponematoses

Anton F.H. Luger

## Definition

"Endemic" diseases persist within certain areas for a long time, usually for decades but in some places even for centuries, and do not disappear spontaneously. The occurrence in distinct territories accounts for a multitude of different local names for one and the same disease.

The endemic treponematoses are transmitted by nonvenereal contact among children. Consequently, the suggestion has been made to replace the term "endemic treponematoses" with "nonvenereal treponematoses" [1–3]. The original expression is still in general use [4–8].

## Causative Organisms

*Treponema pallidum* (endemic syphilis), *T. pertenue* (yaws), and *T. carateum* (pinta) apparently derive from a common ancestor [9–11] and cannot be distinguished from one another morphologically or by laboratory tests. There are minor differences in the DNA [12] and in some protein antigens, but the common determinates prevail by far [13,14].

*T. pallidum* and *T. pertenue* cause slightly different lesions when inoculated into rabbits and hamsters, and *T. carateum* produces lesions only in humans and higher primates.

## Symptoms and Course

The clinical appearance and the chronic course of the three diseases show common features. Initial lesions are followed by early eruptions, comparable to the symptoms of the secondary stage of venereal syphilis. Finally late manifestations evolve. Climate seems to have some influence on the morphology and localization of the lesions.

Prenatal transmission, cardiovascular involvement, and neurosyphilis do not occur in yaws and pinta but may appear under certain conditions in a few areas of endemic syphilis. However, recent investigations suggest the possibility of a development of congenital, cardiovascular, and visceral complications in late yaws, and cerebrospinal fluid (CSF) abnormalities were discovered in 24.9% of 904 patients [15]. Further research is needed before final conclusions can be drawn.

Attenuated forms of endemic treponematoses have reportedly occurred in areas of endemic syphilis [16] as well as in foci of yaws [17]. In these mitigated variants, early lesions appear to be fewer in number, smaller in size, and less persistent, possibly as a result of an improvement in living conditions or a change in the epidemiologic situation after mass treatment campaigns. Both factors decrease the number of cases with communicable lesions and thus reduce the incidence of superinfections, which are held responsible for the development of new lesions and the long persistence of skin eruptions [16,17].

## Immunity

Little is known about cellular (protective) immunity. Cross immunity between the three diseases evidently exists.

The response to superinfections seems to be comparable to the results of experiments with *T. pallidum*. The reinfected host remains either without symptoms upon further inoculation or develops lesions at the site of the renewed invasion that correspond to the stage of the disease. Thus, superinfections evoke papules during the early period and gummata during the late stage, according to the type of immune response in a sensitized individual.

Protective immunity in patients with endemic treponematoses seems to depend on the type of endemicity. The greater the number of children with communicable lesions in an area, the greater is the probability of repeated further infections that might stimulate protective immune reactions (perhaps comparable to vaccination) and thus prevent the development of cardiovascular syphilis or neurosyphilis. This refers particularly to holoendemic and hyperendemic conditions (see Table 4.1).

The occurrence of such late (fatal) complications in areas where treponematoses are mesoendemic or hypoendemic may be explained by a low incidence or lack of superinfections in the area (18; Table 4.1).

The onset, extent, and duration of antibody production are similar to the situation in venereal syphilis (see Chap. 3). The sera of patients with endemic syphilis, yaws, or pinta react to the same antigens in the same assays as used for the diagnosis of venereal syphilis, including tests for the detection of *T. pallidum*-specific IgM [19,20].

The classification of an endemicity by epidemiologic terms is based on the incidence of seroreactivity in children 6 years of age. The interrelations between the degree of the endemicity, mode of living, disease incidence, and occurrence of prenatal transmission, as well as the involvement of the cardiovascular and the central nervous system in endemic syphilis, yaws, and pinta, are shown in Table 4.1 [21].

TABLE 4.1. Epidemiology and occurrence of late manifestations in endemic trenponematoses.

| Epidemiology | | | | Late Manifestations: Occurrence of congenital syphilis, cardiovascular involvement, and neurosyphilis | | |
|---|---|---|---|---|---|---|
| Incidence of seroreactivity among children at 6th year of life | Epidemiologic term | Mode of living | Extent of infection in population | Endemic syphilis | Yaws | Pinta |
| Greater than 90% | Holoendemic | Primitive | Entire populace infected; exceptions very rare | None | None | None |
| Greater than 50% | Hyperendemic | Primitive | Few individuals escape infection | None | None | None |
| More than 10% | Mesoendemic | Some basic hygiene | Disease moderately spread * | Rare[†] | None[‡] | None[‡] |
| Less than 10% | Hypoendemic | Increasing standard of hygiene | Majority of inhabitants escape infection during childhood | Increasing incidence[§] | None[‖] | None[‖] |

* Venereal infections occur sporadically.
† "Mixed forms" of syphilis (venereal and endemic) may be found in some areas.
‡ Yaws and pinta occur less frequently under mesoendemic conditions.
§ Venereal infections occur more frequently.
‖ Yaws and pinta hardly occur in hypoendemic regions.

## Global Incidence

Endemic treponematoses primarily afflict children in remote, socioeconomically poor areas of tropical and subtropical regions. About half of the 400 million people living in the belt between the Tropics of Cancer and Capricorn were likely to be exposed to *T. pertenue* before 1950. About 160 million persons were infected with yaws [7,22], approximately 1 million with endemic syphilis, and 700,000 [22] to 1 million [7] with pinta. More than 40 million victims suffered from symptoms varying from skin lesions to gross destruction of tissue, joints, and bones and facial disfigurement [22].

Mass treatment campaigns with technical support from WHO and material supplies from UNICEF extended to 46 countries between 1948 and 1969 [23]. Around 160 million persons were examined during initial treatment surveys and 300 million reexaminations were carried out during resurveys. About 50 million persons with lesions or latent infections and contacts were treated with PAM (procaine penicillin with 2% aluminum monostearate). These activities almost eradicated the endemic treponematoses.

Unfortunately, a resurgence to high levels has been noted particularly in Central and West Africa as well as in Southeast Asia, whereas in Latin America the incidence of yaws and pinta continues to decline to very low levels. Today there are more than 2.5 million cases of yaws and endemic syphilis, 75% of them affecting children, with an additional 100 million children at risk of infection [24]. The reasons for this renewed increase of communicable cases are manyfold. One of the major factors has been the failure of many countries to integrate active control measures into local health services after the mass campaigns and the lack of interest in a presumably disappearing disease [25]. New strategies have to be applied, and particular emphasis has to be focused on long-term surveillance [23].

## Nonvenereal, "Endemic" Syphilis

### Synonyms

Synonyms for endemic syphilis include bejel, njovera, dichuchwa, frangi, among others.

### Causative Organism

The causative organism is *T. pallidum*.

### Transmission

For a short time, *T. pallidum* can remain virulent outside the mammalian host, provided it stays in a moist carrier under physiologic conditions at body temperature.

The infection occurs early in childhood. Toddlers become infected as soon as they come into contact with communicable lesions of other children, that is, as soon as they can move about by themselves. Flies and household utensils (e.g., drinking vessels) were once considered possible vectors but apparently are not of epidemiologic importance. All evidence suggests that the most common route of infection is a mouth-to-hand-to-hand-to-mouth transfer of communicable saliva.

The treponemes invade through the mucous membranes of the mouth, the tonsils, or the pharynx. The number of transmitted organisms is rather small and the invasion is hardly concentrated to one spot; therefore a chancre develops only very rarely [28].

## Incubation Period

The time interval between infection and the appearance of symptoms is comparable to that in venereal syphilis. Manifestations of the secondary stage (mucous patches, skin eruptions) may be observed about 10 to 12 weeks after exposure to infection.

## Occurrence

Today, endemic syphilis occurs almost exclusively in remote regions with a hot and dry climate; therefore, a suggested new term for the disease is "treponarid" [11]. It exists mainly among nomads and semi-nomads in Western Asia, Pakistan, Saudi Arabia, Sudan, the sub-Saharan regions, Mali, Niger, Upper Volta (Burkina Faso [26]), Mauritania, and Australia.

Limited outbreaks of nonvenereal endemic syphilis, involving a few individuals only, have been observed after World War II where people live in crowded quarters and hygiene is poor in slums of big cities in Europe and the United States [27].

## Clinical Findings

### Early Manifestations

A chancre can be observed in rare exceptions only because of the mode of infection (see above). Occasionally a one-sided firm painless enlargement of the submental or angular lymph nodes may suggest where the treponemes invaded [28].

### Secondary Stage

The first signs are usually on the mucous membranes and/or the skin. They cannot be distinguished from respective lesions of the secondary stage of venereal syphilis. The most common symptoms are mucous patches—shallow, relatively painless erosions covered with a fibrinous coat, thus appearing as white plaques—localized on the oral mucosa, in the mouth angles (angular or split papules), on the tongue, and on the pharynx. They sometimes cause hoarseness if the vocal cords are involved.

Hypertrophic moist papules may form elevated plaques (broad condylomata) and are seen predominantly on intertriginous parts of the skin, that is, in the axillae, the genitocrural clefts, the rima ani, and eventually between the toes. The surface

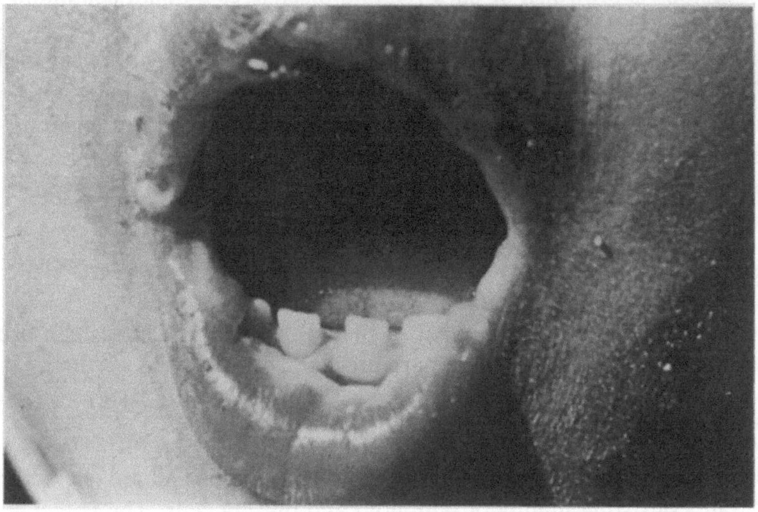

FIGURE 4.1. Mucous patches on the lower lip, angular papules.

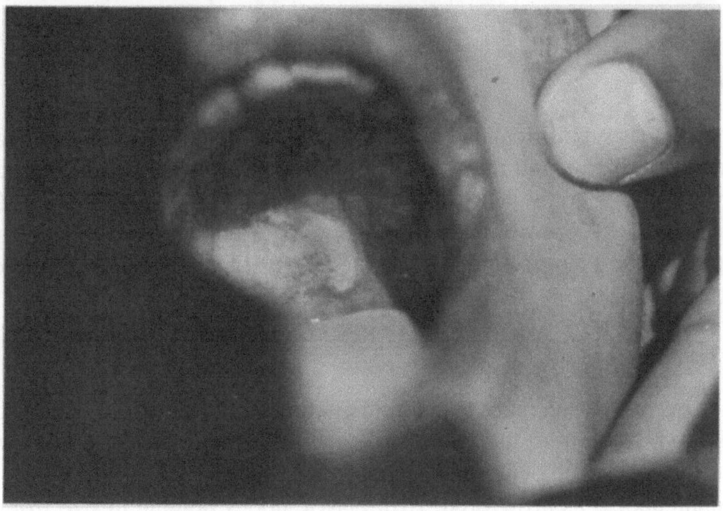

FIGURE 4.2. Mucous patches on the palate.

of these lesions is brownish or dark red and discharges a liquid containing masses of treponemes.

Disseminated macular, papular, or papulosquamous eruptions appear in about 10 to 15% of patients. Annular papules [coinlike plaques, sometimes with elevated margins (circinate syphilids)] seem to occur more frequently in endemic than in venereal syphilis.

Other skin lesions are rarely observed. Visceral involvement (e.g., specific hepatitis or nephritis, etc.) has not yet been reported.

### *Lymphadenopathy*

A generalized moderate enlargement of the palpable lymph nodes can usually be observed as long as early symptoms are present.

### *Histopathology*

Tissue changes are much the same as in venereal syphilis and are characterized by an infiltrate consisting mainly of lymphoid and plasma cells. The vessel walls and the endothelial cells are edematous. Many treponemes are found in the infiltrate, particularly around small vessels. Sometimes granulomas consisting of epithelioid cells and a few multinuclear giant cells can be observed in early lesions [29].

## Late Manifestations

### *Bone Lesions*

Osteo-periostitis syphilitica may develop either in the early or the late stage. It may cause (nocturnal) pain and may sometimes produce a thickening of the bones, particularly of the long bones. The tibia may then appear bowed (sabre tibia). Persistent bone pain occurs frequently in adult inhabitants of endemic syphilis areas, is often associated with radiologic evidence of osteoperiotitis, and may be a consequence of superinfections [16].

### *Skin Lesions*

Nodular, or nodulo-ulcerative syphilids, consist of lentil- to pea-sized, firm, brownish-red, sometimes ulcerating nodules, arranged in arcs or circles with a tendency to healing in the center and extension peripherally.

Gummata appear as brown-red, firm-elastic nodes ranging in size from that of a pigeon egg up to a goose egg or even larger. They usually ulcerate in the center, but may progress at one side of the periphery and thus form arched or scalloped margins. Residual scarring is seen rather frequently among adults in areas of endemic syphilis. A gumma on the septum of the nose might cause destruction and leave behind a saddle nose.

Sometimes a gumma of the palate may progress and destroy the entire nose with the neighboring parts of the maxilla, the palate, and the upper lip. Finally a triangular hole results, which extends from the mouth angles to the root of the nose, exposing the pharynx in the background. Such destructive lesions are called gangosa.

FIGURE 4.3. Mucous patches on the tongue, mouth angle (left side), and upper lip. Circinate syphilids on the shoulders. ►

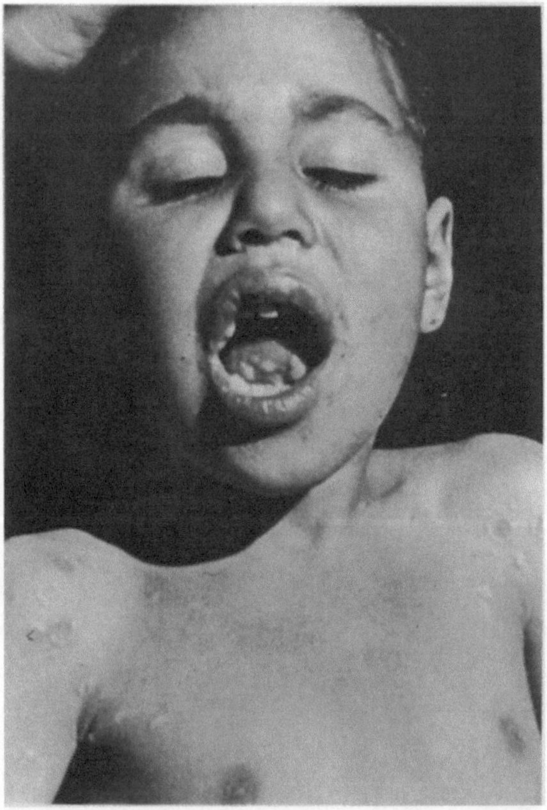

FIGURE 4.4. Circinate syphilide on the scrotum. ▼

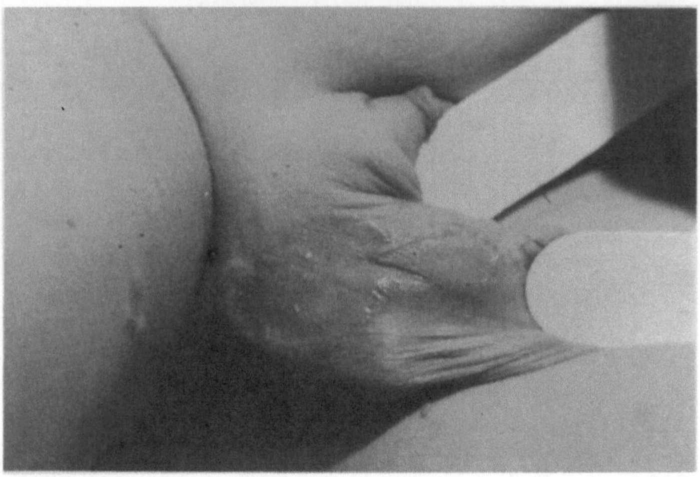

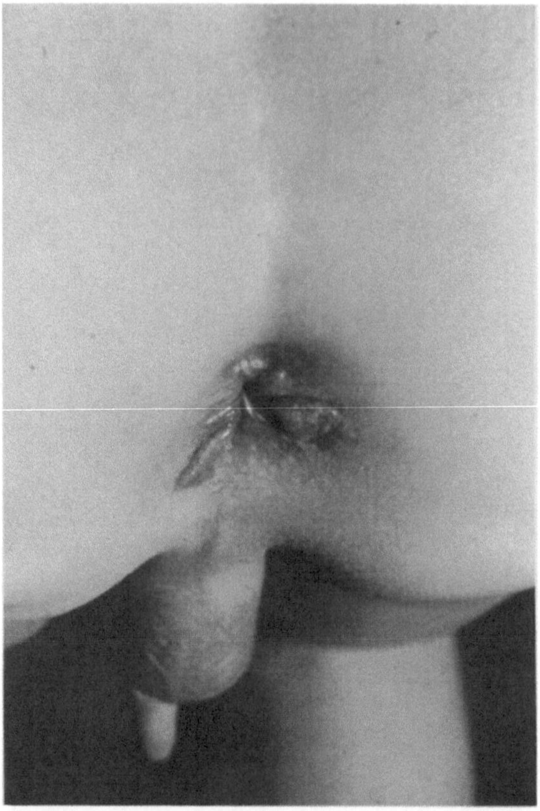

FIGURE 4.5. Hypertrophic papules (broad condylomata) in the perianal region. ◄

FIGURE 4.6. Noduloulcerative syphilid. ▼

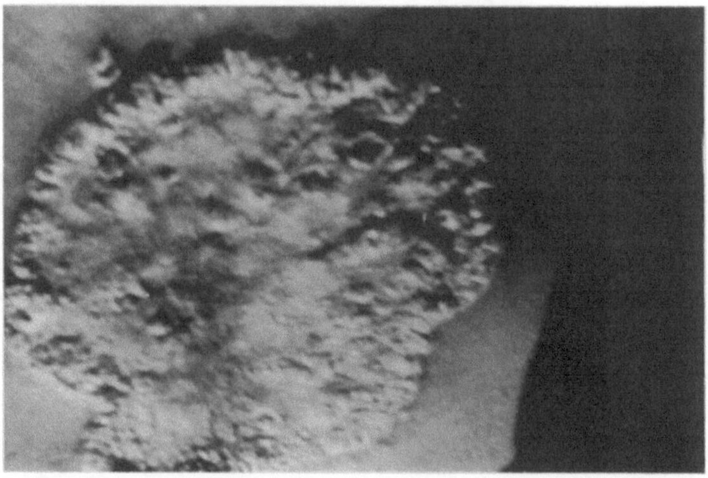

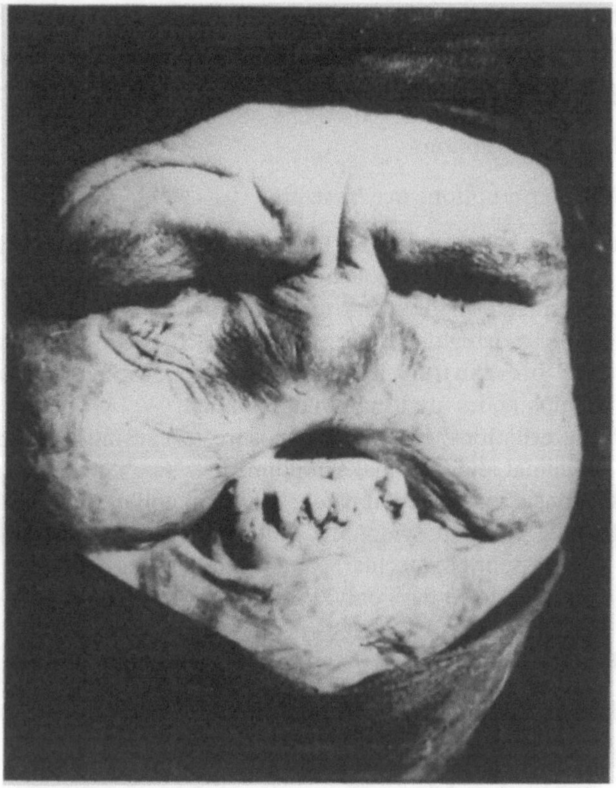

FIGURE 4.7. Gangosa in late endemic syphilis.

*Histopathology.* The histopathology of late skin lesions shows chronic inflammation with infiltrates of lymphoid and plasma cells surrounded by a dense fibrous tissue. Characteristic is the formation of granulomas consisting of epithelioid and multinuclear giant cells with necrosis in the center. The blood vessels may show a thickening of the wall and are encircled by plasma cells. Single treponemes may rarely be seen.

### *Jutaarticular Nodes*

These nodes have been described in textbooks of venerology up to the first half of this century. They were considered symptoms of yaws and of endemic and venereal syphilis, but apparently have not (or extremely rarely) been observed during the past 40 years. Clinically, these lesions appear as firm, round nodules or nodes of different dimensions (usually hazelnut to goose-egg sized) near the joints, preferably near the knees, elbows, or on the wrist and eventually on the feet.

*Histopathology.* Recent nodes appear fairly cellular and show within a dense fibrous tissue granulomatous areas that are composed of epithelioid cells, lymphocytes, and plasma cells with an occasional multinuclear giant cell. Older lesions show an increasing amount of fibrosis and hyalinization. Finally, the node consists of hyalinized collagen with little or no cellular infiltrate [29].

## Differential Diagnosis

### Macular Eruptions

Macular eruptions may resemble

Measles: general malaise; fever 38°–40°C; catarrhal prodrome symptoms with conjunctivitis, white spots on the buccal mucosa (Koplik's spots) which may be few or spread all over the mouth; followed by the skin rash, consisting of pink, blotchy, irregular larger red patches, first appearing on the head, then "descending" over the trunk and the extremities, lasting for 4 to 7 days. Posterior cervical lymph nodes are usually not enlarged.
Drug eruptions: history of exposure to causing substance; rash varying between minimal and maximal symptoms.
Pityriasis rosea: herald patch; marginal collarette of scale; duration 6 to 8 weeks.
Rubella: general symptoms mild or absent; temperature normal; skin eruption small, spotted, macular, papular, sometimes confluent, "descending" like measles but lasts for 3 days only. Posterooccipital lymph nodes regularly enlarged.

### Papular Eruptions

Differentiation may be difficult from

Psoriasis: most frequently affected sites are the elbows and knees. There are scales on top of nodules.
Lichen planus: shiny flat polygonal papules, violaceous color; Wickham's striae; Koebner's phenomenon.
Scabies: typical localization; burrows; demonstration of the mite.

### Eroded Papules

These may be similar to

Impetigo: yellow crusts; no infiltration.
Tinea pedis: interstep erosion; rhagades; no infiltrate; detection of fungi.
Condylomata acuminata: small basis; prominent; darkfield examination negative.
Eroded hemorrhoidal node: single; painful.
Balanitis candidal, circinate, erosive, plasma cellular and others: irregular margins; no lymphadenopathy; darkfield examination negative; negative histopathology.
Herpes simplex: multiple small erosions; regional lymph nodes on one side somewhat enlarged and painful.

### Papules on Palms and Soles

These may look like

Psoriasis: (see above).
Tinea pedis, tinea manum: detection of causative trichophyton.
Palmoplantar keratoderma: hereditary; no symptoms of syphilis.
Corns: (located at areas exposed to pressure).
Plantar warts: thick keratoses, painful, sometimes thornlike.

Papules in Mouth

These have to be distinguished from

Aphthosis: painful erosions grayish yellow, 1 to 10 mm in diameter, hyperemic margin; angular glands somewhat enlarged, painful. Biologic false-positive [bfp] VDRL reactions may occur.
Mononucleosis: fever; membranes on tonsils and pharynx; morbilliform or scarlatiniform skin rashes. Blood examination: leukocytosis; lymphocytosis; immature, vacuolated lymphocytes; bfp reactions in the VDRL may occur.
Angular chelitis (pérleche): localized on mouth angles only; no symptoms of syphilis; serum nonreactive.

Nodular Syphilids

These may appear akin to

Lupus vulgaris: nodules of soft consistency; in relapse nodules in central scars; histopathology sometimes hard to distinguish from that of nodular syphilids; intradermal tuberculin test +++.
Leprosy, tuberculoid form: nodules firm; surface of the lesion dry, hairless, insensitive; sensory nerve thickened; lepromin test +++.
Leishmaniasis cutanea, lupoid form: nodules soft, as in lupus vulgaris, even apple jelly nodules may appear; leishmanin test +++.
Sarcoidosis: nodules firm, resembling a grain of sand; color grayish; opaque; Kveim test +++.

Gummata

A gumma may be confused with

Tropical ulcer: occurs mostly in hot and humid areas; margin undermined, usually painful; fever; constitutional symptoms; *Bacillus fusiformis* and *Borrelia vincentii* in smears.
Leprosy, lepromatous form: multiple lesions; painless; masses of *Mycobacterium leprae* in smears, lepromin test negative.
Carcinoma: single lesion; firm nodular margins; regional lymph nodes enlarged, firm, nodular, adherent.

## Prognosis

Efficient treatment is followed by complete cure, except in cases with late destructive lesions.

# Yaws

## Synonyms

Synonyms for yaws include pian (French), Framboesia (German, Dutch), buba (Spanish), bouba (Portugese), frangi, parru, among others.

## Causative Organism

The causative organism is *T. pertenue.*

## Transmission

The infection occurs by direct contact with communicable lesions under conditions of heat and humidity [30]. Portals of invasion are usually small wounds, abrasions, lacerations, or scratches at insect bites on the lower limbs (more than 90% of patients) or on the forearms. The age peak at manifestation of the first symptom varies between 1 and 14 years, depending on the epidemiologic situation in the respective areas.

## Incubation Period

The time span between infection and the appearance of the first clinical sign varies between 9 and 90 days (average 21 days) and is thus comparable to that of venereal syphilis. A 26-year-old European, who had spent 1 week in a yaws area in Africa, developed a primary lesion 2 months later [31].

## Occurrence

Yaws is endemic almost exclusively in humid tropical areas [32]. At present it occurs in Central and West Africa, in Latin America (Brazil, Colombia, Ecuador, Guyana, Surinam, Dominica, Haiti, Martinique [33]), and in Asia (Indonesia, Papua New Guinea, South Pacific islands, Democratic Kampuchea, and Sri Lanka).

## Clinical Findings

### Primary stage ("mother yaws," "protopianoma," "buba madre," or "mamman pian")

A red papule develops at the site of infection, ulcerates, becomes covered with a yellowish crust, and enlarges by peripheral growth or by confluence with satellite nodules. Proliferation from the base results in a large (5–7 cm or more in diameter) shiny, soft, yellowish-red ulcer with a nodular, granulomatous (raspberrylike) surface. The lesion is painless, sometimes itching. The secretions contain numerous treponemes.

Fever, joint pains, and influenzalike general symptoms may sometimes occur but are usually absent or go unnoticed.

The regional lymph nodes are enlarged, firm, painless, not adherent, and without suppuration.

The primary lesion heals spontaneously within 2 to 6 months, leaving behind a pitted achromic or hypopigmented scar, sometimes surrounded by a darker halo. In about 10% of patients, the primary stage passes without symptoms.

### *Histopathology*

Hyperkeratosis, acanthosis, and a remarkable edema are seen in the epidermis. Copious neutrophils invade and form intraepidermal microabscesses. Dense infiltrates in the dermis consist predominantly of plasma cells but contain also lymphocytes, neutrophils, histiocytes, fibroblasts, and a few eosinophils. In contrast to venereal syphilis, in yaws the endothelium of the blood vessels is unaltered. Numerous treponemes are seen between the epidermal cells, in the infiltrate, and around the blood vessels.

## Secondary Stage

This stage begins 2 to 4 months after the appearance of the primary lesion, occasionally even later. It sometimes overlaps with the primary lesion.

Constitutional symptoms such as headache, fever, pain in the bones and joints, and generalized lymphadenopathy may precede the first eruption (as in venereal syphilis).

Skin manifestations usually consist of scarce or densely disseminated small papules. These lesions proliferate; rapidly become raised, ulcerated, and covered with yellow crusts and discharge serous liquid containing masses of treponemes ("daughter yaws," "pianomas," "framboesiomas"). Sometimes the lesions enlarge to big plaques closely resembling the mother yaws in size and shape, but may well remain small ("miniature yaws"). Peripheral growth and involution in the center may lead to the development of circinate yaws.

The daughter yaws may occur on any part of the skin but are frequently localized around the orifices, the mouth, nose, anus, and vulva. Hyperkeratotic papules on the palms and soles may form painful plaques by peripheral growth and/or confluence ("foot yaws," "crabs," "crab yaws") or may, at periungual localization, cause deformation of the nail ("pianic onychia").

The mucous membranes are not primarily affected but may become partially involved by enlargement of periorificial lesions.

Occasionally lenticular hypochromic macules, which may be covered with thin scales, is all that manifests during the secondary stage. These lesions are considered to be "ide" reactions ("bubides," "framboesides," "pianides"). The skin eruptions usually do not appear in one rash but in successive crops of a few lesions for 6 months to 3 years. Sometimes superficial, soft scars are left behind after spontaneous involution, but more frequently only macular hyperpigmentation remains and disappears spontaneously after some months.

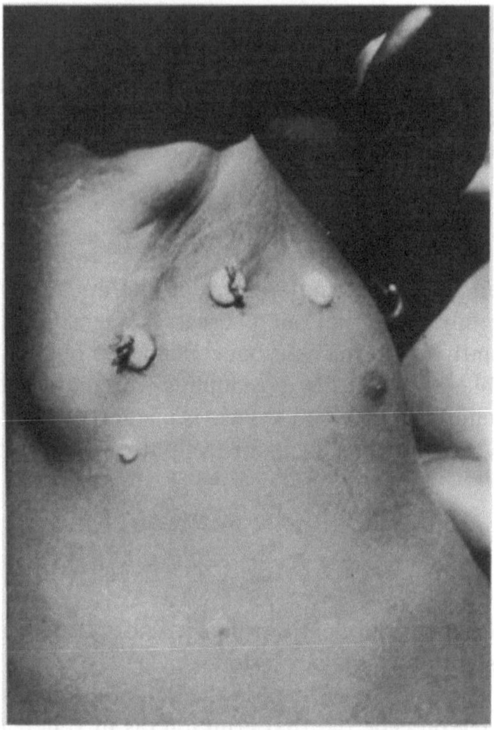

FIGURE 4.8. Daughter yaws (pianomas) in the axillary region.

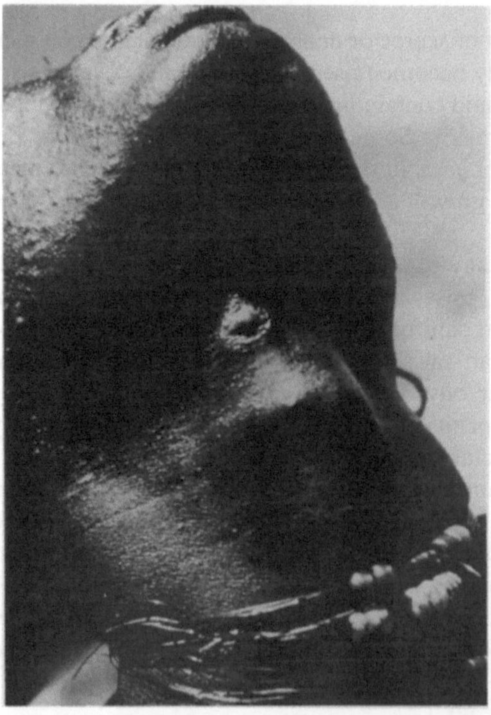

FIGURE 4.9. Yaws plaque in the submental region.

*Histopathology*

Tissue changes in lesions of the secondary stage are the same as in the primary manifestation. The epidermal changes resemble findings in condylomata lata but show a different distribution of the dermal infiltrate, with a diffuse rather than a perivascular arrangement [29].

The secondary period lasts for 3 to 4 years. Some symptoms such as crab yaws, bone lesions, and others may appear in the secondary as well as in the late stage.

## Tertiary Stage

Symptoms of late yaws are usually seen in children older than 5 years of age. Sometimes they overlap with lesions of the early stage or may appear after a period of latency of several years. The late manifestations affect the skin and the bones.

*Skin Lesions*

Nodular or tuberous manifestations usually ulcerate and appear as gummatous lesions. The latter are usually localized on the lower extremities. The first signs are small, firm-elastic, painless, subcutaneous nodes, which then enlarge, involve the overlying skin, and ulcerate. Reinfections or superinfections may be of etiologic importance.

Keratoderma and hyperkeratoses of palms and soles are similar to the respective lesions of the early stage. Keratotic nodules may enlarge and progress to raised, rounded nodes or plaques, which exfoliate from trauma, may occupy most of the plantar or palmar area, and form ill-defined, fissured, crust-covered, painful lesions.

Painless hyperkeratotic plaques without nodes, and minute craters surrounded by hyperkeratotic papules (similar to keratoderma punctatum), called hormiguillo, are sometimes seen.

*Histopathology.* The microscopic appearance of late yaws lesions of the skin is practically the same as in late endemic syphilis (see p. 41). Keratotic lesions of the palms and soles show hyperkeratosis, parakeratosis, acanthosis, and a moderate infiltrate, but no distinctive characteristics.

*Bone Lesions*

Osteitis or periostitis of the secondary or tertiary stage manifests itself in long and small bones (e.g., polydactylitis, resembling spina ventosa in tuberculosis) or may cause saber shin. Rarefaction of the compacta may cause spontaneous fracture [34]. Saddle nose due to partial or total destruction of the cartilaginous and/or osseous parts of the septum, and gangosa and juxtaarticular nodes may occur, as in endemic syphilis (see p. 38, 41).

Gonndou is a rare form of ossifying osteitis that develops in about 1 of 1,000 patients with yaws osteitis. It begins with exostoses at the nasal bones and the frontal processes of the maxilla, and is frequently symmetrical. The lesions grow very slowly to big tumors (2–20 cm in diameter) within 5 to 20 years at both sides of the root of the nose or above the palate, may arrest spontaneously, or may cause complete loss of sight by obstruction of the field of vision. X-ray examination reveals the

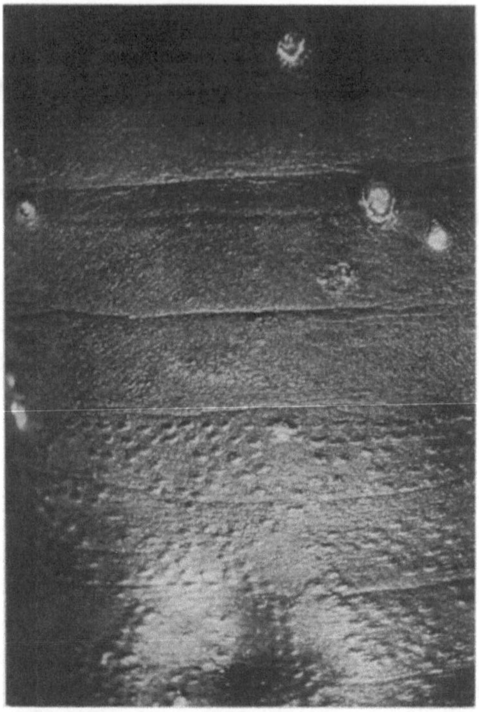

FIGURE 4.10. Yaws papules in the abdominal region.

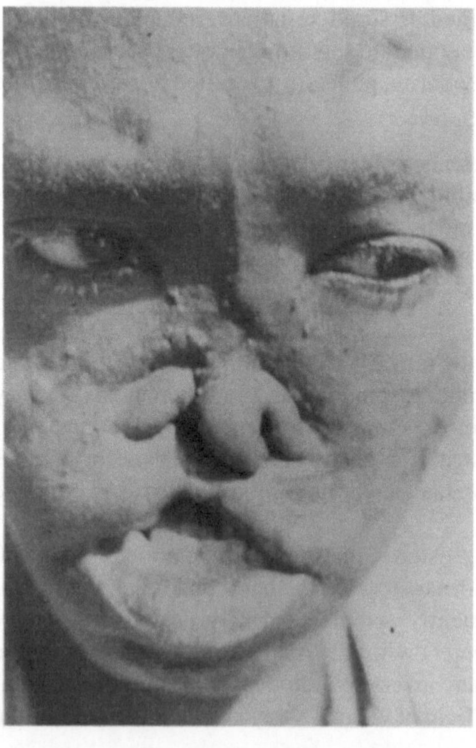

FIGURE 4.11. Gangosa (saddle nose and destruction of the palate) in late yaws.

structure of solid bone but sometimes a spongy composition may be seen in older lesions. Gondou is not universally accepted as being caused by yaws. It has been seen in Africa, Haiti, Jamica, and Venezuela, but not in Brazil or Southeast Asia [35]. It is rarely mentioned in recent reports.

## Differential Diagnosis

### Primary Lesions

Primary lesions may look like

Pyoderma gangrenosum: multiple lesions; immune defect, darkfield examination negative.
Tropical ulcer: see page 43.
Mycobacterium ulcerans infection (Buruli ulcer, searl's ulcer): mild inflammation; lack of granulomatous tissue; margins deeply undermined; clusters of acid-fast bacilli in smears.
Ulcerations due to tuberculosis or sporotrichosis: painful; undermined soft margins; darkfield examination negative.

### Secondary Stage

Cutaneous lesions have to be distinguished from

Framboesiform syphilids: occur in adults in the course of venereal syphilis outside yaws areas.
Framboesoid leishmaniasis: wet type of cutaneous leishmaniasis; multiple lesions after multiple infections or autoinoculation; Leishman-Donovan bodies in the smear, leishmanin (Montenegro) skin test positive.
American leishmaniasis: *Leishmania brasiliensis* in smears.
Paracoccidioidal granuloma (Lutz-Splendore-Almeida disease): regional lymph nodes involved; culture of *Paracoccidioides brasiliensis*.
Tungiasis: located on the soles; demonstration of parasite.
Lepromatous leprosy: see page 43.
Pyoderma vegetans: like pyoderma gangrenosum.

### Pianides

Pianides may resemble

Favus: scutula; culture: *Trichophyton schönleinii*
Pityriasis rosea: see page 42.
Pityriasis alba: scales containing hyphae of *Pityrosporum orbiculare* (*Malassezia furfur*); yellowish fluorescence in Wood's light).
Psoriasis vulgaris: see page 42.
Tinea corporis: circinate forms; fluorescence in Wood's light, culture: *Trichophyton* species.
Crab yaws: see Papules on Palms and Soles, page 42, 43.

### Tertiary Stage

See Nodular Syphilids and Gummata, page 43.

### Prognosis

Proper treatment secures complete restitution except at lesions where tissue destruction has occurred.

## Pinta

### Synonyms

Synonyms for pinta are mal de pinto, carate, cute, and cativa.

### Causative Organism

The causative organism is *T. carateum*.

### Transmission

Pinta is generally acquired in childhood by direct nonvenereal contact with communicable lesions. Portals of infection are small wounds, scratches, and cutaneous abrasions. Favorite areas of invasion are exposed regions of the body, usually the extremities.

The initial lesion appears usually 2 to 3 weeks after exposure.

### Occurrence

The disease once was prevalent in hot, semiarid, coastal regions but was also endemic at altitudes of 2,500 m. It was widespread in Cuba, southern Mexico, Colombia, Venezuela, Guyana, Ecuador, Peru, Bolivia, and Brazil [36–38].

At present pinta is reported from few areas in southern Mexico, Central America, and Colombia. The incidence continues to decline.

### Clinical Findings

Pinta affects the skin exclusively. Bone changes or visceral involvement do not occur. The disease progresses from the early to the late stage; however, it is difficult to differentiate between primary, secondary, and tertiary lesions because the stages are not clearly defined and frequently overlap.

#### Primary Stage

The first symptoms of infection are erythematosquamous plaques or small papules, usually multiple, on uncovered parts of the body, predominantly on the lower limbs

(80%), the forearms (10%), the dorsum of the hands and feet, the face, and the neck. They are rarely on the chest, the loins, or the abdomen. The plaques are small, lenticular, pale red, covered with tenuous scales, and sometimes slightly infiltrated and elevated. They never ulcerate.

The lesions enlarge by peripheral growth and/or by confluence with satellite lesions to plaques up to 20 mm or more in diameter. They last for some months or several years. The plaques may appear psoriasiform, lichenoid, or circinate and may be surrounded by smaller nodules. The color is initially pale red. Pigment changes of varying degrees may occur after the plaque has reached its final size, and hypochromic as well as achromic areas may be seen in the same lesion.

The initial lesions resolve spontaneously, leaving behind a depigmentation in most cases.

*Histopathology*

The epidermis shows slight acanthosis, intracellular and extracellular edema, immigration of lymphoid cells, and hydropic degeneration as well as depletion of melanin in the basal cells. Many melanophores are found in the upper dermis, indicating a gross disturbance of the mechanisms of pigmentation already in the first lesions. Recent ultramicroscopic investigations have revealed that *T. carateum* causes irreversible damage to melanocytes, although the mechanism of this influence is still obscure.

Dense infiltrates consisting of plasma cells, lymphoid cells with occasional histocytes and neutrophils are seen in the upper dermis, particularly around blood and lymph vessels. Generally, the endothelium is not altered except for slight swelling in rare instances, but proliferation never occurs. Numerous treponemes can be demonstrated between the epidermal cells and in the infiltrate [29,38].

Secondary Stage

The phase of cutaneous generalization begins several months or years (usually 3–6 months) after development of the initial manifestation. These first lesions can still be seen; they become indistinguishable from the lesions of the secondary stage.

Three types of skin eruptions, called pintids, may be observed:

1. *Erythematosquamous plaques*. Pale red lesions, usually covered with thin shiny scales, disseminated mainly over the skin of the extensor parts of the extremities. Reports concerning a localization on the palms and soles are controversial.
2. *Hyperchromic lesions*. Characterized by a change from pale red to copper red, slate blue, or bluish black (*carate plombé*) and may become piebald or depigmented in the late stage.
3. *Hypochromic spots*. A vitiligolike depigmentation.

The secondary manifestations are usually extensive. They have a tendency to confluence and to produce hypochromia or achromia, particularly at progression to the late stage.

The pintides may cause progressive atrophy of the skin.

*Histopathology*

Tissue changes are essentially the same as those in the primary lesion, including an abundance of treponemes. The infiltrate may be more intensive, particularly in the papillary dermis. The elastic fibers fade progressively with the duration of the lesion, and finally atrophy occurs.

### Tertiary Stage

The late phase begins 2 to 5 years after infection and is characterized by distinct patches of hyperchromia and achromia as well as by multicolored leukomelanotic areas. Four main symptoms can be observed:

1. *Pigmentation*. Blotches spotted with different colors: grayish, ashy, steel blue, or dark blue according to the depth at which melanin is accumulated in the dermis.
2. *Achromia*. Irregular-shaped areas with complete or partial loss of melanin are frequently observed on the skin close to the bony protuberances, elbows, knees, malleoli, wrists, and dorsum manus.
3. *Hyperkeratoses*. Elevated plaques covered with scaly hyperkeratoses are preferably localized on the extensor parts of the legs and forearms, particularly on elbows, knees, and ankles, sometimes on the palms and soles.
4. *Atrophy.* Pintides may heal with atrophy of the skin, including its appendages (e.g., sweat glands, sebaceous glands, and hair). Favorite localization is the neighborhood of large joints.

*Histopathology*

Hyperpigmented plaques show atrophy of the epidermis and lack of melanin in the basal cells. Accumulations of melanophages with some lymphocytes are seen in the upper dermis. Treponemes are still present in considerable number in the epidermis.

Depigmented splotches, which represent the final stage of the disease, show atrophy of the epidermis, complete absence of melanin even in the dermis, and no signs of inflammation, no infiltrate, and no treponemes.

Electron microscopic examination of lesions of late pinta reveals the absence of basal epidermal melanocytes, but Langerhans cells are still present and some of them contain a few melanosomes within lysosomes [29].

A moderate generalized lymphadenopathy is regularly observed during the secondary and tertiary stages.

*T. carateum* is abundantly present in all lesions of the three stages except in old achromic spots.

## Differential Diagnosis

Pinta lesions might be confused with

Tinea corporis: see page 49.
Psoriasis: see page 42.

Numular eczema: lesions consist of maculae, papulae, and eventually vesiculae; darkfield examination negative; serology negative.
Erythema dyschormicum perstans: occurs outside pinta areas in Latin and North America and Japan; clinical differentiation is hardly possible; darkfield examination negative; serology negative; histopathology facilitates differentiation.
Pityriasis alba: see page 49.
Tuberculoid leprosy: see page 43.
Leukodermas of various types: lesions before depigmentation different from those of pinta; darkfield examination negative; serology negative.
Vitiligo: dark halo at progressing lesions; darkfield examination negative; serology negative.
Pigmentary changes in yaws: limited to yaws areas; presence of other yaws symptoms, bone lesions.

### Prognosis

Total restoration of pigment follows appropriate treatment of primary, secondary, and even tertiary pinta (of short duration). No treatment exists for atrophy and late achromia.

## Diagnosis

In field treatment campaigns, a presumptive diagnosis of endemic syphilis, yaws, or pinta can be based on the features of typical clinical manifestations. Diagnosis may not be difficult in areas of an endemicity; however, confirmation of a clinical diagnosis by darkfield examination and serology tests should be attempted as frequently as possible and should never be neglected in outpatients of dispensaries where facilities for these tests are available.

### Identification of the Causative Organism

Smears from suspected lesions can be taken in the field. They should then be air dried and transported to the laboratory, where staining with monoclonal antibodies provides a safe method for detection of *T. pallidum*, *T. pertenue*, and *T. carateum* [39].

#### Serology

Today, particularly in areas of low prevalence, clinical manifestations may be less characteristic than observed in earlier campaigns and the ratio of latent to infectious cases may be higher. In addition, experience in the identification of endemic treponematoses may have decreased during the years of low incidence. As a result, serodiagnostic tests have assumed a more important role [24].

The sera of patients with endemic syphilis, yaws, or pinta react to the same antigens and assays as used for the diagnosis of venereal syphilis (assays for detection of *T. pallidum*-specific IgM antibodies). The beginning of reactivity after infection and the persistence of positive results after efficient treatment are the same as in venereal syphilis.

The transport of sera in plastic tubes within styropore boxes and storage in a refrigerator at 6° to 8°C during intervals between shipping keeps even a decrease of IgM reactivity within reasonable limits.

Use the filter paper method for collection of finger-prick blood facilitates collecting specimens from children and sampling in remote areas. This method allows examinations by the VDRL and MHA-TP tests and thus provides a means for reliable diagnosis [40,41].

#### Biopsy

Tissue specimens from lesions can easily be obtained by punch biopsy. The sample should be taken from the margin of lesions and fixed in phosphate-buffered saline solution with 10% formalin.

## Management

### Treatment

Endemic treponematoses respond well to treatment with the same antibiotics that have proved effective in the therapy of venereal syphilis (see Chap. 3). Doses and schedules of administration are identical [32]. The main goal of (mass) treatment of endemic treponematoses is to stop further spread by the extinction of sources of transmission, that is, by treatment of patients with communicable lesions and by prophylactic treatment of contacts.

The patient is usually seen once only, and thus single-dose regimens are required. WHO has recommended one injection of 600,000 IU of benzathine penicillin in all active cases and in all contacts who are less than 10 years old; 1.2 million IU of benzathine penicillin is recommended in all patients with communicable lesions and in all contacts older than 10 years of age [2]. Effective serum and tissue levels can be expected to last for at least 10 days. The lesions become noninfective within 18 to 24 hours.

The danger of inefficient treatment is within reasonable limits for patients. Late fatal complications do not occur in yaws and pinta and are exceptionally rare in hypoendemic areas of endemic syphilis. Therefore, the single-dose treatment is justified from the individual point of view as well.

Erythromycin should be given in cases of penicillin allergy (which is extremely rare in the remote areas where treponematoses are endemic). Children under 8 years of age should receive 8 mg/kg of body weight by mouth four times daily. An oral dose of 250 mg four times daily is recommended for children 8 to 15 years of age, and individuals older than 15 years should take 500 mg by mouth four times daily. The regimen should continue for 15 days. Adults might be treated with tetracyclines (500 mg of tetracycline, chlortetracycline, or oxytetracycline four times daily or 100 mg of doxycyline twice daily) for 15 days.

## Control of Endemic Treponematoses

Individual treatment alone cannot prevent a later resurgence of endemic treponematoses. Mass treatment has to be given in a regimen adapted to the epidemiologic condition. Effective control measures must follow. Therefore, successful control of endemic treponematoses is the result of managerial as well as technical effectiveness [42].

## WHO policies for Mass Treatment of Endemic Treponematoses [7]

1. In hyperendemic areas, the entire population should be treated (total mass treatment, TMT).
2. In mesoendemic areas, all active cases, all children under 15 years of age, and all obvious contacts of infectious cases should receive treatment (juvenile mass treatment, JMT).
3. In hypoendemic areas, benzathine penicillin should be given to all active cases, to all persons living in the same household, and to all obvious contacts (selective mass treatment, SMT).

### Possibility of Resurgence of Endemy

It is practically impossible to find all communicable cases in a remote area during one campaign. Table 4.2 shows the estimated number of new cases 1 year after mass treatment under different epidemiologic conditions. These considerations show clearly that careful surveillance measures are indispensable in the control of endemic treponematoses.

TABLE 4.2. Number of new communicable cases 1 year after mass treatment campaign if 1, 3, 5, or 10 cases were missed in a community of 400 inhabitants.*

| | No. of new cases after 1 year if | | | |
|---|---|---|---|---|
| Epidemiologic conditions | 1 Case missed | 3 Cases missed | 5 Cases missed | 10 Cases missed |
| Holoendemic | 0.8 | 3.5 | 5.1 | 10 |
| Hyperendemic | 0.6 | 2.1 | 3.5 | 6.9 |
| Hypoendemic | 0.3 | 0.9 | 1.6 | 3.3 |

*Adapted from Luger [28] and Kranendonk [43].

### Surveillance [7]

Surveillance is the key element in effective control [44]. Periodic resurveys are essential and should begin 6 months after the initial treatment. Timing of subsequent resurveys depends on the incidence of new cases. It should at least be every 2 years.

### Maintenance

After mass treatment, maintenance measures have to be incorporated into primary health care activities [45], thus providing continued facilities for therapy of sporadic new cases and their contacts.

### Selective Epidemiologic Control

In areas where the prevalence of endemic treponematoses is (or has become) low, restricted clinical and serological resurveys should be performed at places or in communities where a resurgence is suspected. At the same time, mass campaigns should be performed or surveillance or maintenance measures should be reinforced.

Failures of eradication programs usually originate from inefficient surveillance or maintenance activities.

## References

1. Rhodes AR, Luger AFH: Syphilis and other treponematoses. In TB Fitzpatrick, AZ Eisen, K Wolff, IM Freedberg, KF Austen (Eds): *Dermatology in General Medicine*. 3rd ed. New York: McGraw-Hill, 1987, vol. 2, pp. 2395–2452.
2. World Health Organization: *Treponemal Infections*. Technical Report Series No. 674. Geneva: World Health Organization, 1982.
3. World Health Organization: *WHO Expert Committee on Venereal Diseases and Treponematoses: Sixth Report*. Technical Report Series No. 736. Geneva: World Health Organization, 1986.
4. Antal GM, Burke JP, Geizer I, et al (Eds): Yaws and other endemic treponematoses. *SE Asian J Trop Med Pub Health* **17** (Suppl.), Dec. 1986.
5. Burke JP, Hopkins DR, Hume JC, et al (Eds): *International Symposium on Yaws and Other Endemic Treponematoses*. Reviews of *Infect. Dis.* **7** (Suppl. 2), 1985.
6. World Health Organization: *Control of Sexually Transmitted Diseases*. Geneva: World Health Organization, 1985.
7. Perine PL, Hopkins DR, Niemel PLA, et al: *Handbook of Endemic Treponematoses*. Geneva: World Health Organization, 1984.
8. World Health Organization: *Yaws and Other Endemic Treponematoses*. Report of a Regional Meeting, Brazzaville, 3–6 Feb. 1986. Regional Office for Africa, Brazzaville: WHO, 1986.
9. Rosebury T: *Microbes and Morals*. New York: Viking Press, 1971.
10. Turner TB: The future direction of research into syphilis. In RD Cattarall, CS Nicol (Eds): *Sexually Transmitted Diseases*. New York: Academic Press, 1976, pp. 221–230.
11. Hackett CJ: *Diagnostic Criteria of Syphilis, Yaws, Treponarid (Treponematoses) and of Some Other Diseases in Dry Bones*. S.B. Heidelberger Akademie der Wissenschaften, math. -nat. Kl. Springer: Berlin, 1976, pp. 1–134.

12. Fieldsteel HA: Genetics of treponema. In RF Shell, DM Musher (Eds): *Pathogenesis and Immunology of Treponemal Infection*. New York, Basel: Marcel Dekker, 1983, pp. 39–55.
13. Bakker-Zander SA, Lukehart SA: Molecular basis of immunological cross reactivity between *Treponema pallidum* and *Treponema pertenue. J Infect Immunol* **42**:634–638, 1983.
14. Thornburg RW, Baseman JB: Comparison of major protein antigens and protein profiles of *Treponema pallidum* and *Treponema pertenue. J Infect Immunol* **42**:623–627, 1983.
15. Roman GC, Roman LN: Occurrence of congenital, cardiovascular, visceral, neurologic and neuro-ophthalmologic complications in late yaws: A theme for future research. *Rev Infect Dis* **8**:760–770, 1986.
16. Pace JL, Csonka GW: Endemic non-venereal syphilis (bejel) in Saudi Arabia. *Br J Vener Dis* **60**:293–297, 1984.
17. Vorst FA: Clinical diagnosis and changing manifestations of treponemal infection. *Rev Infect Dis* 7(Suppl. 2):327–331, 1985.
18. Guthe T, Luger A: Immunitätsverhältnisse bei Treponematosen. *Hautarzt* **22**:329–333, 1971.
19. Merlin S, Andre J, Alacoque, B. et al: Importance of specific IgM antibodies in 116 patients with various stages of syphilis. *Genitourin Med* **61**:82–87, 1985.
20. Schmidt BL, Hutapea NO, Gschnait F, et al: The value of *T. pallidum* specific IgM tests for the diagnosis of latent yaws. *Europ J Sex Trans Dis* **2**:171–174, 1985.
21. Luger A: Sexually transmissible diseases. In JM Beare, LC Parish, R Ruiz-Maldonado: *Textbook of Pediatric Dermatology*. Orlando, Fla: Grune and Stratton, 1987.
22. Schweiker RS: Preface. *Rev Infect Dis* **7** (Suppl. 2):218–219, 1985.
23. Antal GM, Causse G: The control of endemic treponematoses. *Rev Infect Dis* **7** (Suppl. 2):220–226, 1985.
24. World Health Organization: *Programme for the Control of the Endemic Treponematoses*. Geneva: WHO, 1987.
25. Janssen PG: Research: The prerequisite for innovative strategies and technologies. *Rev Infect Dis* **7** (Suppl. 2):289–294, 1985.
26. Baudon D, Saliou P, Bibane L, et al: La syphilis endemique dans une region sahelienne du Burkina Faso: Enquete sero-clinique. *Bull Soc Pathol Exot Filiales* **78**:555–562, 1985.
27. Luger A: Non venereally transmitted "endemic" syphilis in Vienna. *Br J Vener Dis* **48**:356–360, 1972.
28. Luger A: Die Behandlung der endemischen Lues in Entwicklungsländern. *Arch klin exper Dermatol* **219**:211–226, 1964.
29. Lever WF, Schaumburg Lever G: *Histopathology of the Skin*. 6th ed. Philadelphia, London, Mexico City: Lippincott, 1983.
30. Hackett CJ: On the epidemiology of yaws in African miners (1942). *Trans Roy Soc Trop Med Hyg* **78**:536–538, 1984.
31. Schmutz J, Rufli T: Zur Differentialdiagnose indolenter Ulzera bei Tropenrückkehrern: die Framboesie. *Schweiz Med Wochenschr* **114**:880–882, 1984.
32. Willcox RR: Mass treatment campaigns against the endemic treponematoses. *Rev Infect Dis* **7** (Suppl. 2):278–283, 1985.
33. St. John RK: Yaws in the Americas. *Rev Infect Dis* **7** (Suppl. 2):266–272, 1985.
34. Sengupta S: Musculoskeletal lesions in yaws. *Clin Orthop.* **192**:193–198, 1985.
35. Hackett CJ: *An International Nomenclature of Yaws Lesions*. Monograph Series No. 36. Geneva: WHO, 1957.
36. Medina R: Ecology of human treponematoses. *Castellania (Berlin)* **2**:255–256, 1974.

37. Marquez F: Pinta, endemic syphilis. In O. Canizares: *Clinical Tropical Dermatology.* Oxford, London, Edinburgh, Melbourne: Blackwell, 1975, pp. 86–92.
38. Kerdel Vegas F: Yaws, pinta. In A. Rook, DS Wilkinson, FJG Ebling: *Textbook of Dermatology.* 4th ed. Oxford, London, Edinburgh, Melbourne: Blackwell, 1986, Vol. I., pp. 871–883.
39. Perine PL, Nelson UJW, Lewis JO, et al: New technologies for use in the surveillance and control of yaws. *Rev Infect Dis* **7** (Suppl. 2):295–299, 1985.
40. Luger A: Serological diagnosis of syphilis, current methods. In H. Young, and A McMillan (Eds): *Immunological Diagnosis of Sexually Transmitted Diseases*. New York: Marcel Dekker, 1987.
41. Larsen SA, D'Costa JF: Laboratory tests and serologic surveillance for yaws and other diseases and conditions. In GM Antal, JP Burke, I Geizer, SA Lukehart (Eds): *Yaws and Other Endemic Treponematoses. SE Asian J Trop Med Publ Health* (Suppl.) **17**:70–77, 1986.
42. Foege WH: Feasibility of eradicating yaws. *Rev Infect Dis* **7** (Suppl. 2):335–337, 1985.
43. Kranendonk O: *Serological and Epidemiological Aspects in Yaws Control*. Amsterdam: Broos, 1958.
44. Meheus A: Integration of yaws control and primary health care. *Rev Infect Dis* **7** (Suppl. 2):284–288, 1985.
45. Hopkins DR: Control of yaws and other endemic treponematoses: Implementation of vertical and/or integrated programs. *Rev Infect Dis* **7** (Suppl 2):338–342, 1985.

# CHAPTER 5

# Gonorrhea

Daniel S.F. Cheng

## Definition

Gonorrhea is an acute infectious disease of the genitourinary mucous membrane and is almost exclusively transmitted by sexual intercourse. The causative organism is *Neisseria gonorrhoeae*, the gonococcus. The urethra, endocervix, anal canal, conjunctivas, and pharynx can be infected directly. The organism may also cause local or metastatic complications. Local complications in men include infection of the neighboring structures of the urethra such as Tyson's glands, Littré's glands, paraurethral ducts, prostate, vas deferens, seminal vesicles, epididymis, and testis. In women Skene's glands, Bartholin's glands, endometrium, and fallopian tubes can be involved. Metastatic complications of gonorrhea include dermatitis, arthritis, endocarditis, myopericarditis, meningitis, and hepatitis.

## Synonyms

Gonorrhea was a term used by Galen (130–200 A.D.) to describe the syndrome of purulent urethral discharge in acute gonococcal urethritis, in the belief that the urethral exudate was a flow of semen (Greek *gonos* and *rhoea* mean seed and flow, respectively). Descriptions of gonorrhea can be found in the Old Testament and other literatures of ancient civilizations. Descriptive terms such as "running issue" in Leviticus 15 might mean urethral discharge of gonorrhea. Hippocrates (460–335 B.C.) was the first to make scientific observations on gonorrhea, and he used the term "strangury" to depict acute gonorrhea. Perhaps the common name for gonorrhea, the "clap," was derived from the term *clappoir* used for houses of prostitution in Paris in the Middle Ages [1].

## Epidemiology

Gonorrhea has been the most ubiquitous infectious disease of mankind. Its existence may be traced back as far as written records. Its ubiquity is associated closely with sex play. The clinical manifestations of gonococcal infection differ with respect to sex, age, and pattern of sex practice of the patients as well as with relationship to the strains of the infecting gonococcus.

Epidemiologic data of gonococcal infection do not reveal the genuine incidence of the disease. They tend to underestimate the current pandemic of gonorrhea even for countries like the United Kingdom, where a more ideal reporting system is available. In the United Kingdom, about 80 to 90% of cases of gonococcal infection are seen in sexually transmitted disease clinics and are reported regularly through a national system. Patients not seen in these special clinics are not included in the statistics [2].

Gonorrhea has been the most frequently reported communicable disease in the United States since 1965. In 1979 it was reported twice as often as all other notifiable diseases combined. At that time it was estimated that about one third to two thirds of gonococcal infections in the United States were treated in private clinics or by physicians in office practice, but these reported a much smaller percentage of patients than did the public clinics. In 1976 the number of cases reported to the health authorities in the United States was 1,011,014, an underreporting of over 62% of the estimated 2.7 million cases. However, data from countries like the United Kingdom and the United States can cast light on trends in the incidence and pattern of disease transmission. By and large, the number of reported cases of gonorrhea in many developed countries is either stable or decreasing [3]. For example, the number of reported cases of gonorrhea in the United States decreased from 1983 to 1984 by 2.4%, from 900,435 to 878,556. Similarly, gonorrhea rates per 100,000 population declined from 387.6 to 374.8 during the same period [4]. Yet in most developed countries, gonorrhea continued to remain the most frequently reported infectious disease. The reduction in the rate of occurrence of gonorrhea in some countries has been associated with nationwide gonorrhea screening programs, more popular use of condoms, and other social factors. Recently, alterations in male homosexual attitudes and behaviors—reduction in number of different sexual partners, change in criteria for choosing partners, and change in preferred sexual activities—seem to be temporally associated with reduction in the incidence of gonorrhea in this group, a group in whom gonorrhea is one of the most common sexually transmitted diseases. These alterations have been attributed to the alarming and extensive increase in media coverage of the acquired immune deficiency syndrome [5].

Data for the incidence of gonorrhea in developing countries are scarce and inaccurate, but it is speculated that the prevalence rates in Africa may be 5 to 50 times higher than in the United States. Gonorrhea rates are increasing in these countries, while they have leveled off or fallen in most developed countries in the 1980s [3].

Gonorrhea is difficult to eradicate because of its short incubation period, the presence of many asymptomatic carriers of infection, and the emergence of penicillinase-producing *N. gonorrhoeae* and chromosomally mediated resistance to multiple antibiotics. Distributions and trends in incidence of gonorrhea differ greatly in different countries and even in different areas of one country. Successful gonorrhea control programs rely on international cooperation and efforts based upon the perspectives of the clinicians, microbiologists, epidemiologists, and public health authorities.

## Causative Organism

*N. gonorrhoeae* is a nonmotile, gram-negative, aerobic diplococcus that characteristically grows in pairs described as kidney- or bean-shaped, with the concave surfaces facing each other. It was discovered by Albert Neisser (1855–1916) in 1879 and is but one member of the genus *Neisseria*, which includes both pathogenic and saprophytic species. All *Neisseria* species are morphologically indistinguishable one from the other and their differentiation can only be made by special culture and biochemical or immunofluorescent studies. The gonococcus cannot survive long outside the body, as it is rapidly killed by drying, heat, and weak antiseptics.

There are many strains of *N. gonorrhoeae* and their differentiation is of importance in understanding their clinical and epidemiologic features and significance. With methods of typing that include plasmid profile, nutritional requirement (auxotyping), colony morphology, antigenic diversity, and other phenotypic and genotypic markers, we may be able to relate particular auxotypes and "serovars" to complicated infection, to make distinction between reinfection and treatment failure, and to establish molecular epidemiology. This may allow effective control and prevention, in the future if not now.

The outer membrane of the gonococcus is composed of lipopolysaccharide, protein, and phospholipid. There are three major proteins, proteins I, II, and III. Protein I is the most abundant and is present in all gonococci. Serologic classification based on antigenic heterogeneity of protein I has been employed. With the coagglutination method, Sandstrom et al classified the proteins into serogroups WI and WII/WIII [6]. Knapp and co-workers subdivided serogroups WI and WII/WIII into a large number of serovars by means of a battery of monoclonal antibody in a coagglutination assay, namely serovars IA 1 to 18 from WI, and serovars IB 1 to 28 from WII/WIII [7]. Wang and co-workers used microimmunofluorescence to classify gonococcal strains into types A, B, and C with subtypes $A_1$, $A_2$, $A_3$, $B_1$, $B_2$, $B_3$, $C_1$, and $C_2$. Strains $A_2$ and $A_3$ were found predominantly in Seattle, Washington, strains B and C in Southeast Asia [8].

Auxotyping is a method of typing based on genetically determined nutritional requirements of the isolates. Strains that require no supplements are denoted as prototropic, those that require proline as $P^-$, and those that require arginine, hypoxanthine, and uracil as $AHU^-$. Auxotyping has been used to show associations with strain virulence and demographic distribution. For example, $AHU^-$ strains isolated from Seattle are often associated with disseminated gonococcal infection, with asymptomatic urethral gonorrhea in men, and with extreme susceptibility to penicillin but increased resistance to the bactericidal action of normal human serum.

Since the introduction of penicillin for the therapy of gonorrhea more than 40 years ago, increasing resistance of the gonococcus to penicillin has been recognized worldwide [9,10]. Gradual stepwise resistance of gonococcus to penicillin has necessitated ever-increasing single doses for effective therapy. The doses and volume for injection have now reached the maximum that most patients can tolerate. At least two types of resistance to penicillin by the gonococcus are known due to chromosomally mediated resistance *N. gonorrhoeae* (CMRNG) and beta-lactamase resistance due to penicillinase-producing *N. gonorrhoeae* (PPNG). Chromosomally

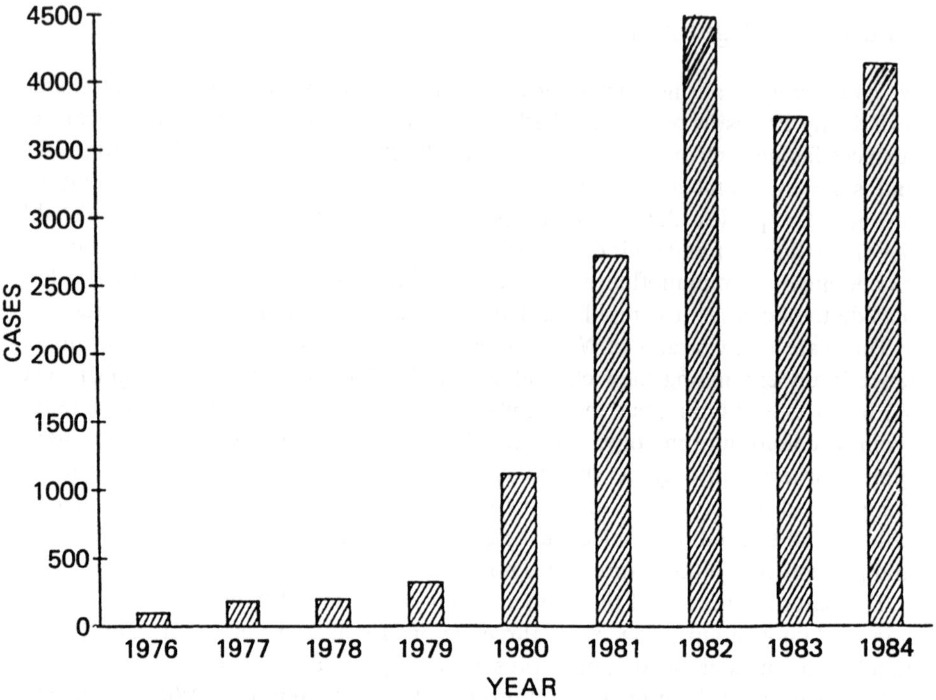


FIGURE 5.1. Reported penicillinase-producing *Neisseria gonorrhoeae* (PPNG) cases, United States, 1976–1984. From Centers for Disease Control [4].

mediated resistance may represent a continuity in the evolution of the resistance of *N. gonorrhoeae* to various antimicrobial agents. The mechanisms involved in such resistance to penicillin may be many: a decrease in the affinity of penicillin-binding proteins for beta-lactam antibiotics; an increase in the concentration of penicillin-binding proteins; or a decrease in the permeability of the gonococcal outer membrane to penicillin [11–13]. There are at least three chromosomal mutations, denoted pen A, pen B, and mtr, and they additively increase gonococcal resistance to penicillin [14,15]. As a result of increasing CMRNG, the Atlanta Center for Disease Control (CDC) in 1972 recommended doubling the currently used dose of procaine penicillin G for gonorrhea therapy from 2.4 to 4.8 million units with concomitant oral probenecid 1.0 g to maintain high serum levels and prolong the serum half-life of penicillin. In 1983 an outbreak of CMRNG in North Carolina was reported for the first time in the United States [16]. Since then more and more cases of CMRNG have been reported involving 23 states [17].

In 1976, PPNG were isolated for the first time in the Far East [18]. Almost simultaneously or shortly afterward they were encountered in the United States and United Kingdom [19,20]. Molecular epidemiology indicated that the U.S. strains were introduced from the Far East, while the U.K. strains were associated closely with the African strain. The Asia strains were originally isolated from the Philippines, and they contained a 4.4 megadalton plasmid and a 24.5 megadalton plasmid. The latter is a conjugative or transfer factor that can transfer the former to other gonococci as well as to other organisms. On the other hand, the African strains contained a 3.2 megadalton plasmid only. Since first isolated, PPNG has spread throughout the world and has become rampant in African and Asian countries like the Philippines, where PPNG prevalence was at least 30 to 40% in the early 1980s. In the United States, PPNG was encountered only sporadically from 1976 to 1979 and more dramatically since then, until in 1982 a peak was reached, totaling 4,457 cases (Fig. 5.1) [4]. Despite this alarming increase of PPNG isolates, their proportion to non-PPNG in 1982 was fortunately less than 0.5% in the United States.

Since February 1985, CDC has identified 12 isolates of *N. gonorrhoeae* with tetracycline resistance of extraordinary high minimal inhibition concentration (24 to 32 μg/ml) but they are all susceptible to penicillin. This is a new phenomenon, and its significance needs further investigation. CDC urges screening for tetracycline resistance by disk diffusion for all positive test-of-cure cultures [21].

## Clinical Findings

### Gonorrhea in Men

Symptoms and signs of acute urethritis usually develop 2 to 5 days after sexual intercourse with an infected partner; however, the incubation period may be as long as 1 month. Symptomatic uncomplicated gonorrhea typically presents as purulent urethral discharge with dysuria and sometimes urinary frequency. The patient may occasionally feel slight malaise. Urethral gonorrhea in men may be completely asymptomatic; it is rare, usually less than 5%. Asymptomatic patients tend to not seek treatment and therefore may transmit the disease to their female sexual partners, who in turn are even less likely to develop or be aware of symptoms. Thus a cycle of transmission is established, which accounts for the high incidence of gonorrhea.

On examination there is a purulent yellow or green-yellow urethral discharge and the lips of the external urethral meatus may be erythematous and swollen (Fig. 5.2). The patient may notice stains on his underclothes. A secondary balanoposthitis with a subpreputial discharge may also be present in the uncircumcised. To confirm that the discharge comes from the urethra and not from under the prepuce, the urethra can be milked forward and more discharge may appear at the meatus. With the two-glass urine test, urine will be hazy in the first glass due to the presence of pus cells and clear in the second glass, indicting that the anterior urethra alone is involved.

If the infection is untreated, the posterior urethra may become involved in about 10 to 14 days. The patient may feel severe pain and burning with urgency and frequency. There may be a few drops of blood at the end of micturition. Both glasses of urine in the two-glass urine test are hazy in appearance. Sometimes constitutional symptoms such as malaise, headache, and pyrexia may develop. There may be slight tender regional lymphadenopathy.

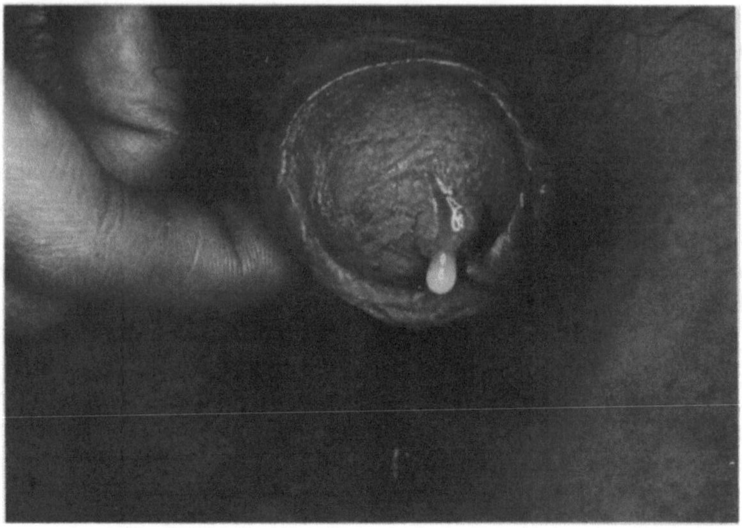

FIGURE 5.2. Acute gonorrhea in a man.

Complications occur when the glands and tissues in close relation to the urethra become involved, but this happens less frequently than previously. Complications tend to occur when symptoms and signs have been ignored and treatment delayed.

## Complications of Anterior Urethritis

The complications of anterior urethritis are infection of Tyson's glands, paraurethral ducts, the preputial sac, Littré's glands, lacunae of Morgagni, subepithelial and periurethral tissue of the urethra, the median raphe, and Cowper's ducts and glands. The parafrenal sebaceous glands of Tyson may occasionally be involved in gonococcal urethritis when the prepuce is long and hygiene is poor. If the ducts of the glands are obstructed, abscesses may develop, and a tender swelling with beads of pustules (Fig. 5.3) will be found next to the frenum. Otherwise there are no additional symptoms and the signs are inconspicuous.

Paraurethral ducts are short mucous channels and run parallel to the fossa navicularis with openings near the meatus. When infected, the paraurethral ducts may present beads of pus at their openings on pressure. Gonococcal balanoposthitis may occur in uncircumcised patients with profuse urethral discharge. Severe phimosis then develops. Infection of Littré's glands occurs inevitably in gonococcal urethritis; in the two-glass urine test, "threads" may appear in the first glass. Littritis itself is asymptomatic, but if ducts of glands are blocked, abscesses may form in the urethral wall.

Lacunae of Morgagni may also be infected, but their contents tend to be undisturbed by urinary flow because their fundi direct backward toward the posterior urethra. The gonococcus invades the submucous tissue of the urethra in gonococcal

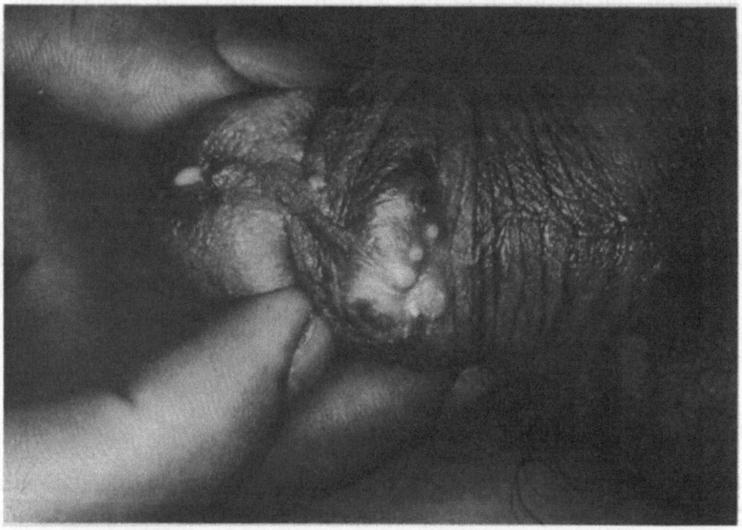

FIGURE 5.3. Acute gonococcal urethritis with abscess of Tyson's glands.

urethritis and causes an inflammatory reaction. When this reaction is severe, inflammatory hyperplasia of the submucous tissue develops, resulting in so-called soft infiltration, which causes fibrous stricture irrespective of antimicrobial treatment. When a number of abscesses in the urethral wall become fused, a large periurethral abscess forms and extends into the subepithelial tissues, with openings into the urethra and sometimes on the surface of the penile shaft or the scrotum. The fossa navicularis and the bulb are the most commonly affected sites. This complication is rarely encountered nowadays. If the ducts of Cowper's glands alone are involved in gonococcal urethritis, there may be no additional symptoms, but when the glands are infected there is likely to be abscess formation. Pain in the perineum is experienced. The skin and raphe of the penis may occasionally be infected in the form of pustular lesions.

## Complications of Posterior Urethritis

The complications of posterior urethritis are prostatitis, epididymitis, vesiculitis, and cystitis. The first two are the most common and are very important complications of gonorrhea, though they too are unusual nowadays. Gonococcal prostatitis may be acute, subacute, or chronic. Acute gonococcal prostatitis causes an exacerbation of the symptoms of urethritis together with pyrexia, general malaise, perineal discomfort, and perhaps suprapubic discomfort. On rectal examination the gland is found to be swollen and tender. This examination should be deferred when acute prostatitis is suspected. Initially the swelling is firm but it becomes fluctuant later as a prostatic abscess forms. The symptoms of acute prostatitis become even worse. The patient may experience pain on defecation and rectal tenesmus. The abscess may rupture into the urethra or rectum with immediate relief of symptoms. In subacute or chronic prostatitis, the symptoms are less severe. It is controversial if gonococcus is the causative agent, because chlamydial infection, which often coexists with gonococcal urethritis, may play an even more important role here. Epididymitis was once a common complication but is now seldom seen (about 1% of cases only). It is now believed that the infection reaches the epididymis as a result of retrograde passage of infected urine along the vas deferens. The condition is usually unilateral. The epididymis and the adjacent testicles are usually infected together, presenting as a painful, hot, red swelling. If the vas deferens is involved, lower abdominal pain may develop, mimicking appendicitis and peritonitis. When the bladder is infected, the trigon is most often involved. The patient may complain of frequency and urgency together with terminal dysuria and hematuria.

## Urogenital Gonorrhea in Women

It is usually believed that one half to three quarters of women infected with gonorrhea either have no symptoms or symptoms are so slight that they are ignored. Perhaps this belief is biased, because it is based on clinical data collected in sexually transmitted disease clinics, which most female patients attend because they are contacts of symptomatic male patients.

The incubation period of gonorrhea in women is usually longer than 2 weeks. Therefore, women are infectious carriers of the pathogen for considerable periods before the diagnosis is made and treatment instituted. When symptoms are present, they are frequently mild or so nonspecific and common that they are neglected. Symptoms include vaginal discharge, dysuria, frequency, backache, pain in the lower abdomen and pelvis, and rectal discharge and bleeding. It is very common for women with urogenital gonorrhea to have coexisting trichomoniasis (about 50% of cases), which accounts for the profuse vaginal discharge. Many women with gonorrhea are seen and treated because their sexual partners have just been diagnosed and treated. Some are discovered in gonorrhea screening programs, others after complications develop.

The endocervical canal is the primary site of female urogenital gonorrhea; urethral infection is present in 70 to 90% of cases. It is possible for the urethra to be infected alone, but this is rare, probably occurring most often in hysterectomized women.

A thorough and systemic physical examination for women with gonorrhea is extremely important. The patient should be placed in the lithotomy position for genital examination and specimen collection for Gram's stain, gonococcus culture, and other investigations. The usual sites for specimen collection are the vagina, cervix, urethra, and rectum. A normal-looking vagina and cervix does not mean the absence of infection. Gram-negative diplococci are found in about one third of infected cases, and therefore culture for gonococcus is mandatory. Many women with urogenital gonorrhea have abnormalities of the cervix, including purulent or mucopurulent discharge, erythema, and friability. Wet films from the vagina for the detection of *Trichomonas* and *Candida* is also important. *Chlamydia trachomatis* should be sought if facilities are available, because of high prevalence of coexisting infection. On pressure, purulent discharge may be expressed from the urethra or Bartholin's ducts.

Local complications of urogenital gonorrhea in women consists of skenitis, bartholinitis, and pelvic inflammatory disease (PID). When the paraurethral ducts of Skene are infected, beads of pus can be expressed from the ducts. Abscess formation of the glands is very rare. Bartholin's glands may be infected unilaterally or bilaterally, causing pain and swelling of the vulva with discomfort and difficulty in sitting and walking. If the duct is blocked, abscess of the gland develops; eventually this may rupture through the skin or mucous membrane. PID is a collective term for the involvement of the fallopian tubes, ovaries, and adjacent peritoneum. It occurs in about 10 to 15% of women with gonorrhea. PID is a serious condition requiring hospitalization and even surgery. Agonizing sequelae such as chronic pelvic pain, dyspareunia, ectopic pregnancy, and sterility may develop eventually even after successful management. Lower abdominal pain, pyrexia, and general malaise are common manifestations that often occur during or within a week after menstruation. Sometimes the patient may have dysuria, vaginal discharge, or abnormal uterine bleeding. Organisms other than gonococcus may also cause PID; frequently the infection is mixed. Gonococcus and *C. trachomatis* are the two most important etiologic agents.

## Other Sites in Men and Women

The rectal mucosa may be infected by the gonococcus in either sex. Most anorectal infection in women is the result of autoinoculation from a urogenital infection, but anorectal gonorrhea in men occurs most often in homosexuals as direct inoculation via rectal intercourse. Symptoms of anorectal gonorrhea range from mild anal pruritus, mucopurulent discharge, and scant rectal bleeding on the one hand to overt acute proctitis manifested as rectal pain, tenesmus, and constipation on the other. It is believed that less than 10% of anorectal gonorrhea in both sexes is asymptomatic, but many symptoms may be so subtle that they are neglected. Rectal mucosa smear for Gram's stain with or without the aid of anoscopy for culture may help in diagnosis. On anoscopy the mucosa looks erythematous, edematous, and friable with mucopurulent discharge.

Gonococcal infection of the pharynx is the result of orogenital sex; it occurs more readily through fellatio than through cunnilingus. Like anorectal gonorrhea, only 10% of pharyngeal gonococcal infections are asymptomatic. Sore throat with pyrexia and cervical lymphadenopathy are the common manifestations. Little is known about transmission of gonorrhea from the pharynx. *N. gonorrhoeae* was isolated from the saliva of 67% of patients with oropharyngeal gonorrhea.[22] Therefore, inoculation with the tongue may not be uncommon, in contrast to the conventional belief that transmission from the throat to another site of the sex partner is not possible.

Gonococcal conjunctivitis is rare in adults. It occurs from direct contamination of the eye with infectious discharge by fingers or towels.

## Disseminated Gonococcal Infection

Disseminated gonococcal infection (DGI) occurs in fewer than 1% of all patients with gonorrhea. It occurs mainly in women, frequently following menstruation. It usually presents with skin rashes, arthritis, arthralgias, or tenosynovitis. Skin lesions usually number fewer than 20 and are generally found on the extremities as small macules, papules, pustules, or vesicles that may be hemorrhagic or necrotic. They heal in 3 or 4 days without scarring. Gram's stain and culture of skin lesions are seldom positive for gonococcus, but direct immunofluorescent studies identify *N. gonorrhoeae* in the majority of cases. Arthritis and tenosynovitis will develop if there is no proper treatment. The hands are most frequently involved, followed by the elbows, ankles, wrists, and small joints of the hands and feet. The arthralgias are characteristically nonmigratory. Gram's stain of synovial fluid may show intracellular gram-negative diplococci in less than half of the cases and cultures will be positive in the same proportion. Blood cultures are more likely to be positive for gonococci in the early stage and rarely positive during the late stage. The diagnosis of DGI is confirmed by isolation of the gonococcus from blood or synovial fluid from commonly infected sites where local symptoms of gonococcal infection are lacking.

Gonococcal endocarditis, myopericarditis, meningitis, and hepatitis are now rare. Meningococcemia may produce an identical clinical picture as DGI and its role in the acute arthritis-dermatitis syndrome has been noted to be even more important than that of the gonococcus [23].

## Gonorrhea in Children

Genital gonorrhea in children is rare, and when it occurs, sexual assault or precocity should be considered. It occurs more often in girls than in boys, directly through sexual contact with an infected adult or indirectly through contact with contaminated body parts or things. Before puberty the vagina mucosa is thin, with poor glycogen content and alkaline pH. Thus it is more susceptible to gonococcal infection, and gonococcal vulvovaginitis may occur. There may be profuse vaginal discharge, dysuria, soreness, swelling, and erythema of the vulva. Complications are uncommon.

Gonococcal ophthalmia neonatorum was formerly a cause of blindness in children, but it is relatively uncommon nowadays. Gonococcus probably accounts for 5 to 15% of cases of ophthalmia neonatorum. The eyes may show infection 1 to 4 days after birth as a result of infection in utero or during parturition through the infected cervix, but the incubation period may be as long as 13 days. Purulent discharge is seen oozing from between swollen and erythematous lids. Care must be taken in parting the lids for examination of the eye, because pus under pressure may spurt out. Without treatment, conjunctivitis may proceed to involvement of the cornea with ulceration and iridocyclitis and eventual blindness. Therefore prevention and proper treatment are very important. The best method of prevention is to diagnose and treat the infected mother during pregnancy. Routine antenatal screening for the disease may be considered in areas with high prevalence.

## Pathology

*N. gonorrhoeae* has a special affinity for columnar epithelium, while the stratified and squamous epithelia are more resistant to attack. Therefore the urethra, its glands, the prostate, seminal vesicles, and epididymis in men, and the endocervix, Skene's glands, urethra, Bartholin's glands, and fallopian tubes in women are particularly susceptible to the gonococcus. The rectal mucosa in both sexes is also at special risk. The gonococcus can penetrate the epithelium easily between the epithelial cells, causing a submucosal inflammation with marked polymorphonuclear reaction within 72 hours of gonococcal inoculation. Infection is manifested clinically as purulent urethral discharge as a result of desquamation together with shedding of white cells. Spread of infection from the anterior to the posterior urethra is by continuity of surface from columnar to transitional epithelium.

The histopathology is similarly submucosal inflammation and desquamation. Untreated anterior urethritis in healthy men resolves as a result of local immune response and adequate drainage; however, in posterior gonococcal urethritis, free drainage is dependent on regular micturition due to two sphincter structures in that part on the urethra. Complications of posterior gonococcal urethritis are closely associated with the sphincters. Natural immunity after an attack of gonorrhea does not occur.

## Diagnosis

The diagnosis of gonococcal infection from clinical manifestations alone can be misleading in male patients and often impossible in female patients. Gram-stained smear and culture of specimens from potentially infected sites with biochemical or special tests such as immunologic studies are necessary for a definite diagnosis. Sometimes it is difficult if not impossible to differentiate gonococcal from nongonococcal urethritis in male patients on clinical grounds alone, though in more than 90% of patients discharge is purulent and 30 to 40% have spontaneous urethral drip, whereas discharge is purulent in only 20 to 25% of patients with nongonococcal urethritis and is rarely spontaneous ($<5\%$) [24]. Many studies have proved that Gram's stain is a safe, simple, inexpensive, and accurate test in symptomatic male patients with gonococcal urethritis, permitting a correct diagnosis in about 95% of cases. False-negative results are common in asymptomatic infections and in female patients, in whom more than 30% of urethral and cervical Gram-stained smears are negative. Gram-stained smears are even more unreliable in rectal and pharyngeal specimens. Therefore, reliable laboratory culture and confirmatory tests are mandatory for a definite diagnosis, and also for cases in which legal action for rape or divorce proceedings might result, for antibiotic sensitivity testing, and for other investigations.

In men with symptomatic gonorrhea and in asymptomatic men who are contacts of patients with gonorrhea, swabs from the urethra for Gram-stained smear and bacteria cultures should be taken. In women, similarly, both urethral and cervical specimens should be obtained for the same purposes. Many physicians recommend rectal tests for women who are presumptive gonorrhea contacts, because occasionally the rectum is the only site infected even if the woman denies rectal intercourse. Rectal smear and culture should be done routinely in passive homosexuals and women admitting to rectal intercourse. In gonorrhea contacts admitting orogenital sex and in homosexuals, throat swab for culture is the only reliable way to make a correct diagnosis. Specimen sites to be included depends on the clinical manifestations and index of suspicion, and repeated tests from sites like the rectum, throat, and female urethra and cervix may be necessary before the diagnosis of gonorrhea can be confidently excluded.

The immediate identification of *N. gonorrhoeae* can be made by means of Gram-stained smears. A bacteriologist's platinum loop sterilized by flame from a Bunsen burner, or a sterile cotton wool swab, is used to obtain material from infected sites. The material is spread evenly and thinly on a clean glass slide. The slide is air dried and fixed by being passed through the flame of a lamp one or two times quickly. The slide is then ready for Gram's stain. Gram's stain has been extensively investigated and modified. The formula and procedures recommended by Lennette's *Manual of Clinical Microbiology* [25] are the following:

| Formula | | Procedure |
|---|---|---|
| 1. Modified Hucker crystal violet | | |
| Crystal violet | 2.0 g | Flood the smear with this solution for 1 minute and then wash the smear briefly with tap water. |
| Ethyl alcohol, 95% | 20.0 ml | |
| Ammonium oxalate | 0.8 g | |
| Distilled water | 80.0 ml | |
| 2. Gram iodine | | |
| Iodine | 1.0 g | Flood the smear with Gram iodine solution for 1 minute and then wash the smear briefly with tap water. |
| Potassium iodide | 2.0 g | |
| Distilled water | 100.0 ml | |
| 3. Decolorizer | | |
| 95% ethyl alcohol or acetone | | Decolorize the smear until the dye doesn't run off the smear. |
| 4. Counter stain | | |
| Stock solution | | |
| Safranin 0 | 2.5 g | Counterstain the smear with freshly prepared working solution for 10 seconds. Then wash briefly with tap water, bolt dry, and examine microscopically with the 2-mm oil immersion lens. Interpretation of result: Gram-positive organisms are blue; Gram-negative organisms are red |
| Ethyl alcohol | 100.0 ml | |
| Working solution | | |
| Stock solution | 10.0 ml | |
| Distilled water | 90.0 ml | |

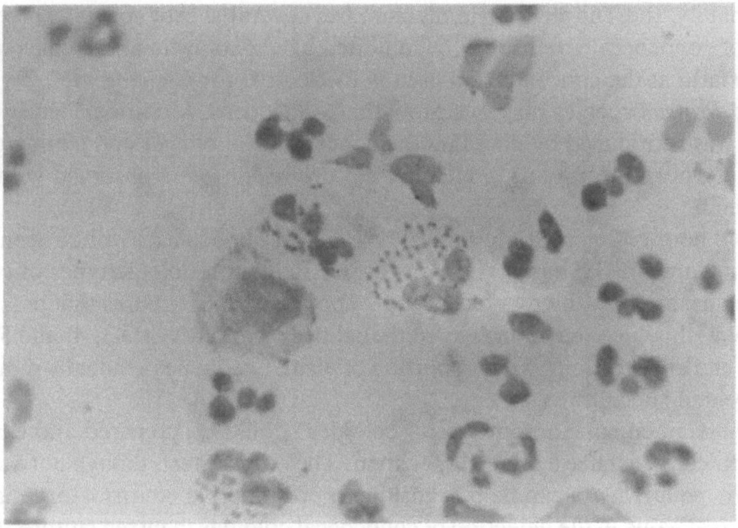

FIGURE 5.4. Gram-stained smear showing gram-negative diplococci intracellularly in polymorphonuclear leukocytes.

A provisional diagnosis can be made by finding gram-negative bean-shaped diplococci with concave surfaces facing each other intracellularly in polymorphonuclear leukocytes (Fig. 5.4). Gram-stained smears have a high degree of sensitivity, 94.5%, in the diagnosis of acute urethral gonorrhea in male patients, but are much less sensitive, about 33 to 66%, in other gonococcal infections [26].

To establish a definite diagnosis of gonococcal infection, culture of the gonococcus and identification of the organism by sophisticated biochemical and immunologic tests are indispensable. The specimens for culture should be plated directly onto culture medium and placed immediately into the incubator at 35° to 36°C with 5% $CO_2$ and at least 70% humidity. When direct plating and immediate incubation are impracticable, transport systems are needed, and many such systems are available. Conventional nonnutrient systems such as Aimes modification of Stuart's medium are replaced by combined systems for transport and isolation at the same time. Transgrow medium is a modified Thayer-Martin medium in a small $CO_2$-containing bottle or tube usable for such purposes.

The most widely used selective medium for primary culture of gonococcus is the modified Thayer-Martin medium. There are two reasons why selective medium is important: (a) It prevents other flora in the sample from overgrowing and masking the presence of any gonococci that may grow and (b) it prevents the growth of several bacterial species that are capable of inhibiting the growth of gonococcus. Examples of these species are *N. meningitidis*, *N. subflava*, *Staphylococcus aureus*, group A streptococci, and *Corynebacterium* species. Thayer-Martin medium contains vancomycin, 3 μm/ml; colistimethate sodium, 7.5 mg/ml; and nystatin, 12.5 mg/ml.

Unfortunately, the Thayer-Martin medium has several shortcomings: Three to ten percent of gonococcal strains may be inhibited by vancomycin at the concentration used; nystatin at the concentration used is ineffective for *Candida albicans* inhibition; and *Proteus* species may overgrow the gonococcus. Modified Thayer-Martin medium was introduced by doubling the concentration of agar and adding glucose and trimethroprim (5 μg/ml), and better culture results were observed with use of this medium.

After 48 hours of incubation, typical colonies of gonococcus will be seen on the plate. They are small, round, and translucent. Five morphologic types of colonies have been described. Colony types 1 and 2 contain virulent strains that possess pili or fibriae with which they attach to epithelial cells. Colony types 3, 4, and 5 do not have pili and are avirulent. The proportion of virulent colonies gradually diminishes after repeated subcultures.

A Gram-stained smear from typical colonies should be prepared and examined microscopically just like a clinical specimen. The oxidase test, though not a specific test for *N. gonorrheae*, can help in making a presumptive confirmatory diagnosis and has great value in the detection of gonococcal colonies in mixed culture. A small amount of freshly prepared oxidase reagent (1.0% aqueous tetramethylparaphenylene-diamine HCl) is applied to suspected colonies. Gonococcal colonies turn pink, purple, and finally black within a few seconds of dye application, and if picked off quickly with a loop can be subcultured. Definite identification of the gonococcus can only be made by sugar fermentation tests. Pure colonies should be inoculated to four hydrocele-agar slopes containing 1% glucose, maltose, sucrose, and lactose, respectively. When the slopes are incubated, a change of color from red to yellow is a positive reaction as acid is formed; a phenyl red indicator in the medium is responsible for the color change. Table 5.1 summarizes the fermentation reaction of the *Neisseria*.

## Treatment

Antibiotic sensitivity of *N. gonorrhoeae* varies geographically. Therefore routine investigation for antimicrobial sensitivity of all isolates is an integral part of a successful gonorrhea control program. In at least 45% of cases of gonococcal urethritis, coexisting chlamydial infection is found if adequate chlamydial cultures are per-

TABLE 5.1. Fermentation reaction of *Neisseria*.

| Species | Glucose | Maltose | Sucrose | Lactose |
|---|---|---|---|---|
| *N. gonorrhoeae* | + | − | − | − |
| *N. meningitidis* | + | + | − | − |
| *N. pharyngis sicca* | + | + | + | − |
| *N. lactamica* | + | + | − | + |
| *N. catarrhalis* | − | − | − | − |

TABLE 5.2. Treatment regimens for uncomplicated gonococcal urethritis.

| Regimen | Special considerations |
|---|---|
| Single-dose | |
| Aqueous procaine penicillin G, 4.8 million units IM PLUS probenecid, 1.0 g PO | Painful; large volume of parenteral injection; possible penicillin anaphylaxis (1 in 10,000); possible procaine reaction (psychosis, 1 in 1,000); no effect on concomitant chlamydial infection; effective for anorectal and pharyngeal gonorrhea; can eradicate incubating syphilis |
| Ampicillin, 3.5 g PO, or amoxicillin, 3.0 g PO, PLUS probenecid, 1.0 g PO | No effect on anorectal, pharyngeal gonorrhea; no effect on concomitant chlamydial infection; can eradicate incubating syphilis |
| Spectinomycin HCl, 2.0 g IM | Recommended for PPNG and CMRNG strains; effective for anorectal gonorrhea; no effect on pharyngeal gonorrhea; no effect on concomitant chlamydial infection; cannot eradicate incubating syphilis |
| Ceftriaxone, 250 mg IM | Recommended for PPNG and CMRNG strains |
| Multiple-day | |
| Tetracycline HCl, 500 mg PO QID for 7 days OR doxycycline, 100 mg PO BID for 7 days | Compliance is needed; ineffective for anorectal gonorrhea in men; effective for susceptible gonococcus and concomitant chlamydial infection; effective for pharyngeal gonorrhea; can eradicate incubating syphilis |
| Combined | |
| Multiple-day therapy with tetracycline/doxycycline for 7 days following any of above single-dose regimens | Compliance is needed; recommended for concomitant chlamydial infection; erythromycin stearate or base, 500 mg PO QID, can be used when tetracycline is contraindicated |

Adapted from CDC information.

formed. Homosexual men are less likely than heterosexual men to have coexisting chlamydial infections.

A single-dose regimen for gonorrhea is ideal for the problem of patient compliance. A multiple-day tetracycline/doxycycline regimen for the coexisting chlamydial infection following the antigonorrhea regimen is favored by many venereologists. But routine use of the combined regimen has not yet been critically evaluated. No attempt has been made here to list all possible treatment regimens. With any regimen, considerations must include efficacy, safety, ease of administration, and cost.

## Uncomplicated Gonococcal Infection

The regimens recommended by the Atlanta Centers for Disease Control (CDC) for uncomplicated gonococcal infection are summarized in Table 5.2 [27]. Aqueous procaine penicillin G–probenecid, ampicillin–probenecid, and amoxicillin–probenecid are regimens of choice for uncomplicated infection caused by non-beta-lactamase gonococci, which is still common in the United States. If beta-lactamase gonococci exceed 5% in most gonococcal infections in an area, penicillin and related agents are not drugs of choice [28]. For infection due to PPNG, the current drugs of choice are spectinomycin and third-generation cephalosporins such as ceftriaxone. Other antimicrobials such as clavulanic acid and sulbactam in combination with penicillin or ampicillin, quinolone derivatives, and monobactam derivatives have been investigated in the treatment of gonorrhea with successful cure rates both in penicillin-susceptible and penicillin-resistant strains [29].

The fluorinated 4-quinolone derivatives are a subgroup of quinolones that include nalidixic acid. The quinolones include rosoxacin, norfloxacin, enoxacin, ofloxacin, and ciprofloxacin. Ciprofloxacin, as low as 250 mg once, or enoxacin, as low as 400 mg once, will provide an almost 100% cure. A single 300-mg dose of rosoxacin has a cure rate of 78 to 100% for gonococcal infection in adults. A two-dose regimen of rosoxacin, 150 mg 4 hours apart, has yielded a 100% cure rate. Norfloxacin, in a single oral dose of 400, 600, or 800 mg, has produced cure rates approaching 100%. Ofloxacin, at 100 mg to 600 mg given in a single dose, is almost 100% effective. Adverse effects for these drugs include dizziness, headache, nausea, malaise, giddiness, and euphoria; they are not dosage dependent.

## Disseminated Gonococcal Infection

The patient should be hospitalized and endocarditis and meningitis ruled out.

| |
|---|
| Aqueous crystalline penicillin G, 10 million units IV QD for at least 3 days or until improvement occurs, followed by amoxicillin or ampicillin, 500 mg PO QID, to complete at least 7 days of therapy—OR |
| Amoxicillin, 3.0 g, or ampicillin, 3.5 g, each with probenecid, 1.0 g, by mouth followed by amoxicillin or ampicillin, 500 mg PO QID, for at least 7 days—OR |
| Cefoxitin, 1.0 g IV QID × 7 days—OR |
| Cefotaxine, 500 mg IV QID × 7 days—OR |
| Ceftriaxone, 1.0 g IV QD × 7 days—OR |
| Tetracycline HCl, 500 mg PO QID, OR doxycycline, 100 mg PO BID, for at least 7 days each |

Gonococcal endocarditis and meningitis require high-dose penicillin therapy IV, 10 to 14 days for the latter and 1 month for the former. An expert should be consulted for the treatment of PPNG- or CMRNG-related endocarditis or meningitis.

## Gonococcal Pelvic Inflammatory Disease

### Severe

| |
|---|
| Hospitalization |
| Aqueous crystalline penicillin G, 20 million units/day IV in divided doses, until significant clinical improvement occurs, followed by ampicillin, 0.5 g orally QID × 10 days |
| OR |
| Tetracycline HCl, 2.0 g/day IV, OR doxycycline, 100 mg IV Q12h until significant clinical improvement occurs, followed by tetracycline HCl, 0.5 g orally QID × 10 days |

### Mild or Moderate

No hospitalization
Procaine penicillin G, 4.8 million units IM, and probenecid, 1.0 g PO, in a single dose followed by ampicillin, 0.5 g PO QID × 10 days

OR

Ampicillin 3.5 g PO, and probenecid, 1.0 g PO, in a single dose followed by ampicillin, 0.5 g PO QID × 10 days

OR

Tetracycline HCl, 1.5 g PO, followed by 0.5 g PO QID × 10 days

## Gonorrhea in Pregnancy

Use regimens as shown in Table 5.2 except that tetracyclines be replaced by erythromycin. Patients with acute salpingitis and disseminated gonococcal infection should be referred to appropriate sections for management.

## Gonococcal Ophthalmia

### Adults

Hospitalization
Aqueous crystalline penicillin G, 10 million units IV QD × 5 days
For PPNG strains:
Cefoxitin, 1.0 g IV QID × 5 days,

OR

Cefotaxime, 500 mg IV QD × 5 days,

OR

Ceftriaxone, 1.0 g IM QD × 5 days

The eyes should be irrigated with saline or buffered ophthalmic solutions as adjunctive therapy. Topical antibiotics have no place here. All patients should be followed carefully for ocular complications.

### Neonates

Hospitalization and isolation for 24 hours after beginning of treatment
Aqueous crystalline penicillin G, 100,000 units/kg/day in four divided doses × 7 days.

The rest of the principle of management is similar to that of gonococcal ophthalmia in adults.

## Infants Born to Mothers with Untreated Urogenital Gonorrhea

Aqueous crystalline penicillin G: for full-term infants, 50,000 units IM or IV in a single dose; for low-birth-weight infants, 200,000 units IM or IV in a single dose.

To assist prompt and satisfactory recovery from gonococcal infection, patients should be advised to refrain from alcohol and vigorous exercise for at least 2 weeks. All patients infected with gonorrhea should refrain from sexual intercourse until they have recovered completely from the infection and from associated non-gonococcal infections.

## Prognosis

With present diagnostic tools and therapeutic modalities, uncomplicated gonococcal infection treated early has an excellent prognosis for complete recovery. Problems may occur from neglect in seeking proper advice and from concomitant nongonococcal infection, especially chlamydia. Catastrophic complications such as gonococcal meningitis and endocarditis are rare nowadays, but pelvic inflammatory disease due to *N. gonorrhoeae* and/or *C. trachomatis* may lead to recurrent morbidity if diagnosis and treatment are delayed.

## Follow-Up

Patients treated for gonorrhea should be followed regularly for test-of-cure and coexistent infections, particularly syphilis and chlamydial infection. However, more than half of patients do not come back for close observation and tests after relief of their symptoms.

Patients treated for gonorrhea should be seen 3 to 7 days after treatment. Tests including Gram's stain, culture for gonococcus, two-glass urine test, and tests for chlamydia (if facilities are available) should be performed. Men should be seen again 1 or 2 weeks later and women twice more at weekly intervals, with the last visit preferably after a menstruation. Serologic test(s) for syphilis should be done before treatment and repeated after 3 months.

## References

1. Morton RS: Gonorrhoea. London: WB Saunders, 1977.
2. Nicol CS: World trends in sexually transmitted diseases: The situation in the United States. In: RD Catteral, CS Nicol (Eds): *Sexually Transmitted Diseases*. London: Academic Press, 1976, pp. 13–25.
3. Barnes RC, Holmes KK: Epidemiology of gonorrhea: Current perspectives. *Epidemiol Rev* **6**:1–30, 1984.
4. Centers for Disease Control: Annual Summary-1984: Gonorrhea. *MMWR* **33**:24–26, 1986.
5. Weller IVD, Hindley DJ, Adler MW: Gonorrhoea in homosexual men and media coverage of the acquired immune deficiency syndrome in London 1982-3. *Lancet* **2**:1041, 1984.
6. Sandstrom EG, Chen KCS, Buchanan TM: Serology of *N. gonorrhoeae*: Coagglutination serogroups WI and WII/WIII correspond to different outer membrane protein I molecules. *Infect Immunol* **38**:462–470, 1982.

7. Knapp JS, Tam MR, Nowinski RC, et al: Serological classification of *N. gonorrhoeae* with use of monoclonal antibodies to gonococcal outer membrane protein. I. *J Infect Dis* **150**:44–48, 1984.
8. Wang SP, Holmes KK, Knapp JS, et al: Immunologic classification of *N. gonorrhoeae* with micro-immunofluorescence. *J Immunol* **119**:795–803, 1977.
9. Reyn A: Sensitivity of *N. gonorrhoeae* to antibiotics. *Br J Vener Dis* **37**:145–157, 1961.
10. Marin JE, Lester A, Price EV, et al: Comparative study of gonococcal susceptibility to penicillin in the United States, 1955–1969. *J Infect Dis* **122**:459–461, 1970.
11. Dougherty TJ, Koller AE, Tomasz A: Penicillin-binding proteins of penicillin-susceptible and intrinsically resistant *N. gonorrhoeae*. *Antimicrob Agents Chemother* **18**:730–737, 1980.
12. Dougherty TJ: Peptidoglycan biosynthesis in *N. gonorrhoeae* strains sensitive and intrinsically resistant to beta-lactam antibiotics. *J Bacteriol* 429–435, 1983.
13. Dougherty TJ, Koller AE, Tomasz A: Competition of beta-lactam antibiotics for penicillin-binding proteins of *N. gonorrhoeae*. *Antimicrob Agents Chemother* **20**:109–114, 1981.
14. Jaffe HW, Schroeter AL, Reynolds GH, et al: Pharmacokinetic determinants of penicillin cure of gonococcal urethritis. *Antimicrob Agents Chemother* **15**:587–591, 1979.
15. Sparling PF, Sarubbi FA Jr, Blackman E: Inheritance of low-level resistance to penicillin, tetracycline, and chloramphicol in *N. gonorrhoeae*. *J Bacteriol* **124**:740–749, 1975.
16. Center for Disease Control: Penicillin-resistant gonorrhea-North Carolina. *MMWR* **32**:273–275, 1983.
17. Rice RJ, Biddle JW, JeanLouis YA, et al: Chromosomally mediated resistance in *N. gonorrhoeae* in the United States: Results of surveillance and reporting, 1983–1984. *J Infect Dis* **153**:340–345, 1986.
18. Ashford WA, Golash RG, Hemming VG: Penicillinase-producing *N. gonorrhoeae*. *Lancet* **2**:657–658, 1976.
19. Philips I: Beta-lactamase-producing, penicillin-resistant gonococcus. *Lancet* **2**:656–658, 1976.
20. Percival A, Riwlands, Corkill JE, et al: Penicillinase-producing gonococci in Liverpool. *Lancet* **2**:1379–1382, 1976.
21. Center for Disease Control: Tetracycline-resistant *N. gonorrhoeae*-Georgia, Pennsylvania, New Hampshire. *MMWR* **34**:563–570, 1985.
22. Hutt DM, Judson FN: Epidemiology and treatment of oropharyngeal gonorrhea. *Ann Intern Med* **104**:655–658, 1986.
23. Rompalo AM, Hook III EW, Roberts PL, et al: The acute arthritis-dermatitis syndrome. *Arch Intern Med* **147**:281–283, 1987.
24. Jacobs NF, Kraus SJ: Gonococcal and non-gonococcal urethritis in men: Clinical and laboratory differentiation. *Ann Intern Med* **82**:7–12, 1975.
25. Lennette EH, Balows A, Hausler WJ, et al (Eds): *Manual of Clinical Microbiology*. 4th ed. Washington, D.C.: American Society for Microbiology, 1985, pp. 1102–1103.
26. Goh BT, Varia KB, Ayliffe PF, et al: Diagnosis of gonorrhea by Gram-stained smears and cultures in men and women: Role of the urethral smear. *Sex Trans Dis* **12**:135–139, 1985.
27. Center for Disease Control: *Sexually Transmitted Diseases Treatment Guidelines*. Atlanta: CDC, 1985.
28. Editorial: Penicillinase-producing *N. gonorrhoeae*-a retrospective. *N Engl J Med* **307**: 438–439, 1982.
29. Rice RJ, Thompson SE: Treatment of uncomplicated infections due to *N. gonorrhoeae*. *JAMA* **255**:1739–1746, 1986.

CHAPTER 6

# Chancroid

Allen R. Ronald

## Overview and Definition

Chancroid is a sexually transmitted infection, clinically manifested by acute ulcers on the external genitalia and inguinal lymphadenopathy with bubo formation. Although it was initially described by Ricord in 1838, it was first differentiated from syphilis by Bassereau in 1852. Ducrey described the etiologic agent in 1889, but its cultivation on solid media was difficult and unpredictable. As a result, controversy about *Haemophilus ducreyi* and its role in chancroid continued until recently. Newer technologies that facilitate the culture of *H. ducreyi* now permit a specific diagnosis.

Chancroid is epidemic in many countries in the developing world. In some it is the second most commonly diagnosed sexually transmitted disease. In Western countries, chancroid appears sporadically in clusters that result in limited epidemics. Sporadic importation of cases is also seen, particularly at sea ports.

The definitive diagnosis of chancroid requires isolation of *H. ducreyi* in culture. The supposedly classic chancroidal ulcer can be mimicked by other sexually transmitted diseases. Also, about 25% of patients with chancroid have lesions that mimic donovanosis, herpetic ulcers, or primary syphilis. Laboratory investigation is essential to establish an etiologic diagnosis [1].

Several treatment regimens have been shown to eradicate *H. ducreyi* and cure chancroid. Short-term and single-dose regimens have now been proven to be effective. *H. ducreyi* has been able to acquire plasmid-mediated resistance readily from other bacteria, and increasing resistance can be anticipated in the future.

Control and prevention of chancroid can be accomplished by programs to diagnose and treat ulcers in prostitutes and by measures to encourage condom usage in men who engage in high-risk sexual activity.

Recent evidence that chancroid increases the risk of concomitant infection with human immunodeficiency virus (HIV-1) should encourage increasing efforts to control chancroid.

## Synonyms

Common synonyms for chancroid are ulcus molle, soft sore, soft chancre, and chancre mou.

## Etiology

*H. ducreyi* is a small, gram-negative, bipolar-staining rod. Its requirement for hemin classifies it within the genus *Haemophilus*. Although the organism shares some antigenic relationships with other members of the genus *Haemophilus*, bacterial genetic studies suggest that it is only distantly related.

*H. ducreyi* has no unique immunologic or biochemical characteristics that permit specific identification; however, on primary isolation, its colonies are distinctive. They vary in size and opacity and give the impression of a mixed culture. Most colonies are 0.5 to 1.0 mm in diameter, yellow-gray in color, dome shaped, and extremely cohesive when nudged with a straight wire [2].

*H. ducreyi* require a unique environment for primary isolation. Two primary selective media, gonococcal agar base and Mueller-Hinton agar base with vancomycin added to prevent overgrowth of gram-positive contaminating bacteria, are incubated at 33°C in $CO_2$ in a humid environment. Typical colonies are apparent only at 48 hours. The organism is very susceptible to temperature, not growing at incubator temperatures above 36°C. It requires 100% humidity and $CO_2$. Many laboratories continue to have difficulty with isolation of *H. ducreyi* because they fail to recognize its fastidious requirements [3].

No serotyping system has yet been designed for *H. ducreyi*.

Plasmids are commonly found in *H. ducreyi*; 11 specific plasmids have been described since 1978. These can mediate antibacterial resistance to ampicillin, tetracycline, chloramphenicol, streptomycin, kanamycin, sulfonamides, and trimethoprim. The plasmids are similar to and, in some cases, identical to those found in *Neisseria gonorrhoeae* or in other *Haemophilus* species [4].

## Epidemiology

In an industrialized society, chancroid occurs in clusters frequently at major ports of entry. Five discrete outbreaks have been described in the United States and Canada during the past 12 years. Endemic chancroid is presently occurring in New York City and in South Florida. In these outbreaks, prostitutes are implicated as a reservoir for chancroid. Epidemiologic investigation and treatment of prostitutes ended an outbreak in Winnipeg in 1977 [5] and one in Orange County, California, in 1982 [6]. Chancroid continues to occur sporadically among individuals who have traveled to endemic regions. Although investigators in Sheffield, England, reported that *H. ducreyi* was endemic in their region and was co-infecting herpetic ulcers, this has not been confirmed by other investigators and was presumably an incorrect observation [5,7].

In Third World societies, chancroid is endemic. Prostitution again appears to be the reservoir for ongoing disease in men. In an epidemiologic study carried out in East Africa, the source contacts of 10 men with chancroid were investigated, and all 10 women had genital ulcers. Among 29 secondary contacts of men with culture-proven chancroid, 17 had ulcers. We, and others, have not been able to prove that *H. ducreyi* exists in an asymptomatic reservoir in either men or women, and it is presumed that individuals capable of transmitting the infection to others have ulcers;

however, particularly in women, ulcers may often be subclinical and patients continue to be sexually active [8,9].

The incubation period of chancroid ranges from 3 days to 3 weeks, with an average incubation period in men of about 7 days. Presence of the foreskin increases susceptibility to infection; the incidence of chancroid is about 3 to 1 in uncircumcised compared with circumcised men.

Historically, chancroid has been presumed to be a disease of individuals with low standards of cleanliness. Recent studies from East Africa have shown that prostitutes with limited health care have a very high prevalence of genital ulcer disease. These women become an efficient reservoir for continued dissemination of *H. ducreyi* throughout the community of sexually promiscuous men and women. In Western societies, prostitutes make a more limited contribution to the epidemiology of sexually transmitted diseases. This may explain the infrequency of chancroid in such societies.

## Clinical Findings

The chancroidal ulcer begins as a tender papule that ulcerates within 24 hours. The papule is never vesicular.

Most patients do not present themselves for care until 1 to 2 weeks after the appearance of the ulcer. In an outbreak of 101 men, 77 presented themselves because of the genital ulcer and 11 because of painful inguinal lymphadenopathy, 8 had gonococcal urethritis with an ulcer detected only during examination of the genitalia, and 5 were identified as a result of contact tracing after being named as sexual partners by women with ulcers [5]. In this series of men, most of whom were uncircumcised, fully one quarter were unaware of the genital ulcer when they presented for the initial examination. Among women, an even smaller proportion (5 of 34) presented with symptomatic ulcer disease. Thirteen women presented with primary symptoms related to the urinary tract, and seven presented because of pain on defecation. Nine women with genital ulcers were identified only by contact tracing, and five of these denied knowledge of ulcers when examined. Rarely do women present with a primary complaint of inguinal lymphadenopathy. Presumably, chancroid in women is often subclinical because of the slow progression of ulcers, the lesser visibility of lesions on female genitalia, and the minimal discomfort of ulcers in some women.

Among men, about two thirds have classic chancroidal ulcers. The lesions are painful, irregular, undermined, not indurated, and sharply demarcated. Very little inflammation of the surrounding skin is apparent. The base of the ulcer is covered by gray-yellow purulent exudate and bleeds during sampling for culture. Although an unpleasant odor is often described, this is not particularly characteristic and is more associated with inadequate cleanliness. It is often exacerbated in uncircumcised men by the presence of painful ulcers that prevent retraction of the foreskin [10].

In men, chancroid presents in one of six sites. Although the site of infection presumably relates in some way to the site of the ulcer in the female contact, this has not been investigated. In uncircumcised men, about one half of all ulcers occur on the prepuce. Edema of the prepuce is common and may create phimosis or make it impossible to retract the foreskin. Lesions occur on the external skin on the prepuce, either singly or as multiple lesions clustered together. A ring of small ulcers numbering 6 to 20 on the distal margin of the prepuce is a unique clinical presentation of chancroid. In only about 20% of uncircumcised men do lesions occur on the inner skin of the prepuce; frequently at this site they are paired with an ulcer on the glans ("kissing ulcers"). The second most common site for genital ulcers is the coronal sulcus. A single ulcer or a partial to complete ring of ulcers is commonly seen at this site.

The frenulum is the next most common site for ulcers. It has been postulated that with penile movement during intercourse, the frenulum sustains minor abrasions that facilitate inoculation of *H. ducreyi*. The glans and meatus are the next most common sites. Internal urethral lesions are rare, but have been described in men who present primarily with pain on urination. The penile shaft is the fifth most common site, and ulcers occur in about 15% of patients. On the shaft, the ulcers are frequently less painful and more indolent. Increased condom use may also result in more ulcers appearing at the base of the penile shaft. A minority of ulcers, less than 5%, occur on the scrotum and on the skin surrounding the genitalia, including the perineum and thighs. Two cases of extragenital lesions on the fingers were described in a series of 101 men, but these locations are rare [5]. Ulcers frequently satellite and new ulcers may appear due to infection from the primary ulcer. Anal ulcers due to *H. ducreyi*, have been reported but are unusual. Chancroid may present with unique and atypical features. In about 5% of men in Nairobi, chancroid is first manifest as a septic sore, characterized by an abscess of the foreskin that may contain several milliliters of pus. Other presentations include herpetiform ulcers that mimic genital herpes, pustular chancroid that resembles a folliculitis, and giant serpiginous ulcers due to the merger of several spreading ulcers. About 10% of ulcers are indurated and have many of the features of the primary chancre of syphilis. Suprainfection with necrotizing anaerobic bacteria can produce a progressive destructive foul-smelling ulcer.

*H. ducreyi* can cause purulent urethritis. Studies in Kenya have shown that 1 to 2% of men who present with acute purulent urethritis are infected with *H. ducreyi* and that this is a concomitant presentation in 2 to 3% of men with genital ulcer disease.

Among women, the most common site for ulcers are the labia majora, the forchette, the perineum, the medial aspects of the thighs, the clitoris, and around the anus, in descending order of importance. Women tend to have multiple ulcers; a mean of 4.5 discrete lesions was reported in one study. Cervical ulcers and extragenital ulcers each occur in about 10% of women. Ulcers on the vaginal wall are unusual. In several studies, about one half of women were unaware of the ulcers at the time of genital examination.

Ulcers in women tend to be purulent, superficial, nonindurated, irregular, and tender. In general, they are less painful than in men.

Within 1 week of ulceration, inguinal lymphadenopathy appears in about 40% of men and 25% of women. The lymph nodes are initially discrete, very tender, and bilateral in about one half of patients. If untreated, the lymphadenopathy

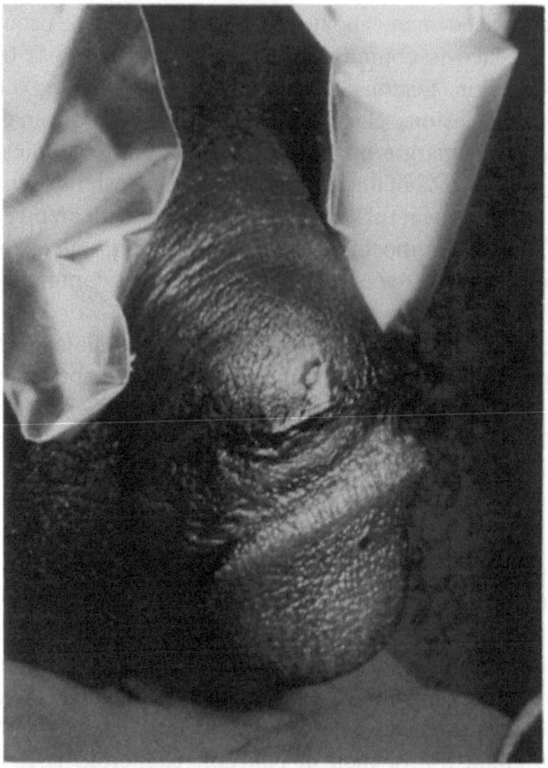

FIGURE 6.1. A septic sore. Over 1 ml of pus was present in the skin of the penile shaft. A culture of the pus yielded a pure growth of *H. ducreyi*. No ulcer is present.

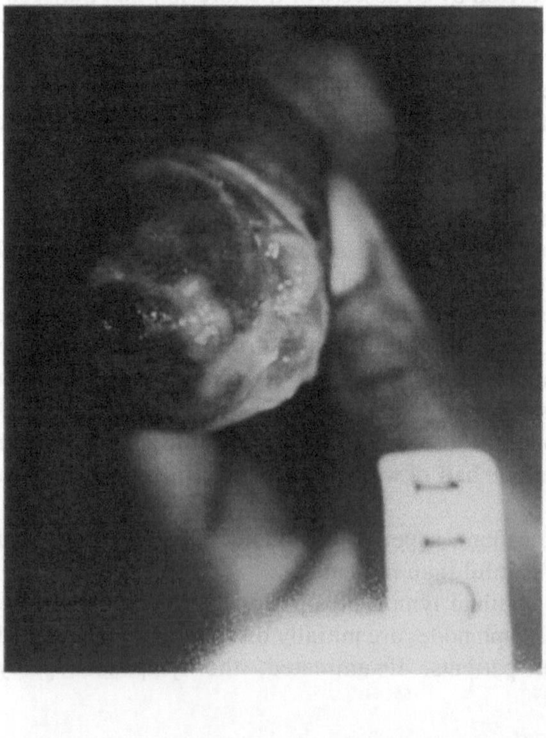

FIGURE 6.2. Three small ulcers on the glans with three additional ulcers present on the coronal sulcus and on the frenulum. Culture was positive for *H. ducreyi*.

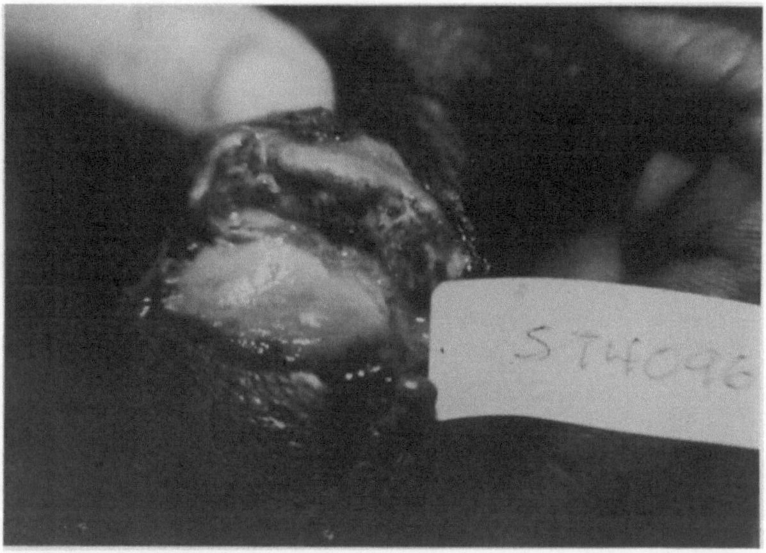


FIGURE 6.3. Large necrotic penetrating ulcer on the coronal sulcus. Necrotic base culture was positive for *H. ducreyi*.

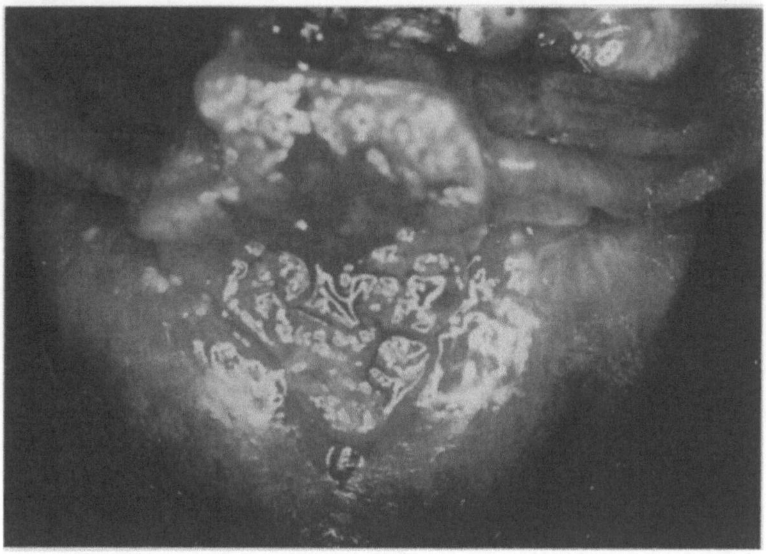

FIGURE 6.4. Painful ulcer on the frenulum extending onto the glans.

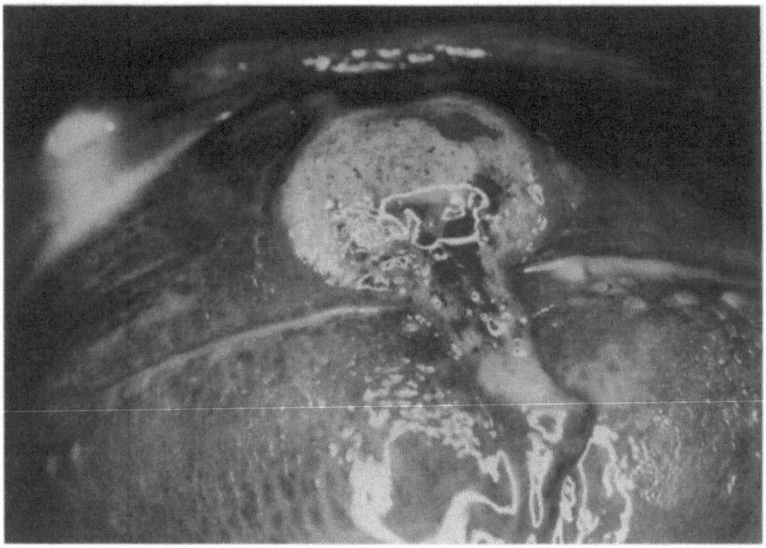

FIGURE 6.5. Painful ulcer on the frenulum extending onto the glans.

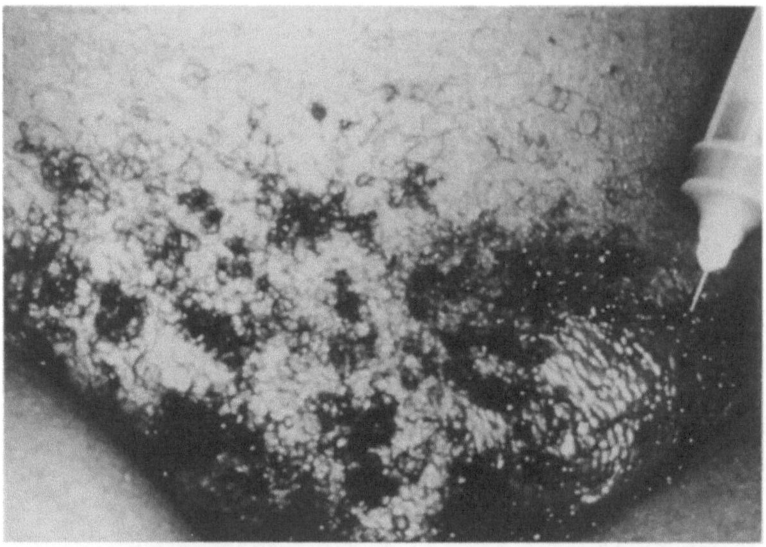

FIGURE 6.6. Aspiration of a left inguinal bubo in a woman. Cure quickly occurred following aspiration. An ulcer had healed but the bubo had progressed following treatment with a single dose of trimethoprim/sulfamethoxazole 5 days earlier. No additional therapy was required.

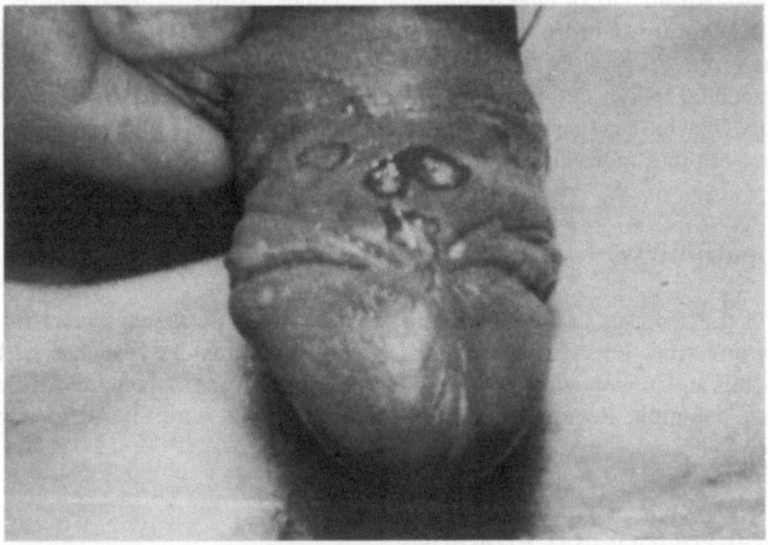

FIGURE 6.7. Four superficial ulcers on the anterior surface of the penile shaft, herpetiform in appearance. However, they were culture positive for *H. ducreyi*. *Herpes simplex* was not recovered.

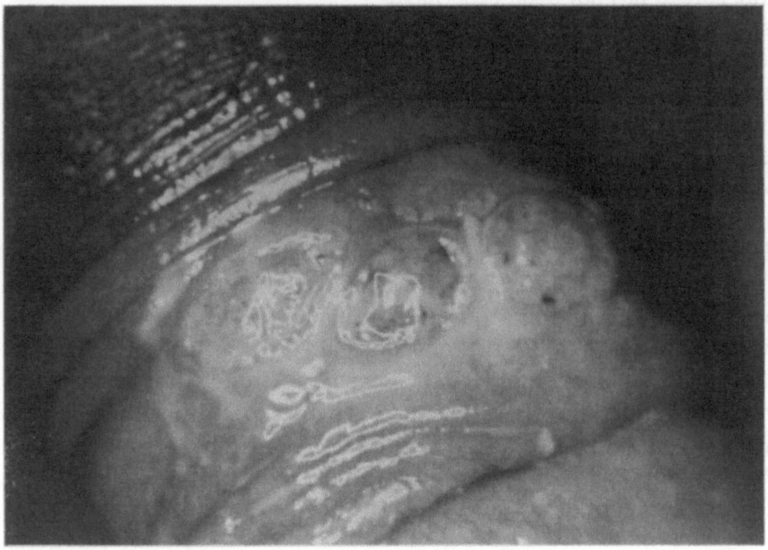

FIGURE 6.8. Three painful ulcers on the coronal sulcus. Culture positive for *H. ducreyi*.

progresses within 3 to 14 days to suppurative bubos. With continued nontreatment, the bubos rupture and form inguinal abscesses that drain pus and penetrate deeply into the groin.

Extragenital lesions in the oropharynx or on the skin have been described, but are unusual. They have no particular characteristic features other than the concomitant presence of other more classic genital lesions.

## Histopathology

None of the features of the chancroid ulcer are specific or characteristic of *H. ducreyi* infection. Interstitial edema or intense inflammatory response with both neutrophils and mononuclear cells, and disruption of normal subcutaneous architecture, are common. Regional lymph nodes are involved with microabscesses that coalesce to become large pyogenic abscesses.

## Natural History and Prognosis

In the absence of treatment, ulcers in men persist for 3 to 8 weeks with a median duration of 5 weeks. In women, however, ulcers are known to persist for 4 to 6 months. Progressive destruction of genital tissue can lead to urethral fistulas, cicatrization of tissue with sexual dysfunction, and chronic draining inguinal abscesses. Systemic spread has not been described.

Relapse occurs in about 5% of patients after complete healing, both in those who do not receive treatment and in those who are cured with antimicrobial agents. Relapse occurs at the site of the original infection and is presumably due to persisting organisms within the skin.

A recently recognized complication of genital ulcer disease is concomitant infection with human immunodeficiency virus (HIV-1). In retrospective studies in both men and women, a history of genital ulcer disease is associated with an increased prevalence of HIV-1 seropositivity. In a prospective study of men who acquired chancroid from sexual contacts who were infected with HIV-1, the risk of seroconversion in the 12 weeks after acquisition of chancroid was over 15%. This risk was significantly greater than the risk of acquiring HIV-1 following gonococcal infection also dually acquired from HIV-1-infected prostitutes. It is postulated that the presence of a genital ulcer may facilitate egress of HIV-1 into genital secretions, increasing the risk of HIV-1 being acquired from the sexual partner, concomitantly with *H. ducreyi* [11].

## Differential Diagnosis

The clinical diagnosis of genital ulceration is frequently erroneous. As many as 50% of ulcers will be incorrectly categorized if laboratory confirmation of the etiology is not accomplished. The recent advances in techniques for the culture of *H. ducreyi* permit an exact diagnosis and now should be routine in Western societies [10].

In studies in Detroit, Atlanta, Nairobi, and Winnipeg, series of men and women with genital ulcers have been investigated to determine the sensitivity, specificity, and predictive value of clinical findings. In Atlanta, among 33 patients who presented with "chancroidal ulcer," herpes simplex was isolated from 16 and *H. ducreyi* from only 1. This study confirmed the earlier studies that suggested that herpes can present with lesions that mimic chancroid. Culture for herpes simplex is essential to exclude herpes in patients with chancroidal ulcers [1].

Chancroid can mimic granuloma inguinale (GI). The "beefy" exuberant granulomatous response of GI occurs occasionally in patients with chancroid. As the course of treatment is different, an exact diagnosis of GI should be made [12]. A smear for Donovan bodies can usually rapidly sort out this differential diagnosis.

The primary chancre of syphilis is typical in about 50% of patients. In at least 10% of patients with primary syphilis, the lesion can be readily confused with the classic chancroid ulcer. Also, in the same proportion of patients with chancroid, induration is present and suggests a syphilitic lesion. Darkfield examination and serial serology, in addition to culture of *H. ducreyi*, can usually rapidly identify the etiologic agent and avoid confusion.

Other spirochetal diseases occur from time to time concurrently with *H. ducreyi* infection. Spirochetes can usually be differentiated from *Treponema pallidum* and they respond to penicillin.

Dual infections with herpes simplex and *H. ducreyi* occur in Kenya in about 3% of patients. In our judgment, this is usually reactivation of herpes simplex in a patient who has recently acquired chancroid. Dual infections with *T. pallidum* and *H. ducreyi* are seen in 2 to 3% of patients. Differing incubation periods should prevent this, but it does happen. All patients with genital ulcer disease should routinely have darkfield examination and serial serology to exclude *T. pallidum* infection, regardless of the presence of other etiologic agents of genital ulcer disease.

In societies in which syphilis cannot be excluded, we suggest that all patients be treated concurrently with benzathine penicillin. The nonspecificity of clinical diagnoses and the consequence of untreated luetic infection demand that all genital ulcers be assumed to be due to syphilis until this diagnosis is excluded by laboratory investigation.

## Treatment

In 1938, Hanschell reported his successful treatment of chancroid with sulfonamides. Treatment rapidly eradicates *H. ducreyi* from the ulcer, and pain disappears. The ulcer base becomes granulomatous and healing proceeds. The average duration after successful therapy to complete healing occurs is 9 days in men and 5 days in women [13].

In addition to the sulfonamides, the tetracyclines, streptomycin, kanamycin, and chloramphenicol have all been used successfully to treat chancroid.

Resistant strains of *H. ducreyi* were first reported in 1978; however, clinical resistance was noted during the previous decade. Only since 1980 have prospective studies demonstrated the correlation between clinical failure and in vitro resistance. Plasmids have now been shown to mediate resistance to the sulfonamides, the penicillins, kanamycin, streptomycin, tetracycline, chloramphenicol, and trimethoprim. As a result, treatment regimens have been undergoing continuous change [4].

Combinations of trimethoprim and sulfonamides have continued to be an excellent treatment regimen in most countries. In Thailand and Southeast Asia, however, isolates are now generally resistant to both sulfonamides and trimethoprim, and these regimens can be anticipated to fail in patients who have acquired infection in these countries [14].

Studies in Kenya have shown that the optimal duration of treatment is about 48 hours. Several short-course treatment regimens have been shown to be effective.

The U.S. Centers for Disease Control in Atlanta presently recommend 500 mg of erythromycin four times each day for 7 days as a standard treatment regimen. Two studies have shown that a single 250-mg dose of ceftriaxone administered intramuscularly is a very effective regimen [14,15]. More recent studies have shown that amoxicillin combined with clavulinic acid is also effective when prescribed for 3 days [16]. Also, the new fluorinated 4-quinalone, ciprofloxacin, prescribed in a dosage of 500 mg twice daily for 3 days, cures chancroid in essentially all patients [17].

These treatment regimens give considerable latitude to physicians. All regimens are equally successful in curing ulcers and bubos. Frequently, the bubo will reaccumulate pus and will require two or three needle aspirations before resolving. This is not due to failure of the treatment regimen, but rather appears to be the natural course of the infection. Bubos should only be aspirated; they do not require surgical drainage.

## Prevention and Control

Widespread treatment of prostitutes with ulcers and prostitutes named as sexual contacts of men with genital ulcer disease has been effective in eradicating chancroid during large outbreaks in Winnipeg and in California. Condoms can also markedly reduce the acquisition of *H. ducreyi* infection.

Control strategies need to be introduced into societies in which chancroid is endemic to reduce the risk of infection with this pathogen and concurrently with HIV-1. Control strategies need to be evaluated to determine if widespread screening of prostitutes for ulcers and ongoing treatment will reduce the epidemic of chancroid in these countries.

## References

1. Salzman RS, Kraus SJ, Miller RG, et al: Chancroidal ulcers that are not chancroid: Cause and epidemiology. *Arch Dermatol* **120**:636–639, 1984.

2. Sturm AW, Zanen HC: Characteristics of *Haemophilus ducreyi* in culture. *J Clin Microbiol* **19**:672–674, 1984.
3. Dylewski J, Nsanze H, Maitha G, et al: A laboratory diagnosis of *Haemophilus ducreyi*: Sensitivity of culture media. *Diag Microbiol Infect Dis* **4**:241–245, 1986.
4. McNicol PJ, Ronald AR: The plasmids of *Haemophilus ducreyi*. *J Antimicrob Chemother* **14**:561–573, 1984.
5. Hammond GW, Slutchuk M, Scatliff J, et al: Epidemiologic, clinical, laboratory and therapeutic features of an urban outbreak of chancroid in North America. *Rev Infect Dis* **2**:867–879, 1980.
6. Blackmore CA, Limpakarnjanarat K, Rigau-Perez JG, et al: An outbreak of chancroid in Orange County, California: Descriptive epidemiology and disease-control measures. *J Infect Dis* **151**:840–844, 1985.
7. Kinghorn GR, Hafiz S, McEntegart MG: Pathogenic microbial flora of genital ulcers in Sheffield with particular reference to herpes simplex and *Haemophilus ducreyi*. *Br J Vener Dis* **58**:377–380, 1982.
8. Plummer FA, D'Costa LJ, Nsanze H, et al: Clinical and microbiologic studies of genital ulcers in Kenyan women. *Sex Trans Dis* **12**:193–197, 1985.
9. Plummer FA, D'Costa LJ, Nsanze H, et al: Epidemiology of chancroid and *Haemophilus ducreyi* in Nairobi. *Lancet* **2**:1293–1295, 1983.
10. Chapel TA, Brown WJ, Jeffries C, et al: How reliable is the morphological diagnosis of penile ulcerations? *Sex Trans Dis* **4**:150–152, 1977.
11. Cameron DW, Plummer FA, Simonsen JN, et al: Female to male heterosexual transmission of HIV infection in Nairobi. 3rd International Conference on AIDS, Washington, D.C., 1987.
12. Kraus SJ, Werman BS, Biddle JW, et al: Pseudogranuloma inguinale caused by *Haemophilus ducreyi*. *Arch Dermatol* **118**:494–497, 1982.
13. Hanschell HM: Sulphanilamide in the treatment of chancroid. *Lancet* **1**:886–888, 1938.
14. Tayler DN, Pitarangsi C, Echeverria P, et al: Comparative study of ceftriaxone and trimethoprim-sulfamethoxazole for the treatment of chancroid in Thailand. *J Infect Dis* **152**:1002–1006, 1986.
15. Bowmer MI, Nsanze H, D'Costa LJ, et al: Single dose ceftriaxone for chancroid. *Antimicrob Agents Chemother* **31**:67–69, 1987.
16. Ndinya-Achola JO, Nsanze H, Karasira P, et al: Three day oral course: Augmentin in the treatment of chancroid. *Genitourin Med* **62**:202–204, 1986.
17. Naamara W, Plummer FA, Greenblatt R, et al: Treatment of chancroid with ciprofloxacin: A prospective randomized clinical trial. *Am J Med* **82**(Suppl. 4A):317–320, 1987.

CHAPTER 7

# Lymphogranuloma Venereum

Fulvio Allegra

## Overview

Although the first description of Lymphogranuloma Venereum (LGV) dates from 1833 by Wallace, its complete nosographic pattern was extensively studied by Durand, Nicolas, and Favre in 1913 [1]. An important date is 1925, when Frei [2] first reported "a new cutaneous reaction for lymphogranuloma inguinale." The name "lymphogranuloma inguinale" was accepted by the American Medical Association, as reported by Favre and Hellerström [3] in 1954, and is still used in some statistical reports (ISTAT). The discovery of the etiologic role of *Chlamydia trachomatis* is attributed to Gay-Prieto (1927) (quoted by Hart [4]). *Chlamydiae* were demonstrated to be the causative agent of LGV, after intracerebral inoculation in monkeys, by Favre and Hellerström. Sulfonamides were the first effective drug used in the treatment of LGV.

## Definition

LGV is a systemic infectious disease usually transmitted by sexual contact and caused by one of the three specific immunotypes of *Chlamydia trachomatis*.

A primary, transitory lesion is followed by an acute, suppurative regional lymphoadenitis. During this primary phase, constitutional symptoms are evident and apparent recovery occasionally follows. After a latency period, anorectal strictures and elephantiasis in the genital area may eventually develop, due to obstruction of the lymphatic vessels. In female patients, lymphoedema produces the so-called esthiomene, a debilitating and disfiguring condition.

## Synonyms

Synonyms of LGV are lymphogranuloma inguinale, lymphopathia venereum, inguinal poradenitis, poradenolymphitis, climatic or tropical bubo, Durand-Nicholas-Favre disease, Frei's disease; fourth venereal disease, and Nicolas-Favre disease.

This last eponymic denomination is still widely used in France and other Latin language countries, originating with the first description of the condition, by Durand, Nicolas, and Favre in 1913 [1] and exhaustively treated by Nicolas and Favre in 1936 [5].

Some of the above synonyms are definitely misleading and should be abandoned. They serve only to increase an already existing confusion between LGV and another sexually transmitted disease, granuloma inguinale, otherwise known as donovanosis.

## Epidemiology

Until recently, LGV seemed to be ubiquitous, occurring in all climates and countries. This was the conclusion of a detailed epidemiologic study published in 1954 by Favre and Hellerström [3]. Presently, however, official reports, for the most part inadequate, make the exact evaluation of LGV incidence again controversial. While LGV is endemic in Southeast Asia, Africa, South America, and West India, in the United States it predominantly affects black people with a low economic status. The number of reported cases and the case rate per 100,000 population in the United States and its neighboring countries from 1974 to 1979 (STD Statistical Letter, no. 129), showed a maximum of 651 cases in 1974 and a minimum of 54 cases in 1984, with an average rate per 100,000 population of 0.2 to 0.1 cases. This tendency was confirmed by the U.S. Department of Health and Human Services (CDC, Atlanta). The states of New York, Florida, Georgia, and Texas had the greatest number of cases, as did big cities such as Washington, D.C., New York and Atlanta.

Data on the epidemiologic situation of LGV in Europe are unreliable. An average of 5 to 9 cases was reported by the Italian Health Central Authorities (ISTAT). An unusual outbreak of six LGV cases was accurately documented by Panizza et al [6] in Sicily, probably due to the large number of African immigrants in the Sicilian community.

The frequency of LGV seems to be increasing in homosexual men with anorectal infections [7]. Others [8] believe that since many epidemiologic studies are founded on serologic tests, they are unreliable. This is due to the frequent existence of other *C. trachomatis* infections in the general population.

LGV can appear sporadically anywhere in the world. Actually, however, higher prevalence seems to be confined to the tropical countries [9].

## Etiology and Pathogenesis

LGV is due to an infection by one of the following strains of *C. trachomatis*: L1, L2, or L3.

*C. trachomatis* can no longer be considered a virus. Recent knowledge about its morphology, life cycle, and physicochemical properties has clearly demonstrated that *C. trachomatis* is a bacteria and belongs to the *Rickettsiae* family [10].

Since *C. trachomatis* has already been described in this volume, the present section will only elucidate its pathogenetic aspects and the sequence of events that occur during the natural history of LGV.

Among the various infectious agents that afflict mankind, *C. trachomatis* is one of the most common causes of bacterial infection. Infection by *C. trachomatis* is limited to humans; it is transmitted in the mucosal secretions present during intimate or traumatic contact, for example, during sexual intercourse or delivery of a child, or by means of insect vectors, as is the case in true trachomatous conjunctivitis. The majority of chlamydial infections remains localized on the mucosal surface; however, the strains that give rise to LGV are extremely aggressive. They invade and spread from the regional lymphatic channels to the surrounding deeply located structures and internal organs throughout the body, according to the following schema:

| Epithelial damage(*) | *C. trachomatis* serotypes | Lymphatic system damage(*) |
|---|---|---|
| +++ | D, E, F, G, H, I, J, K (genital) | + |
| ++ | A, B, Ba, C (trachoma) | ++ |
| + | L1, L2, L3 (LGV) | +++ |

(*)+++ = Maximal damage.
++ = Moderate damage.
+ = Minimal damage.

Epithelial involvement, which occurs on the genital or nasopharyngeal and laryngeal mucosae and occasionally gives rise to pneumonitis in the newborn, is maximum when serotypes D through K are involved. These serotypes are only occasionally found in cases of LGV. On the contrary, serotypes L1, L2, and L3 are found almost exclusively in patients suffering from LGV. These strains have a greater tendency to compromise the lymphatic structures and permit infection to spread from the regional lymph nodes to the surrounding tissues. *C. trachomatis* L1, L2, and L3 strains can be differentiated both in vivo and in vitro from other strains by their greater virulence. LGV strains prefer mononuclear cells, specifically macrophages, and apparently ignore the squamocolumnar cells preferred by other *C. trachomatis* strains. Such a restricted host range may be a result of the fact that they have less specialized receptor requirements than the other strains. LGV strains are capable of unrestricted multiplication in vitro, and are considered to be a junior antigen, capable of extensive cross-reactions [11].

Since the inflammatory process involves the majority of the regional lymph nodes and ends in necrosis, a purulent fusion of the entire bubo is eventually followed by skin ulceration and discharge of necrotic material. Fortunately, however, a purulent fusion of the deeply situated iliac lymph nodes rarely occurs. As the inflammatory process subsides, the affected lymph nodes are overwhelmed by a fibrotic process that is responsible for the subsequent obliteration of the lymphatic channels and the formation of a relevant scar, which extends to the pelvis, rectum, lower sigmoid, and other organs.

The diffusion of *C. trachomatis*, in the case of LGV, is not limited to the genital and perigenital areas but has even been found in the bloodstream and cerebrospinal fluid. Furthermore, the well-known Frei skin test positivity and the possibility of demonstrating both the presence of delayed hypersensitivity and circulating antibodies proves that LGV is a systemic disease and that many of its symptoms are caused by a cell-mediated hypersensitivity reaction [8].

## Clinical Findings

### The Primary Lesion

After an incubation period of 1 to 6 weeks, the primary lesion usually manifests in the form of a painless, herpetiform abrasion or ulceration. In rare cases it has been possible to follow the evolution starting from the first manifestation, a small, papular lesion that soon acquires vesicular and pustular features. The lesion is usually solitary and its dimension small; however, multiple lesions can occur in the same subject. They are always limited to the same cutaneous or mucosal area.

In male patients, the primary lesion most commonly occurs on the balanopreputial sulcus (Fig. 7.1) and therefore on the frenulum, penile skin, glans penis, and scrotum. Anorectal primary lesions have been diagnosed in male homosexuals and in women, using a proctoscope [9].

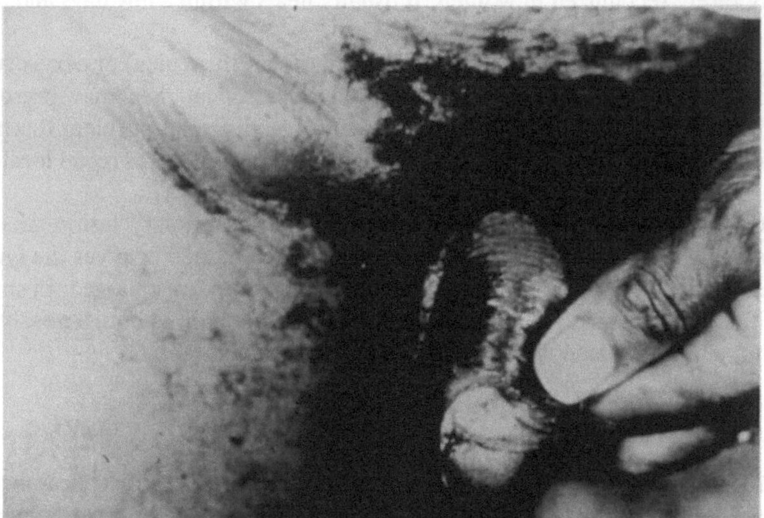

FIGURE 7.1. The primary preputial erosion and the inguinal bubo. Courtesy of Prof. E. Alessi, Milan, Italy.

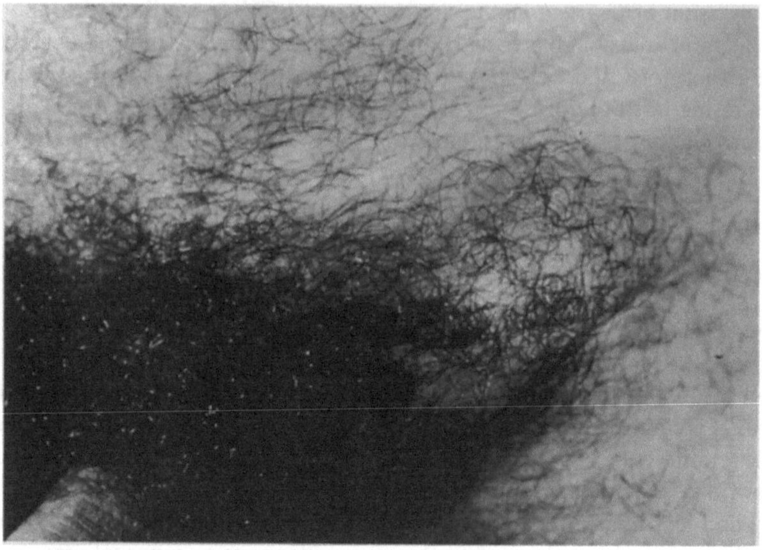

FIGURE 7.2. The inguinal bubo before ulceration. Courtesy of Prof. A. Rebora, Genoa, Italy.

In female patients, similar lesions can be observed on the posterior wall of the vagina and/or on the cervical and vulvar mucosa; however, due to the fact that there are few subjective symptoms and that the lesion is a transient one, the initial lesion is only rarely recognized in women. It usually heals within a few days and does not leave a scar.

A mucopurulent discharge originating from the urethra (men) or cervix (women) has been observed. Moreover, women and homosexual men may present with hemorrhagic proctitis, accompanied by rectal bleeding and purulent discharge. It has been postulated that intraurethral and endocervical as well as rectal localizations are probably much more common than reported.

After a few days without proper management, the primary lesion generally is accompanied by a concomitant lymphangitis, which in men involves the lymphatic vessel of the dorsum penis. This lymphatic channel appears enlarged; in some portions the skin may ulcerate, creating the so-called bubonuli. In both sexes, lymphangitis may be associated with edema of the external genitalia.

## The Secondary Period

The secondary period of LGV begins 1 to 4 weeks after the disappearance of the primary lesion. It gives rise to local and systemic symptoms. Male patients complain of pain in one or both of the inguinal lymph nodes, which are enlarged and tender (Fig. 7.2). Lymphadenopathy first occurs in the medial lymph nodes and progresses laterally. Its progression produces a swelling in the entire inguinal region and the

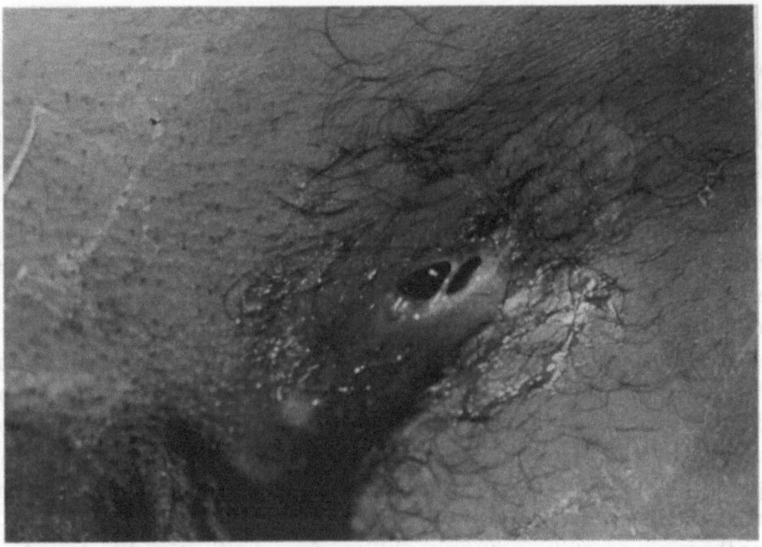

FIGURE 7.3. The same inguinal bubo as in Fig. 7.2, after ulceration. Courtesy of Prof. A. Rebora, Genoa, Italy.

"groove sign," extremely characteristic in this phase of the disease, due to the presence of Poupart's ligament, which separates the swollen lymph nodes into two portions.

Depending on the location of the primary lesion, similar lymph node swelling may become evident in other contributing territories, such as the iliac lymph nodes. This is the case in female patients, in whom the primary lesion is generally found in the deep genital mucosa.

Laterocervical lymph node involvement is evident when the primary lesion occurs in the oral mucosa. After 1 or 2 weeks of harsh pain, a few of the involved bubos become fluctuant and the overlying skin ulcerates (Fig. 7.3), releasing a dense, purulent, yellow material. Coincidentally, the local and constitutional symptoms gradually disappear.

## Constitutional Symptoms

Since LGV is a systemic disease, local adenopathy can be accompanied by systemic symptoms: headache, malaise, myalgia, anorexia, and fever, accompanied or not by chills and profuse sweating. Since the infectious agent invades the bloodstream and the cerebrospinal fluid, symptoms of hepatitis, pneumonitis, arthritis, erythema nodosum, and/or polymorphic meningitis and encephalitis have been reported in many cases.

### Late Manifestations

Late manifestations of LGV are much more common in female than in male patients, due to the fact that the appearance of the primary lesion in women is frequently missed. These late symptoms constitute the "anogenital and rectal syndrome." This complication can develop in both sexes and is a direct consequence of an infection that starts in the rectal mucosa and, in men, follows a primitive involvement of the posterior urethra. In both sexes, the rectal mucosa is gradually invaded by a chronic, inflammatory granuloma, which initiates from the bowel wall and manifests itself by anal itching and a mucopurulent discharge. As a result of the granulomatous process, all the layers of the bowel wall are gradually replaced by scar tissue, and the retraction of this fibrous tissue can give rise to an incomplete or complete reduction of the rectal lumen. The presence of a stricture, habitually located 2 to 5 cm above the anus, causes chronic constipation and ribbonlike feces to be passed. In the few cases where digital exploration of the rectum is possible, one can appreciate ulcerative and granular lesions below the stricture, while the mucosa above the stricture is of a normal firmness.

Under these circumstances, the possibility of a complication like bowel perforation followed by acute peritonitis has to be feared; this is the most common direct cause of death in LGV patients. The perianal skin and the rectal mucosa below the stricture are frequently the sites of perirectal or rectal-vaginal fistulae and anal fissurations. Moreover, the presence of protruding masses of lymphatic tissues may cause formation of the so-called lymphorrhoids, similar to hemorrhoids. When an abrasion or ulceration appears on these surfaces, a more or less important lymphorrhea occurs. In the chronic stage of lymphatic stasis, even correct therapy effects no or little change in the lesion [4]. Elephantiasis of the vulvar structures is called *esthiomene*, from the Greek word "eaten or eroded." In fact, this condition is commonly observed in female patients, although genital elephantiasis also affects men, in particular the penis and scrotum. Occasionally, elephantiasis of one or both legs has been described [12].

Development of cancer following rectal strictures and/or genital elephantiasis has been reported by Rainey [13]. A rapidly fatal case of immunoblastic lymphoma was described in a young man affected by LGV that evolved by progressive losses in immunologic competence [14].

## Differential Diagnosis

The differential diagnosis of LGV must take into consideration all the known conditions that begin at the genital level and are characterized by a primary complex. Special attention must be paid to the site of entry and the presence of satellite adenopathy. Therefore, herpes simplex, primary syphilis, and chancroid must be systematically ruled out. Extragenital lesions require that a complete case history be taken regarding where the patient lives and comes from or/and awareness that the same condition possibly exists in the sexual partner.

With late symptoms, in both male and female patients radiographic examination of the bowel and rectum may be needed to detect the presence of perianal or anovaginal fistulae. LGV rectal strictures have a characteristic radiologic pattern that is very different from that of rectal cancer [15].

## Diagnosis

Laboratory tests constitute the major diagnostics protocol in LGV. The recent introduction on the market of specific, reliable, and reproducible tests, relatively inexpensive and easily performed in any hospital laboratory, has greatly simplified the diagnostic protocol for chlamydial infections. The Frei test deserves today only historical interest, though for years it was considered the most reliable procedure in the diagnosis of LGV.

### Frei Test

Originally, Frei obtained the antigen from a pus collection of uncontaminated, unruptured bubos and injected it intradermally after dilution with saline and heat sterilization. A cutaneous reaction, however, was incapable of detecting the existence of an actual infection. The Frei test is not specific and becomes positive 2 to 8 weeks after the infection in only 95% of the tested subjects. For these reasons, the commercial production of a standardized antigen, obtained from the yolk sac of chick embryo culture (Lygranum), was discontinued in 1974.

### Direct Demonstration

In past years, the use of Giemsa's or Macchiavello's stain or of Lugol solution was claimed to allow direct demonstration of *C. trachomatis* in tissue and/or smears of pathologic material obtained from a bubo or any of the other late manifestations of LGV. Unfortunately, this method proved to be extremely unreliable, due to frequent contamination of the specimen by bacteria, cellular debris, and other artifacts. Direct demonstration of *C. trachomatis* in smears or tissues was recently achieved using monoclonal antibodies (discussed below).

### Serologic Tests

Currently existing serologic tests include complement fixation (CF) neutralizing antibodies, microimmunofluorescence, and the radioisotope precipitation test.

The CF test, although more sensitive than the Frei test, has low specificity, giving cross-reaction with the antigen of psittacosis. Low-titer positive results persist for years and may indicate that at some point in life the patient suffered from LGV. Since other chlamydial infections are also common, a positive CF test does not definitely establish the diagnosis of LGV, despite the fact that a positive test for chlamydial urethritis rarely has a titer greater than 1:16.

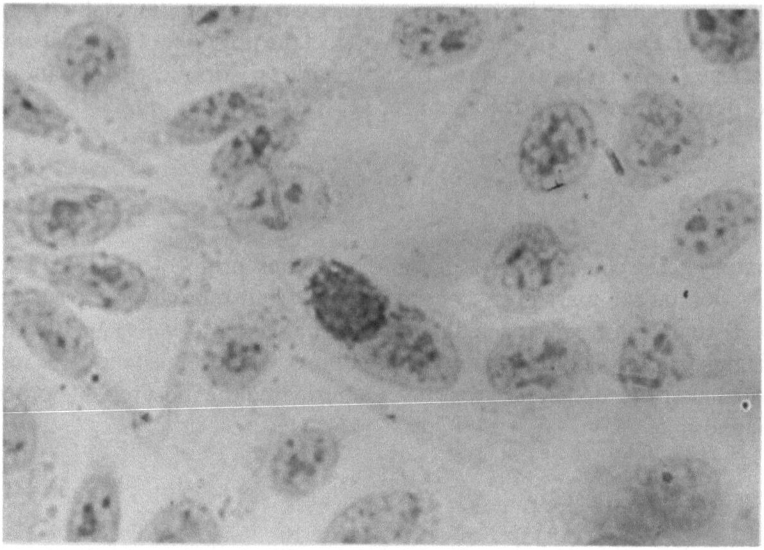

FIGURE 7.4. Jodophilic intracytoplasmic inclusions of *C. trachomatis* stained with Lugol solution in McCoy cell culture. Courtesy of Dr. C. Medici, Parma, Italy.

The microimmunofluorescence test seems to be one of the most sensitive and specific tests available. In fact, with this test it is possible to identify individual strains carrying a particular antigen. Unfortunately, the complexity of this technique makes its widespread use an impossibility.

The radioisotope precipitation test [16] gives high titers (up to 1024) in serum from patients with LGV. However, it also has low specificity, and it can only be performed in specialized laboratories.

## Culture and Other Methods

Previous studies have demonstrated that it is possible to isolate *Chlamydia* after inoculation of pathologic material in mouse brain, yolk sac, or tissue culture. One of the most useful and reliable methods of culture was proposed by Hobson in 1977 [17]. This procedure utilizes the McCoy cell line tissue culture: *Chlamydia* reproduction occurs after inhibition of cell replication by means of cycloheximide. After incubation, the stratified cultures are stained with Lugol solution (Fig. 7.4) or Giemsa's stain (Fig. 7.5) and/or are observed in a dark field (Fig. 7.6). They show characteristic intracellular inclusions.

Commercially available fluorescein-labeled monoclonal antibodies that detect *C. trachomatis* are now available [18]. These are used for the detection of *Chlamydia* in both tissue-culture and smears of material obtained from any source. This test offers no apparent advantages over Giemsa's stain in tissue culture, but with it the detection of elementary bodies in smears is quicker and more sensitive than isola-

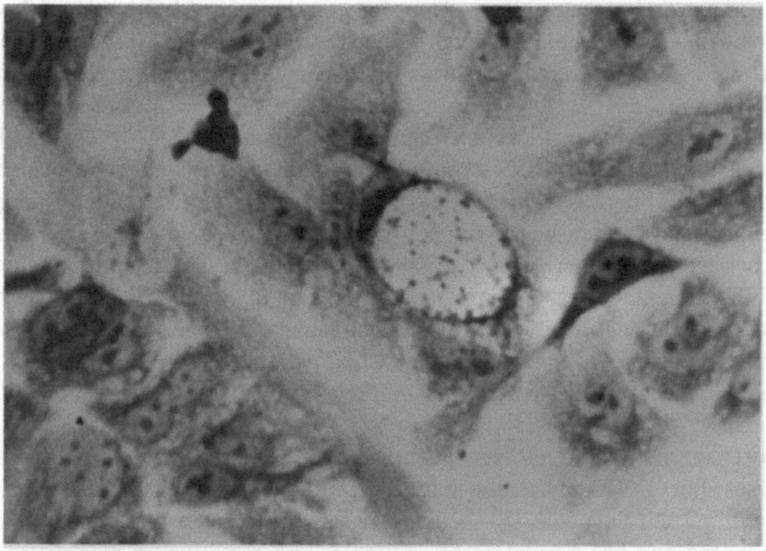

FIGURE 7.5. Intracytoplasmic microcolonies of *C. trachomatis* in McCoy cells, stained with Giemsa. Courtesy of Dr. C. Medici, Parma, Italy.

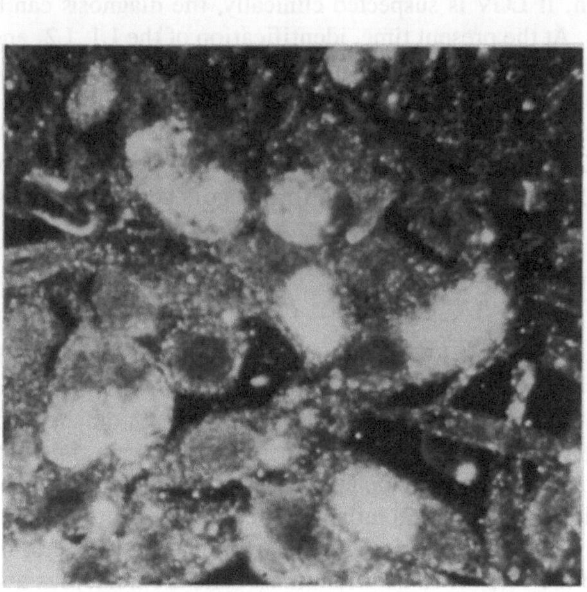

FIGURE 7.6. Intracytoplasmic inclusion of *C. trachomatis* (Giemsa's stain, darkfield).

tion of *Chlamydia* in tissue culture. Therefore, in the case of LGV, this method also seems to be the most reliable, especially since few clinicians have access to laboratories that offer cell culture confirmation of suspected *C. trachomatis* genital infections [19].

The Chlamydiazyme test (Abbott Laboratories) is an alternative enzymatic test that claims to have good specificity (94.2%). No data are available about this test in LGV patients, but because Chlamydiazyme is a chromogenic reaction developed to detect chlamydial antigens in urethral and cervical swab specimens, it seems reasonable to believe that this method could also be useful in LGV laboratory screening. One of the advantages of Chlamydiazyme is that it detects *Chlamydia* antigens irrespective of the viability of the microorganisms, while culture isolation requires living bacteria [20]. On the other hand, Chlamydiazyme requires almost 4 hours to be performed, and the kits on the market are available for a minimum of 90 specimens.

Ortho-Diagnostic Systems has recently introduced the DNA Probes method, which uses short DNA chains able to localize and quantify the genomes of infective agents within their host cell. On the basis of this principle, a Patho-Gene II kit has been prepared and has proved useful, reliable, and sensitive on monolayer tissue culture cells, smears, and biopsy specimens containing cells with viable microorganisms. The entire procedure requires not more than 45 minutes and the company offers a positive control.

In conclusion, if LGV is suspected clinically, the diagnosis can be obtained by many methods. At the present time, identification of the L1, L2, and L3 serotypes is not yet possible in common laboratories and it is my opinion that the monoclonal antibody system represents the most reliable and simplified test for *Chlamydia* infection. On the other hand, Perine and Osoba [8] have reported that the percent diagnosis of LGV from pathologic material (bubo, genital or rectal mucosal tissues) is remarkably lower than that reported for nongonococcal urethritis.

## Histopathology

The histologic changes of LGV are not pathognomonic. Small, stellate abscesses surrounded by histiocytes and arranged in a palisade pattern are visible in the primary stage of the disease. In the late stage (vulvar esthiomene, according to Alacoque et al [21], epidermal acanthosis and papillomatosis are apparent. The papillary dermis is edematous, and the lymphatic vessels are dilated. The reticular dermis is densely fibrotic and contains an inflammatory cell infiltrate (lymphocytes, plasma cells, and a few multinucleated giant cells) arranged in clusters, most frequently located around the vessels. In addition, mast cells are numerous and disseminated inside the granuloma. They contain small, spherical blue granulations in the cytoplasm. Some of these acidophilic granulations are visibly disseminated in the tissues. The cytoplasm of the macrophages are filled with large granulations, 0.4 to 3 mμ in size, irregularly shaped and dark blue when stained with Giemsa's stain. The above granulations were first described by Favre [22] and by Gamma [23] in 1924.

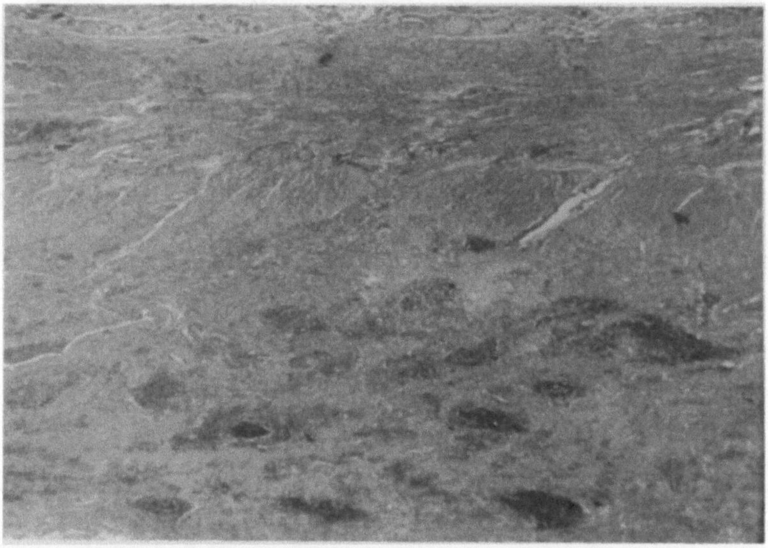

FIGURE 7.7. Histopathology of lymphogranuloma venereum-affected rectal mucosa: a follicular lymphohistiocytic infiltrate, with predominant lymphocytes in the central zone. Courtesy of Prof. G.M. Hutchins, Baltimore, MD.

Ultrastructural studies showed evidence of the specificity of these intracytoplasmic granulations, which proved to be *Chlamydiae* [21].

The histopathologic lesions of the intestinal wall have been extensively studied [24]. A follicular lymphohistiocytic and plasma cell infiltrate has been found in the submucosa, muscularis propria, and serosa: Lymphocytes predominate in the central zone of the follicular proctitis (Fig. 7.7); lymphocytes, plasma cells, and histiocytes are predominant in the peripheral zone. Neuromatous hypertrophy and hyperplasia with perineural chronic inflammation are visible in the muscularis propria of the rectum (Fig. 7.8). The presence of lesions limited to the rectum seems to be the criterion on which the histopathologic diagnosis between LGV and Crohn's disease is based.

## Therapy

Genital, inguinal, and anorectal LGV should be treated with tetracycline HCl, 500 mg by mouth four times a day (2 g/day) for a minimum of 3 weeks.

Sulfisoxazole can be used as an alternative drug. Felman (1986) recommends 4 g initially, followed by 1 g four times daily for 3 weeks, or sulfamethoxazole 2 g, followed by 1 g two times daily for 3 weeks. An epidemiologic treatment of the sexual partner(s) of the patient should be undertaken even in the absence of clinical symptoms or positive laboratory tests, using one of the above recommended regimens.

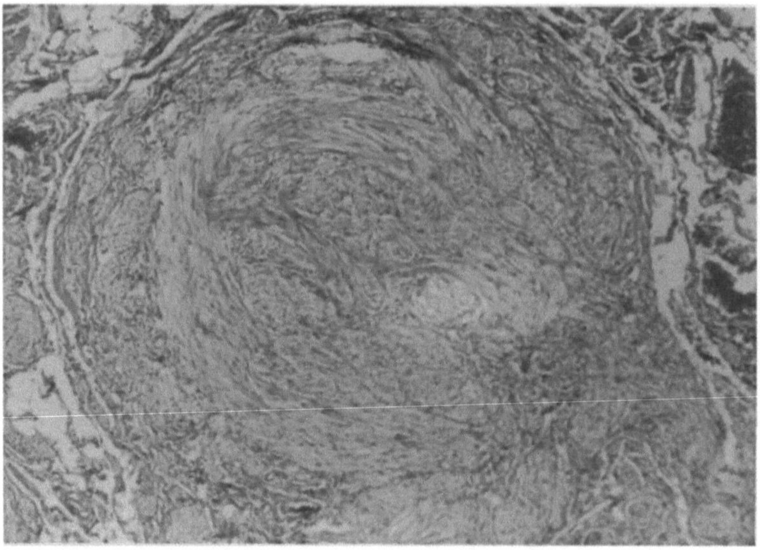

FIGURE 7.8. Histopathology of the LGV rectal affected mucosa: neuromatous hypertrophy. Courtesy of Prof. G.M. Hutchins, Baltimore, MD.

Other drugs known to be effective on LGV serotypes in vitro, but which have not been extensively evaluated in culture-confirmed cases, are doxicycline, 100 mg by mouth two times daily for at least 2 to 3 weeks, or erythromycin, 500 mg by mouth four times daily for at least 2 to 3 weeks. No agreement exists regarding the duration of the treatment. Felman [25] recommends that the above therapeutic regimen be continued until the adenopathy and inflammatory lesions have subsided and are healed, while the U.S. Department of Health and Human Services from the Atlanta Centers for Disease Control recommends a 2-week treatment program.

Management also includes surgical treatment of fluctuant lymph nodes. They should be aspirated through the adjacent healthy skin, avoiding incision and drainage or excision of the bubo(es), which often results in delayed healing.

Rectal strictures, esthiomene, and anorectal fistulae cannot be completely healed by medical treatment and frequently require surgical intervention.

If prevention and treatment of LGV are not serious problems in highly civilized countries, the control of the disease in endemic areas is, because diagnostic facilities are often lacking or rudimental, long-term treatment is too expensive, and patient follow-up is problematic.

## Prognosis

If accurately diagnosed and properly treated, all primary LGV lesions can be completely cured. Complete recovery is also possible for lesions in the second stage of the disease, provided that a correct diagnosis is made and therapy instituted.

Spontaneous healing of the primary lesion has been reported in men [26]. Furthermore, it seems reasonable to believe that after healing, men are no longer infectious.

On the contrary, no data are available regarding the duration of the female infectious period. Regarding this nosographic aspect of LGV, it is interesting to note that this condition is more commonly observed in men than in women, with a 2:1 ratio. The probability that women are asymptomatic LGV carriers is suggested by the fact that *C. trachomatis* was isolated in 0.5 to 8% of asymptomatic women. The prognosis when there are systemic symptoms is directly related to the making of an immediate and correct diagnosis. Prospects for complete recovery in cases with late manifestations are poor. Indeed, after medical therapy, the rectal strictures and chronic lymphedema do improve, but some of the sequelae can be only partially influenced, and the threat of bowel obstruction, perforation, and lethal peritonitis exists throughout the patient's life. Perianal and rectovaginal fistulae may be the sites of repeated superinfection, followed by periodic flashes of systemic and aspecific symptoms. Moreover, as previously mentioned, evolution of the chronic, granulomatous lesion toward cancer is always a possibility.

## References


1. Durand M, Nicolas J, Favre M: Lymphogranuloma inguinale subaigue d'origine genitale probable peut-être venerienne. *Prov Med* (Paris) **24**:55–62, 1913.
2. Frei W: Eine neue Hautreaktion bei Lymphogranuloma inguinale. *Klin Wschr* **4**:2148–2152, 1925.
3. Favre M, Hellerström S: The epidemiology, aetiology and prophylaxis of lymphogranuloma inguinale. *Acta Derm Venereol* (Stockh) **34**(suppl 30):1–68, 1954.
4. Hart G: *Chancroid, Donovanosis, Lymphogranuloma Venereum*. Atlanta: U.S. Dept. of Health, Education and Welfare, 1979.
5. Nicolas J, Favre M: *Maladie de Nicolas-Favre. Nouvelle Pratique Dermatologique*, Vol. 4. Paris: Masson, 1936, p. 477.
6. Panizza E, Nigro M, De Pasquale R, et al: Considerazioni epidemiologiche a proposito di 6 casi di linfogranuloma venereo in Sicilia, in un anno. *Giorn Ital Dermatol Venereol* **122**:11–14, 1987.
7. Levine JS, Smith PD, Brugge WR: Chronic proctitis in male homosexuals due to lymphogranuloma venereum. *Gastroenterology* **79**:563–565, 1980.
8. Perine PL, Olu Osoba A: Lymphogranuloma venereum In Holmes H, Märdh PA, Sparling PF, et al (Eds): *Sexually Transmitted Diseases*. New York: McGraw-Hill, 1984, p. 281.
9. Laurijssens MT: Early proctoscopic aspects of lymphogranuloma venereum. *Riv Ital Colo-Proctol* **4**:14, 1985.
10. Lennette EH, Schmidt MJ: *Diagnostic Procedures for Viral and Rickettsial Infections*. New York: American Public Health Association, 1969, p. 871.
11. Schachter J, Osoba HO: Lymphogranuloma venereum. *Br Med Bull* **39**:151–154, 1983.
12. King A, Nicol C: *Venereal Diseases*. 3rd ed. London: Balliére Findall, 1975, p. 243.
13. Rainey R: The association of lymphogranuloma inguinale and cancer. *Surgery* **35**: 221–235, 1954.

14. Senitzer D, Gibbon J, Gohara A, et al: Infectious antecedents of immunoblastic lymphoma: Progressive immunosuppression in a patient with lymphogranuloma venereum. *Am J Med* **78**:163–167, 1985.
15. Annamunthodo H, Marryat J: Barium studies in intestinal lymphogranuloma venereum. *Br J Radiol* **34**:53–57, 1961.
16. Philip RN: Study of *Chlamydia* in patients with lymphogranuloma venereum and urethritis attending a venereal disease clinic. *Br J Vener Dis* **47**:114, 1971.
17. Hobson D: Tissue culture procedures for the isolation of *Chlamydia trachomatis* from patients with nongonococcal genital infections. In Hobson D, Holmes KK (Eds): *Nongonococcal Urethritis and Related Infections*. Washington, D.C.: American Society for Microbiology, 1977, p. 286.
18. Thomas BJ, Evans RT, Hawkins DA, et al: Sensitivity of detecting *Chlamydia trachomatis* elementary bodies in smears by use of a fluorescent labelled monoclonal antibody: Comparison with conventional Chlamydial isolation. *J Clin Pathol* **37**:812–816, 1984.
19. Stamm WE, Harrison HR, Alexander LD, et al: Diagnosis of *Chlamydia trachomatis* infections by direct immunofluorescence staining of genital secretions: A multicenter trial. *Ann Intern Med* **101**:638–641, 1984.
20. Amortegui AJ, Meyer MP: Enzyme immunoassay for detection of *Chlamydia trachomatis* from the cervix. *Obstet Gynecol* **65**:523–526, 1985.
21. Alacoque B, Cloppet H, Dumontel C, et al: Histological immunofluorescent and ultrastructural features of lymphogranuloma venereum: A case report. *Br J Vener Dis* **60**:390–395, 1984.
22. Favre M: Sur l'étiologie de la lymphogranulomatose inguinale subaigue. *Presse Méd* **62**:651–652, 1924.
23. Gamma C: Sur l'étiologie de la lymphogranulomatose inguinale subaigue. *Presse Méd* **37**:404–405, 1924.
24. de la Monte SM, Hutchins GM: Follicular proctocolitis and neuromatous hyperplasia with lymphogranuloma venereum. *Hum Pathol* **16**:1025–1032, 1985.
25. Felman JM: Lymphogranuloma Venereum. In: Maddin S (Ed): *Current Dermatologic Therapy*. Philadelphia: WB Saunders, 1986, p. 295.
26. Noble RC: *Sexually Transmitted Diseases*. Garden City, N.Y.: Medical Examination, 1979, p. 139.

CHAPTER 8

# Granuloma Inguinale

Virendra N. Sehgal

## Overview

Granuloma inguinale, a mildly contagious, autoinoculable granulomatous condition, was described in 1882 by McLeod [1] as serpiginous ulceration. Its causative organism was recovered from oral lesions by Donovan [2] in 1905, as intracellular protozoans. The organism was subsequently demonstrated in large numbers in large mononuclear cells; however, Aragao and Vianna are credited with naming it *Calymmatobacterium granulomatis*. Goldzieher and Peck [3] identified Donovan bodies in histologic sections and narrated the classic clinical description.

The specific histology of granuloma inguinale was described by Pund and Greenblatt [4], including its pathognomonic name (cell of Greenblatt). Greenblatt et al. [5] later produced the disease experimentally in volunteers by injecting material from an unruptured bubo and also described pseudobubo formation as its clinical manifestation.

Several efforts to recover the organism in vitro were unrewarding, until Anderson [6] succeeded in cultivating the organism on the yolk sac of developing chick embryos. He described it as bacteria (*Donovania granulomatis*). Subsequently, Dienst and colleagues [7] introduced an artificial culture medium. Granuloma inguinale is now considered a sexually transmitted disease, and its occurrence has been reported from endemic as well as from so-called nonendemic areas [8].

## Definition

Granuloma inguinale is a chronic, mildly contagious, sexually transmitted disease characterized by granulomatous ulceration of the genitalia and neighboring sites. It is caused by *Calymmatobacterium granulomatis* [9].

## Synonyms

Some synonyms for granuloma inguinale are donovanosis, granuloma venereum, serpiginous ulcer of the groin, ulcerating granuloma of the pudenda, chronic venereal sore, and granuloma inguinal tropicum.

## Clinical Findings

Granuloma inguinale is endemic in many parts of the world, sporadic in certain places, and rarely epidemic [10]. Presently, the disease is sparingly reported from Europe, Japan, and other temperate zones. China, Jamaica, and some parts of Papua New Guinea have shown a sizable decline in endemicity in the recent past, while in Vietnam, Indonesia, Africa, southern Papua New Guinea, and southern India the disease continues to be endemic. Racial susceptibility, hot and humid climate, low socioeconomic status, lack of personal hygiene, poor educational standards, and sexual promiscuity are all factors in its occurrence and transmission. Generally, prostitutes are the reservoir of the disease.

Onset of the disease is marked by formation of a firm papule. This may erode to form an ulcer, expressed as an ulcerogranulomatous, hypertrophic, sclerotic, or necrotic variant [8].

1. *Ulcerative/Ulcerogranulomatous Variant.* A single well-defined, friable, beefy-red, nontender, nonindurated ulcer with profuse granulation tissue, bleeding on touch and showing no necrosis on the surface (Fig. 8.1). Atypical variants may be encountered. Secondary infection of the ulcer may cause it to become tender, with necrotic slough and regional lymphadenopathy. Multiple lesions may occasionally be encountered. Ulcers of longer duration have a tendency to spread slowly, leading to the formation of a well-marked, raised margin at the edge of the ulcer. They often exhibit less granulation tissue. Chronicity may result in mild induration.
2. *Hypertrophic.* An irregular, friable raised growth bleeding on touch or an ulcer with a well-defined raised edge and an elevated granulomatous base is the usual presentation (Fig. 8.2).
3. *Sclerotic.* A deep, nontender, nonindurated ulcer with a clean floor and straight to undermined, nonbleeding edges, with waxing and waning of the activity. Atypical forms may be encountered.
4. *Necrotic.* A large foul-smelling, tender, nonindurated, irregular ulcer developing rapidly in the course of a few days, resulting in destruction of the genitalia.

A true bubo is generally not formed in granuloma inguinale. Sometimes, however, the subcutaneous tissue of the groin is affected, probably through lymphatics, leading to a fluctuant swelling. This has been named by Greenblatt et al. [5] a "pseudobubo." This swelling usually ruptures, forming a clean, raised granulomatous ulcer (Fig. 8.3).

### Other Sites of Disease

The perianal region can be affected following homosexual contact [11]. Dissemination of the disease to other parts of the body, such as the oral cavity [12] lip, gums, pharynx, cheeks, eyelid, sternum, thorax, abdomen, ribs, clavicles, and colon may also occur [13].

Metastatic lesions of granuloma inguinale in bones have also been reported. Of the 11 cases of bone disease thus far recorded [14], 10 were in women with lesions

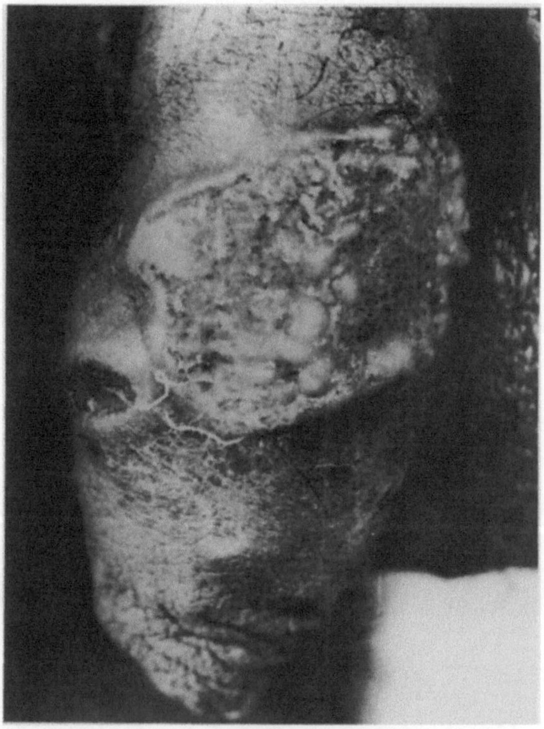

FIGURE 8.1. A well-defined nontender, nonindurated ulcer with everted edges over the shaft of the penis. Base of the ulcer shows exuberant granulation tissue.

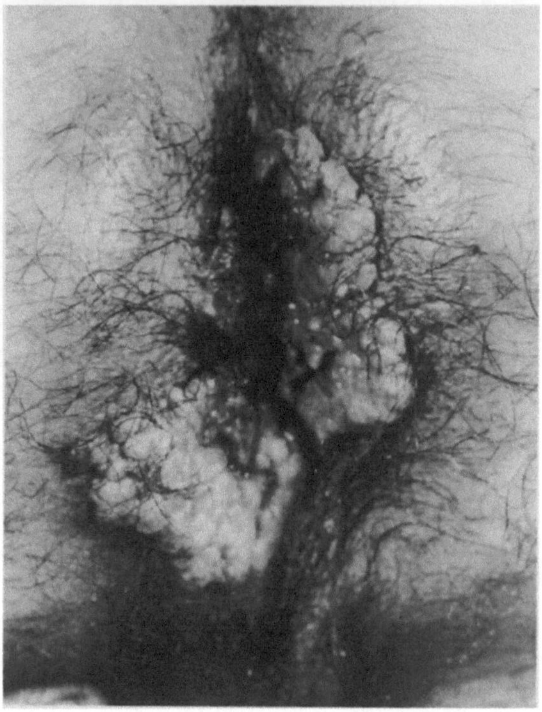

FIGURE 8.2. Hypertrophic ulcer. Tender, necrotic, well-defined lesion with irregular everted margins over the perianal region.

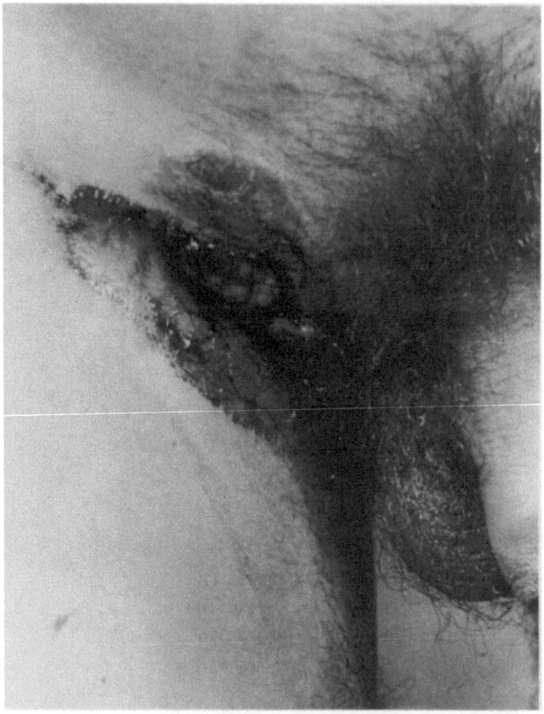

FIGURE 8.3. A burst inguinal pseudobubo. ◄

FIGURE 8.4. Cells of Greenblatt. ▼

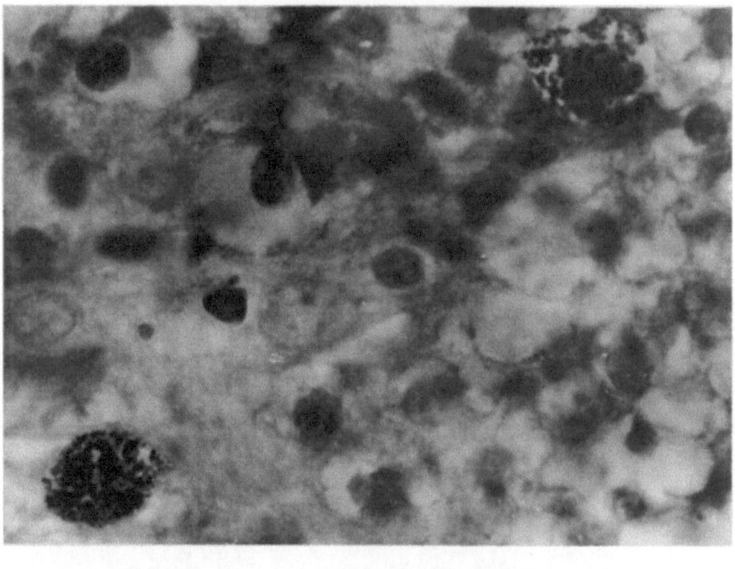

on the cervix. Osteolytic lesions are the usual presentation in the skeletal system [15].

## Histopathology

Initially it was believed that the histopathologic changes of granuloma inguinale were nonspecific, and not sufficiently characteristic to permit a diagnosis on tissue section. Pund and Greenblatt [4] indicated, however, that a massive cellular reaction surcharged with plasma cells, a paucity of lymphocytes, a diffuse sprinkling as well as focal collections of polymorphs in papillae, pseudoepitheliomatous changes, and pathognomic mononuclear cells filled with intracytoplasmic cysts containing darkly staining bodies were unique enough to make the diagnosis. Recently, Sehgal et al. [16] have emphasized the distinctive histopathologic features that affect the dermis as well as the epidermis.

The dermal changes are primarily inflammatory. They consist of a dense infiltrate, formed predominantly of large numbers of plasma and mononuclear cells throughout the dermis. In addition, histiocytes are seen in varying numbers. A few large cells containing cystic spaces, often with nuclei pushed to one side, and darkly staining inclusions (cells of Greenblatt) are conspicuous (Fig. 8.4). The number of neutrophils and lymphocytes is insignificant in most sections. Donovan bodies have different morphologic features: coccoid, coccobacillary, or bacillary. Mature forms surrounded by a capsule are seen in some sections. They are easily identified in slow (overnight) Giemsa-stained tissue sections [17]. The organisms in the tissue section are primarily intracytoplasmic clusters of coccobacillary forms taking a purplish to pink stain. They stand prominently over the background of faint blue cytoplasm surrounding the deep blue nuclei of the mononuclear cells. In addition, enlarged mononuclear cells with multiple cystic spaces containing Donovan bodies and eccentrically situated nuclei are uniformly conspicuous. They are difficult to identify in hematoxylin and eosin-stained sections [17]. Vascular changes (dilation, proliferation, or both) are predominant. Endothelial proliferation is a common feature, and proliferation of the tunica media may be seen.

The tissue sections show discontinuity in the epidermis, with ulcerations varying from mild to severe. Proliferation of the stratum spinosum (acanthosis) in the form of elongation of rete ridges is a constant feature of the hypertrophic variety. This, however, may also be seen in some of the ulcerative lesions. Similarly, pseudoepitheliomatous hyperplasia may also be a feature of the hypertrophic variant. Evidence of malignancy in the form of horn pearls, atypia of individual cells, or numerous mitotic figures is usually lacking. Neutrophilic sprinkling of both upper dermis and the epidermis is seen regularly; these occasionally form microabscesses. The adnexae, fat, and muscle are conspicuously spared.

## Natural History

A major breakthrough came when Donovan [2] recognized intracellular bodies from an oral lesion of the disease as the incriminated agent. These are now called

Donovan bodies. Goldzieher and Peck [3] recognized these bodies in histologic sections of the tissue. Their observations, the first of their kind, helped considerably in alleviating existing doubts. However, their claim of having cultivated an intracellular capsulated bacillus was unconvincing.

DeMonbreun and Goodpasture [18] succeeded in isolating a bacillus of the aerogen group from lesions and feces of patients with granuloma inguinale. They could demonstrate a morphologic resemblance to Donovan bodies in culture, but they failed to transmit the infection to animals. They documented that the disease was a chronic intestinal infection by the aerogen group of bacilli, with secondary fecal contamination of the skin. McIntosh [19] was the first to successfully transmit the disease experimentally. He also had reported that Donovan bodies were the causative organism of the disease and demonstrated changes in agglutinins, serum proteins, and skin sensitivity, suggesting production of antibodies against Donovan bodies.

Until the end of the 1930s, the controversy regarding the nature of the etiologic organism remained unsolved. Greenblatt et al. [5] were successful in producing granuloma inguinale in three human subjects. They were of the view that the Donovan bodies were sporozoans because of their affinity for mononuclear cells. Histologic examination of lymph nodes revealed Donovan bodies, from which it was surmised that lymphatics could also be affected, Anderson [6] was able to culture *C. granulomatis* on the yolk sac of chick embryos. Later, Anderson et al. [20] described the process in detail. They inoculated the yolk sac of a chick embryo with contaminant-free tissue from a patient with granuloma inguinale. The first embryo with a positive culture was obtained after 17 days having been inoculated 6 days previously. Serial cultures in 9-, 10-, or 11-day-old embryos produced for the most part unencapsulated organisms. Encapsulated organisms were produced if propagation was done on 4- to 6-day-old chick embryos. On the basis of their successful culture of the organism, they proposed a new genus, *Donovania granulomatis*.

The aforementioned attempts showed that previous so-called cultures of the Donovan microorganism were highly doubtful and were probably not of the organism itself but of contaminants. Encouraged by the culture of *D. granulomatis* on the yolk sac of chick embryo, other investigators tried to discover an artificial medium for cultivation. Only partial success was achieved by Dunham and Rake [21]. Following this, Goldberg et al. [22] defined and demonstrated the bacteriologic behavior of *D. granulomatis*. Goldberg [23] pointed out that factors such as a low O-R potential, which can be achieved by a thioglycollate medium and a factor (or factors) present in egg, were necessary for the growth of *D. granulomatis*. The egg factor could be substituted by the enzymatic digestion of bovine albumin or soya meal. Goldberg [23] also succeeded in isolating a bacterium resembling *D. granulomatis* from the feces of a patient with granuloma inguinale. Recently, study of basic hematologic profile and lymphocyte subpopulations (T lymphocytes with subsets T4 helper/inducer, T8 suppressor/cytotoxic, and B lymphocytes) showed its general increase. In addition, an overall increase in B lymphocyte and immunoglobulin levels was also evident. It is envisaged that distribution of T cell subsets and immunoglobulin-synthesizing B lymphocytes in the tissues, and their ultimate correlation with blood findings, may substantially add to further elucidation of the bacterium's natural history [24].

## Complications and Sequelae

The most important sequel of granuloma inguinale, which has been studied quite extensively, is its relationship to squamous cell carcinoma of the penis. Pund and Greenblatt [4] in a histopathologic study of the disease found pronounced epithelial proliferation, simulating early epitheliomatous changes. Beerman and Sonck [25] graded pseudoepitheliomatous hyperplasia seen in the disease into grades I, II, and III. They concluded that when hyperplasia extended deeply enough, a diagnosis of carcinoma of the penis could be made.

Rajam and Rangiah [9] emphasized that the resemblance between granuloma inguinale and carcinoma can be close, on both clinical and histologic grounds. A true epitheliomatous change can occur as a complication or sequel to granuloma inguinale but seems to be an infrequent occurrence.

Besides carcinoma, other complications are adhesions to the scrotum and penis, destruction of the penile shaft, pseudobubo [26], and pseudoelephantiasis [27]. Stenosis of the urethral, vaginal, or anal orifice is a complication of the sclerotic variety of the disease [9]. Pseudoelephantiasis is an unusual, sparingly reported entity. It occurs in both men and women and is characterized by morphology simulating that of elephantiasis of the genitals. Differentiation from the latter is made on the basis of conspicuous ulcer(s) preceding the swelling (Fig. 8.5) and absence of constitutional symptoms of fever, weakness, and arthralgia. Mechanical obstruction of the lymphatics following scarring may cause this condition [27]. Other unusual sites are the gingiva, uterus, fallopian tubes, ovary, buttock, lymph node, and epididymis [28]. Sehgal et al. [29] presented an extremely rare case of primary extragenital disseminated cutaneous granuloma inguinale.

## Differential Diagnosis

The diagnosis of granuloma inguinale may appear simple if it is suspected whenever ulcers appear over the genitalia. Confirmation should, however, be through demonstration of Donovan bodies in the tissue smears.

Donovan bodies are identified in smears as mature and/or immature organisms present inside the cytoplasm of mononuclear cells. These cells may exhibit vacuolation inside the cytoplasm. The mature organism is ovoid or bean shaped, varying from 1 to 1.5 μ in length and 0.5 to 0.7 μ in thickness, with a well-defined pinkish material surrounding a blue bacillary body. In addition, it has a dark-blue chromatin inclusion arranged at the poles. The capsule may remain unstained or stain bright pink. The morphology of the immature organism may conform to a coccoid, diplococcoid, or bacillary form. The organism varies in size from 0.6 to 1.0 μ. The

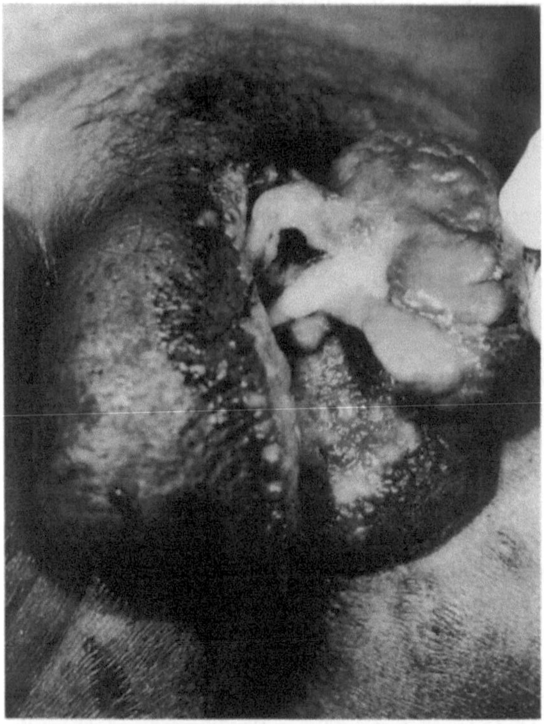

a

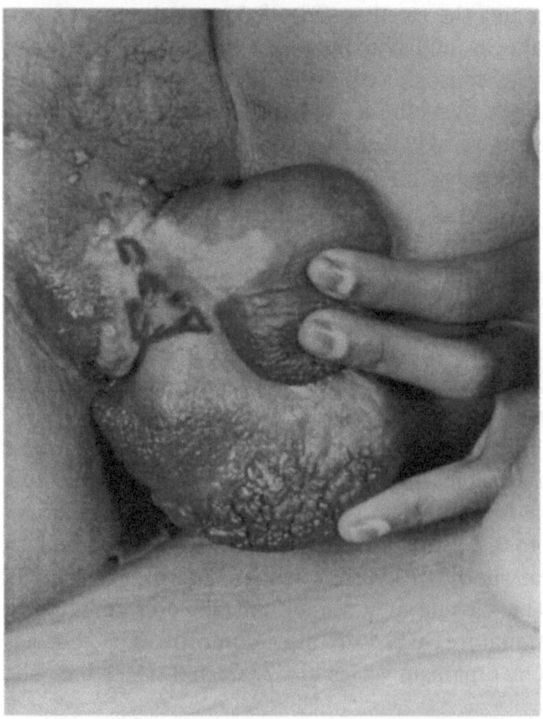

b

FIGURE 8.5a,b. Pseudoelephantiasis with a classic ulcerogranulomatous lesion (hematoxylin and eosin; × 1,000).

diplococcoid forms in particular are interesting, resembling a closed safety pin (Fig. 8.6).

Tissue smears cannot be overemphasized, even though they may be negative in up to one third of cases ulcerogranulomatous, necrotic, and sclerotic variety [17]. Other ulcerative lesions of venereal or nonvenereal origin may have to be excluded.

## Other Sexually Transmitted Diseases

### Chancroid

Chancroid is characterized by multiple, small, superficial, painful, dirty necrotic ulcers of varying sizes. The edges of the ulcers are undermined and surrounded by a narrow zone of erythema and edema. They are tender and bleed on touch. Inguinal bubo may be an accompaniment. Usually the bubo is a unilateral, unilocular, fluctuant, tender swelling with overlying taut and erythematous skin. The incubation period varies from 2 to 7 days. Dwarf chancroid is characterized by a small superficial ulcer. Giant chancroid is a large granulomatous ulcer as a consequence of a ruptured bubo extending to involve the surrounding skin. Follicular chancroids are seen in association with the hair follicles, while serpiginous chancroids are characterized by multiple ulcers coalescing to form a serpiginous pattern. Its phagedenic variant may cause extensive destruction of the genitals, associated with a foul-smelling discharge. Demonstration of *Haemophilus ducreyi* in a Gram-stained smear is diagnostic. Recovery of the organisms in vitro is, however, imperative for diagnosis.

### Chancroidal Ulcers

These ulcers have recently been defined [30]. They are single ulcers with the morphology of chancroid. Their incubation period is longer, 8 to 11 days, and they show an absence of lymphadenopathy. Modern culture techniques [31], which can be used to isolate *H. ducreyi* in a majority of chancroid cases, fail to demonstrate the organism from chancroidal ulcers. Instead, a polymicrobial flora may be isolated [32].

### Herpes Progenitalis

Only rarely can this viral infection be mistaken for granuloma inguinale. It presents classically as grouped vesicular lesions on an erythematous base. The vesicles rupture in a day or two to form superficial, tender, polycyclic erosions on the genitalia. There may be a long history of recurrences and remissions. In early cases, scraping the floor of a vesicle gently with a scalpel, putting the material on a clean glass slide, and staining with Giemsa's stain reveals characteristic multinucleated giant cells in the smear. Cell culture technique is used to isolate the causative virus. The condition heals spontaneously.

### Syphilis

Early syphilis comprises primary and secondary stages. The incubation period of the primary chancre varies from 10 to 90 days. It is a painless, erythematous,

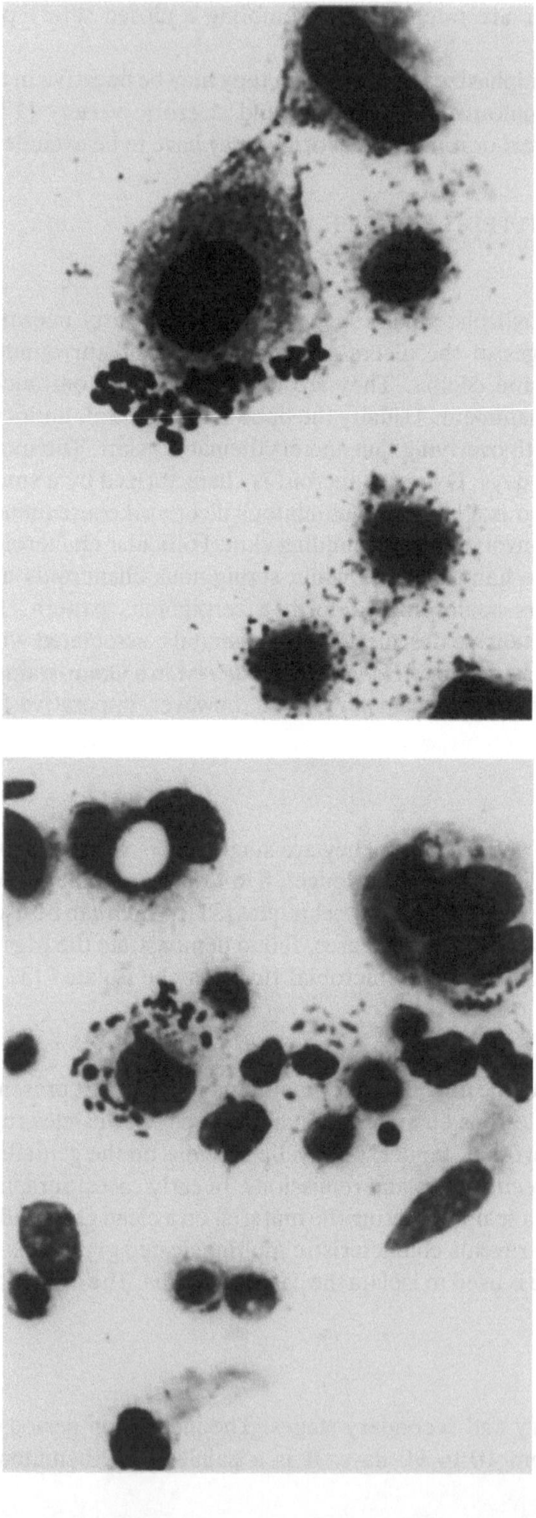

a

b

FIGURE 8.6a,b. Tissue smear depicting intracellular and extracellular Donovan bodies.

indurated papule that erodes to form an ulcer. The ulcer is painless, clean, well defined, and indurated and has a raw exuding surface. It resembles a button glued to the skin or the mucous membrane. The secondary stage is recognized by an asymptomatic polymorphic bilateral and symmetrical rash, mucous patches, snail track ulcers, and generalized lymphadenopathy with the classic features just listed. Distinct clinical variants comprising syphilides of various morphology, namely macular, papular, pustular, follicular, annular, psoriasiform and condylomata lata may be found. The condylomalata, in particular, are quite frequent and are evident as flat-topped, grayish-white eruptions with oozing of serum, primarily on the genitals, anus, and axillae. Demonstration of *Treponema pallida* from the secondary lesions is confirmatory.

Tertiary syphilis is rarely seen nowadays. The ulcerative variety has a punched-out appearance with sharp vertical edges and a dull-gray, chamoislike slough base. The nodular and psoriasiform type are unlikely to be mistaken for granuloma inguinale.

### Lymphogranuloma Venereum (LGV)

Granuloma inguinale and LGV are morphologically distinct from each other; however, the earlier nomenclature (granuloma venereum vs. lymphogranuloma venereum) may be a cause of confusion. LGV presents initially as transient, herpetiform vesicular lesions on the genitalia. These heal within a week. After 2 to 8 weeks, the patient has inguinal lymphadenitis and constitutional manifestations. The adenitis is multilocular, tender, and nonfluctuant. The overlying skin is usually normal unless suppuration occurs, in which case multiple discharging sinuses are formed. Lymph nodes above and below the inguinal ligament are involved (groove sign), with the inguinal ligament appearing as a groove between the two lymph node masses. A positive intradermal Frei test and the modern serologic techniques of complement fixation and microimmunoassay further differentiate LGV from granuloma inguinale. *Chlamydia trachomatis*, the causative organism, may also be cultured from material taken from a bubo or from the genital. The late manifestations of LGV due to lymphatic obstruction may be very similar to those seen in granuloma inguinale-induced pseudoelephantiasis. Elephantiasis, leading to enormous hypertrophy of the genitalia, is the usual feature in such cases.

### Candidosis

This common condition is due to *Candida albicans*, an opportunistic yeast. It presents in men as balanoposthitis with fissuring of the prepuce. A moist, sodden, whitish plaque is seen. Its removal reveals an erythematous erosive area. There may be isolated, peripheral vesiculopustules. Demonstration of the fungus is simple. A surface scraping of the lesions mounted in 10% potassium hydroxide solution shows budding pseudohyphae in abundance. There is frequently concomitant diabetes mellitus.

### Traumatic Ulcers

These are seen in men in the form of sharply demarcated, usually linear cuts on the genitalia. The history is that the condition developed or was noticed immediately after sexual intercourse. The tendency is spontaneous healing, if further intercourse is avoided. However, if a sexually transmitted condition is superimposed, the lesion changes its morphologic characteristics.

## Non-Sexually Transmitted Diseases

### Squamous Cell Carcinoma

Squamous cell carcinoma of the penis may pose a diagnostic problem. The resemblance to granuloma inguinale can be close, both conditions exhibiting a granulomatous, ulcerated growth with hypertrophic rolled-over edges. In later stages, of course, involvement of the inguinal lymph nodes occurs in carcinoma. These are firm to hard and subsequently become fixed to deeper structures. In the earlier stages, both a tissue smear and a biopsy are prerequisites. Histopathologically, although epidermal changes can be similar, the presence of numerous mitoses, irregularity, bizarre patterns of nuclei, and horn pearls in carcinoma help to differentiate the two conditions.

### Skin Tuberculosis

Scrofuloderma may present in the inguinal region as discharging sinuses and ulcers. Usually, however, the underlying lymph nodes can be felt as a matted mass to which the sinuses are fixed. They are necrotic and friable, have undermined edges, and have a bluish margin. Tuberculosis verrucosa cutis may, very rarely, present in the genitoinguinal region. In such cases, confusion with the hypertrophic variant of granuloma inguinale may arise. Histopathology provides the answer: skin tuberculosis shows areas of caseation necrosis with a surrounding granuloma of epithelioid cells and lymphocytes. An admixture of polymorphonuclear cells may be present. Special staining with Ziehl-Neelsen stain will reveal acid-fast bacilli.

### Filariasis

The late stage of filaria presents as elephantiasis of the genitalia. However, the absence of genital ulcerations in the past, an initial acute episode of fever with (usually) scrotal swelling, and microfilaria seen on a peripheral blood smear taken at night all distinguish it from granuloma inguinale.

### Fixed Drug Eruption

This can be diagnosed by its salient morphologic features, namely, single, well-defined, superficial, erosive lesions with no regional lymphadenopathy. The lesion is preceded or accompanied by itching and burning. Patients often do not relate their complaints to the use of drugs. Drug eruption is especially important in developing countries. A drug history should, therefore, be pursued thoroughly and systematically. In cases where the nature of the drug is not known to the patient, eliciting the complaint for which the drug was taken may be helpful. Provoking the lesion(s) with the suspecting drug confirms the diagnosis and may help to prevent recurrences in

TABLE 8.1. Treatment schedule for granuloma inguinale.

| Drug | Daily dosage | Total dose* | Duration |
|---|---|---|---|
| Tetracyclines (oral) | | | |
| Terramycin | 2 g in four equal doses | 20–40 g | 10–20 days |
| Aureomycin | Same as Terramycin | | |
| Streptomycin (intramuscular) | 2 g in two equal doses | 20–40 g | 10–20 days |
| Cotrimoxazole (oral) (trimethoprim, 80 mg, plus sulfamethoxazole, 400 mg) | 2 tablets two times a day | 20–30 tablets | 10–15 days |

*Treatment may be prolonged if recovery is partial/incomplete.

the future. It also allays the patient's anxiety regarding the venereal origin of the signs [33].

## Management

Granuloma inguinale has long presented difficulties in treatment. Until the early part of this century, surgery was employed to excise the lesion, along with the margin of normal tissue. The resulting scar often broke down to cause a recurrence. Earlier, potassium antimony tartrate was used in a 1 to 2% solution in normal saline or in 5% dextrose and given intravenously, repeated on alternate days. Although this was successful for disease in the early stages, chronic cases were very resistant. Fouadin, a trivalent antimony preparation [34], was also used, as were other antimonials. The toxicity and antimony fastness (recurrent lesions developing resistance) were the main drawbacks of antimonial therapy.

### Drugs

#### Streptomycin

Barton et al. [35] first used this drug in the treatment of granuloma inguinale. Greenblatt et al. [36] organized the first large-scale trial of streptomycin and attempted to rationalize the dosage schedule. A dosage of 4 g per day in divided doses for 5 days was found to be optimal. Donovan bodies disappeared from the lesions an average of 6 days after initiation of therapy, while healing occurred 1 to 2 weeks after cessation of treatment. There were a few relapses. In another well-documented study. Kupperman et al. [37] found that streptomycin in total dose of more than 20 g resulted in cure in all cases, while recurrences were experienced with smaller dosages. Rajam and Rangiah [9], however, had commendable results with smaller (1–2 g) daily doses over a period of 10 days; however, failure of streptomycin later was reported from India and abroad. The high risks of side effects has further discouraged its use.

### Tetracyclines

Oxytetracycline was found to be effective in optimal doses of 2 g per day by mouth over a period of 10 to 14 days [38]. Chlortetracycline was found to be equally effective [39,40], the optimal dosage being the same as that for oxytetracycline. Low cost, high efficacy, and ease of administration make tetracyclines the drug of first choice in granuloma inguinale [10].

### Cotrimoxazole

Although sulfonamides are ineffective in the treatment of granuloma inguinale, a combination of sulfamethoxazole and trimethoprim has been found useful [41]. In a subsequent follow-up, only 2 of 116 patients had recurrence after administration of two tablets twice a day for 10 to 15 days. This was confirmed by Rosen et al. [42], Subramanian [43], and Spagnole et al. [44]. The treatment schedule is given in Table 8.1.

### Chloramphenicol

This drug also is highly effective in the treatment of granuloma inguinale, both orally and parenterally [37,45]. The optimal oral dose is 2 g per day in divided doses for 10 to 14 days; however, the serious (although rare) side effect of bone marrow depression caused by this drug ensures that it should be used only sparingly.

## Other Drugs

Ampicillin, in doses of 1 to 2 g per day for 14 days, was effective in two studies [46] but ineffective in another [47]. Triacetyloleandomycin was extremely efficacious in a single study [48]. Erythromycin, both parenterally and orally, is useful [49,50]. Gentamicin, in a dosage of 1 mg/kg three times a day, was found effective in all nine cases treated with this drug [51]. Penicillin [52] has been found to be ineffective.

## Surgery

Appropriate surgical intervention may be needed in pseudoelephantiasis and other complications.

## References

1. McLeod K: Précis of operations performed in the wards of the first surgeon, Medical College Hospital during the year 1881. *Ind Med Gaz* **11**:113–123, 1882.
2. Donovan C: Medical cases from Madras General Hospital. *Ind Med Gaz* **40**:414–415, 1905.
3. Goldzieher MA, Peck SM: *Virchows Arch. Path. Anat.* **259**:795 Quoted by Rajam and Rangiah.
4. Pund ER, Greenblatt RB: Specific histology of granuloma inguinale. *Arch Pathol* **23**:224–230, 1937.

5. Greenblatt RB, Dienst RB, Pund ER, et al: Experimental and clinical granuloma inguinale. *JAMA* **113**:1108–1116, 1939.
6. Anderson K: An etiologic consideration of *Donovania granulomatis* cultivated from granuloma inguinale (three cases) in embryonic yolk. *J Exp Med* **81**:25–46, 1943.
7. Dienst RB, Reinstein CR, Kupperman HS, et al: Studies on the causal agent of granuloma inguinale. *Am J Syph* **31**:614–617, 1947.
8. Sehgal VN, Prasad ALS: A clinical profile of donovanosis in a non-endemic area. *Dermatologica* **168**:273–278, 1984.
9. Rajam RV, Rangiah PN: *Donovanosis*. WHO Monograph Series No. 24. Geneva: World Health Organization, 1954.
10. Anonymous: *Nongonococcal Urethritis and Other Sexually Transmitted Diseases of Public Health Importance.* WHO Technical Report Series No. 660. Geneva: World Health Organization, 1981.
11. Milton Marmell MA: Donovanosis of the anus in the male – an epidemiological consideration. *Br J Vener Dis* **34**:213–218, 1958.
12. Lal S, Arunthathi S, Sawhney KL: Oral granuloma venereum. *Ind J Derm Vener Lepr* **37**:19–20, 1971.
13. Rajam RV, Rangiah PN, Anguli VC: Systemic donovanosis. *Br J Vener Dis* **30**:73–80, 1954.
14. Sieber PE: Granuloma inguinale with bone involvement. *J Radiol* **95**:515–517, 1965.
15. Kirkpatrick DJ: Donovanosis: A rare cause of osteolytic bone lesions. *Clin Radiol* **21**:101–106, 1970.
16. Sehgal VN, Prasad ALS, Beohar PC: The histopathology of donovanosis. *Br J Vener Dis* **60**:45–48, 1984.
17. Sehgal VN, Jain MK: Tissue section Donovan bodies: Identification through slow Giemsa (overnight) technique. *Dermatologica* **174**:228–231, 1987.
18. DeMonbreun WA, Goodpasture EW: Further studies on the etiology of granuloma inguinale. *Am J Trop Med* **13**:447–463, 1933.
19. McIntosh JA: The etiology of granuloma inguinale. *JAMA* **87**:996–1002, 1926.
20. Anderson K, Goodpasture EW, DeMonbreun WA: Immunologic relationship of *Donovania granulomatis* to granuloma inguinale. *J Exp Med* **81**:41–50, 1945.
21. Dunham W, Rake G: Culture and serologic studies on granuloma inguinale. *Am J Syph* **32**:145–149, 1948.
22. Goldberg J, Weaver RH, Packer H: Studies on granuloma inguinale. I. Bacteriologic behaviour of *D. granulomatis. Am J Syph* **37**:60–70, 1953.
23. Goldberg J: Studies on granuloma inguinale. IV. Growth requirements of *Donovania granulomatis* and its relationship to the natural habitat of the organism. *Br J Vener Dis* **35**:266–268, 1959.
24. Sehgal VN, Jain MK, Sharma VK: Lymphocyte subpopulation determined by monoclonal antibodies, and immunoglobulins in donovanosis. *Genitourin Med* **63**:274–276, 1987.
25. Beerman H, Sonck CE: The epithelial changes in granuloma inguinale. *Am J Syph* **36**:501–510, 1952.
26. Sehgal VN, Jain MK: Patterns of epidemics of donovanosis in "so-called" non-endemic regions. *Int J Dermatol* **27**, 1988.
27. Sehgal VN, Jain MK, Sharma VK: Pseudoelephantiasis induced by donovanosis. *Genitourin Med* **63**:54–56, 1987.
28. Sehgal VN, Prasad ALS: Donovanosis: Current concepts. *Int J Dermatol* **25**:8–16, 1986.
29. Sehgal VN, Sharma NL, Bhargava NC, et al: Primary extragenital disseminated cutaneous donovanosis. *Br J Dermatol* **101**:353–356, 1979.

30. Sehgal VN, Shyam Prasad AL: Chancroid or chancroidal ulcers. *Dermatologica* **170**:136–141, 1985.
31. Borchardt KA, Hoke AW: Simplified laboratory technique for the diagnosis of chancroid. *Arch Dermatol* **102**:188–192, 1970.
32. Chapel T, Brown WS, Jeffries C, et al: The microbiological flora of penile ulcerations. *J Infect Dis* **137**:50–56, 1978.
33. Sehgal VN, Gangwani OP: Genital fixed drug eruptions. *Genitourin Med* **62**:56–58, 1986.
34. Rajam RV: A note on the treatment of infective granuloma with Fouadin. *Ind Med Gaz* **69**:372-375, 1934.
35. Barton RL, Craig RM, Schwemlein GX, et al: Granuloma inguinale treated with streptomycin. Report of 3 cases. *Arch Dermatol Syph* **56**:1–6, 1947.
36. Greenblatt RB, Dienst RB, Cupperman HS, et al: Granuloma inguinale: Streptomycin therapy and research. *J Vener Dis Inform* **28**:183–188, 1942.
37. Kopperman HS, Greenblatt RB, Dienst RB: Streptomycin in the therapy of granuloma inguinale. *JAMA* **136**:84–89, 1948.
38. Wright LT, Prigot A, Dilorenza JC, et al: Oral terramycin in rapid treatment of gonorrhoea and other venereal diseases. *Am J Syph* **35**:490–495, 1951.
39. Greenblatt RB, Barfield WE, Dienst RB, et al: Terramycin in the treatment of granuloma inguinale. *J Vener Dis Inform* **32**:114–115, 1951.
40. Greenblatt RB, Barfield WE, Dienst RB, et al: A five year study of antibiotics in the treatment of granuloma inguinale. *Am J Syph* **36**:180–191, 1952.
41. Milton Marmell MA, Santora E: Donovanosis—granuloma inguinale. Incidence, nomenclature and diagnosis. *Am J Syph* **34**:83–96, 1950.
42. Rosen T, Tschen JA, Ramsdell W, et al: Granuloma inguinale. *J Am Acad Dermatol* **11**:433–437, 1984.
43. Subramian S. Sclerosing granuloma inguinale. *Br J Vener Dis* **57**:210–212, 1981.
44. Spagnolo DV, Coburn PR, Cream JJ, et al: Extragenital granuloma inguinale (donovanosis) diagnosed in the United Kingdom: A clinical, histological and electromicroscopical study. *J Clin Pathol* **37**:945–949, 1984.
45. Robinson RC, Cronk B: Granuloma inguinale: Further observations on results of treatment with aureomycin and chloramphenicol. *Am J Syph* **35**:378–382, 1951.
46. Thew MA: Ampicillin in the treatment of granuloma inguinale. *JAMA* **210**:866–867. 1969.
47. Davis CM: Granuloma inguinale: A clinical, histological and ultrastructural study. *JAMA* **211**:632–636, 1970.
48. Kerdel-Vegas F, Convit J, Soto JM: Treatment of granuloma inguinale with triacetyloleandomycin. *Arch Dermatol* **84**:248–255, 1961.
49. Ghosh S, Ghosh R: Donovanosis treated with erythromycin parenterally. Report of a first case. *Br J Vener Dis* **35**:260–261, 1959.
50. Robinson HM, Cohen MM: Treatment of granuloma inguinale with erythromycin. *J Invest Dermatol* **20**:407–409, 1953.
51. Maddocks I, Anders EM, Dennis E: Donovanosis in Papua New Guinea. *Br J Vener Dis* **52**:190–196, 1976.
52. Nelson RA: Penicillin in the treatment of granuloma inguinale. *Am J Syph* **28**:611–614, 1944.

CHAPTER 9

# Nonspecific Urethral Infections and Reiter's Syndrome

Angelika Stary and Friedrich Gschnait

## Part 1. Nonspecific Urethal Infections

## Definition and Overview

Nongonococcal urethritis (NGU) is defined as sexually or nonsexually transmitted urethral inflammation not due to *Neisseria gonorrhoeae.* Its causes are many established, suspected, or unknown infectious agents. Clinical manifestations include urethral discharge, dysuria, and urethral irritation revealing erythema of the terminal urethra. Objective findings such as an increase in number of inflammatory cells in urethral smears (four polymorphonuclear leukocytes [PMNL] per high-power field) or in the urine sediment indicate urethral infection.

NGU is one of the most common sexually transmitted diseases (STD) in men. It may be followed by complications such as epididymitis and infection of female sexual partners, who then may develop salpingitis and may even transmit the infectious agent to newborns.

## Synonyms

Synonyms for nonspecific urethral infections are nongonococcal urethritis, and nonspecific urethritis.

## Signs and Symptoms; Complications

NGU develops about 2 weeks after contact. The incubation period is longer in *Chlamydia trachomatis*-induced NGU than in other types [1].

Clinical symptoms include urethral discharge and dysuria ranging from mild pruritus to severe burning pain. In contrast to gonorrhea, in NGU the discharge is usually mucoid, white, and scant and may be detected in the early morning only (Table 9.1). Due to the mild symptoms, less than 50% of NGU patients seek medical treatment.

TABLE 9.1. Signs and symptoms of nongonococcal urethritis.

| Sign, symptom | Percent of patients |
|---|---|
| Discharge and dysuria | 38 |
| Dysuria alone | 15 |
| Discharge alone | 47 |
| Only in morning | 29 |
| Profuse | 3 |
| Moderate | 12 |
| Scant | 12 |
| Purulent | 6 |
| Nonpurulent | 21 |

No clinical symptom is characteristic for NGU caused by *C. trachomatis* [2]; symptoms may be severe or mild [3,4]. Furthermore, clinical overlap often exists between NGU and gonorrhea. NGU may also be asymptomatic, which is an important aspect in contact tracing.

So far, the causative agent of NGU cannot be diagnosed or suspected on clinical grounds alone. Laboratory testing thus is necessary, so that specific and effective therapy for NGU can be given.

If NGU is caused by chlamydial infection, complications are frequent and may lead to severe disturbances. They are discussed in detail in chapter 20.

Complications in NGU not due to chlamydia, such as epididymitis, rarely develop. Prostatic enlargement seems not significantly more common among patients with NGU than in healthy persons [4]. In 1 to 2% of NGU patients, sexually acquired reactive arthralgia (SARA) is described and may be a part of Reiter's syndrome (see the second part of this chapter). In a small number of persons with NGU, autoinoculation may be followed by conjunctivitis.

## Etiology

Several infectious agents have been implicated as causes of NGU. Practical interest is focused on *C. trachomatis* and on genital mycoplasmas, herpesviruses, and *Trichomonas vaginalis*.

### C. Trachomatis

The association of *C. trachomatis* and NGU has been established in many studies, which indicates that this organism may be the most important and most common cause of NGU. Its leading role is based on clinical, microbiologic, and serologic studies as well as on animal trials and treatment results.

That *C. trachomatis* is a major cause of NGU was initially recognized by Dunlop in 1965 [5]. His results and others have led to the conclusion that *C. trachomatis* (serotypes (D–K) is a urethral pathogen and causes a variety of genitourinary disorders in both sexes. *C. trachomatis* is discussed in detail in chapter 20.

TABLE 9.2. Colonization of *Mycoplasmas* in neonates and adults.

| Population | Percent affected | |
|---|---|---|
| | *M. hominis* | *U. urealyticum* |
| Neonates | | |
| Pharynx | 3 | 10 |
| Vagina | 1 | 23 |
| Male urethra | 1 | 7 |
| Adults* | | |
| Men | 0–14 | 3–81 |
| Women | 0–31 | 8.5–77.5 |

*Depending on number of partners and sexual experience.

## GENITAL MYCOPLASMAS

Mycoplasmas are the smallest free-living microorganisms. Serologic, cultural, and genetic data show that mycoplasmas constitute a heterogeneous group of microorganisms. Three species have been found to cause symptoms in humans. *Mycoplasma pneumoniae* is associated with atypical pneumonia. *M. hominis* and *Ureaplasma urealyticum* are common inhabitants of the genital mucous membranes. *M. hominis* has been demonstrated to be a possible etiologic agent of pelvic inflammatory disease (PID). The role of *U. urealyticum* in the etiology of NGU remains controversial [6–8]. *M. genitalium*, a new species of mycoplasmas, is also regarded as a potential pathogen in the male and female urogenital tract.

The frequency of colonization with mycoplasmas increases with sexual experience and the number of different sexual partners and is higher in women than in men (Table 9.2) [9,10]. Genital mycoplasmas are reported to have a higher prevalence among blacks. This, however, may be due to different patterns of sexual behavior [11].

### Pathogenicity of Mycoplasmas

At this time evidence is insufficient that *M. hominis* causes NGU, either from isolation studies, from serology, or from therapeutic trials. The pathogenic role of *U. urealyticum* in NGU is also controversial. Several data support the potency of *Ureaplasma* to cause NGU: Therapeutic studies have correlated clinical improvement of urethritis with anti-*Ureaplasma* treatment, suggesting a pathogenic role of this microorganism in NGU [12–14].

Intraurethral self-inoculation with strains of *U. urealyticum* isolated from patients with NGU and subcultured several times has led to urogenital symptoms with dysuria and micturition accompanied by pyuria and pyrexia [15]. These clinical symptoms were combined with a high titer response in the metabolism inhibition test to *U. urealyticum*. Treatment was followed by amelioration of symptoms in one of the two men tested; the other one developed persistent urinary and prostatic discomfort.

Arguments against an etiologic role for *Ureaplasma* in NGU include identical isolation rates in NGU patients and healthy controls [16], lack of clear correlation between seroconversion and the clinical situation [17], and the ubiquity of *Ureaplasmas*. These controversial data may be explained by the assumption that only certain serotypes of ureaplasmas have a definite pathogenic potential.

NGU may develop after the first exposure to *U. urealyticum*, and its development may be related to the number of microorganisms inoculated by sexual contact. Host factors such as local immunity may influence the development of NGU and cause susceptibility for clinical symptoms only in a small proportion of men.

### Isolation and Identification of Mycoplasmas

Mycoplasmas are gram negative but cannot be recognized on microscopic examination of Gram-stained clinical specimens. They grow well in broth medium under atmospheric conditions. *M. hominis* metabolizes arginine to ammonia, raising the pH of the medium. Ureaplasmas possess the enzyme urease, which changes urea to ammonia. This chemical reaction leads to a color change of the medium. In a second step the microorganisms are subcultured onto agar medium. This liquid-to-agar technique has proven to be the most sensitive method for the isolation of both groups of genital mycoplasmas [18].

Colonies of *M. hominis* have a characteristic "fried egg" appearance. Ureaplasmas produce small, dark-colored colonies (Fig. 9.1).

At least 7 serotypes of *M. hominis* and 14 serotypes of *U. urealyticum* have been identified. No data, however, exist that any serotype is associated with particular disease.

## Other Bacteria

Bacteria other than *C. trachomatis* and *U. urealyticum* play a minor role in the development of NGU [12,19]:

*Staphylococcus saprophyticus* is documented as a possible etiologic agent of the urethral syndrome in women and is more frequently diagnosed in men with NGU than in symptomless controls [20].

*Corynebacterium genitalium* type 1 has been suggested as a cause of NGU, though controversial data have been obtained by different investigators [21].

## Herpes Simplex Virus (HSV)

Primary genital herpes in more than 30% of men is complicated by herpetic urethritis. NGU due to recurrent herpes infection is rare, and HSV has not been isolated more frequently in patients with NGU than in control groups [4].

## Parasites and Yeasts

*Trichomonas vaginalis* seems to play no significant role in the development of NGU; the majority of men harboring *T. vaginalis* are asymptomatic. This organism may,

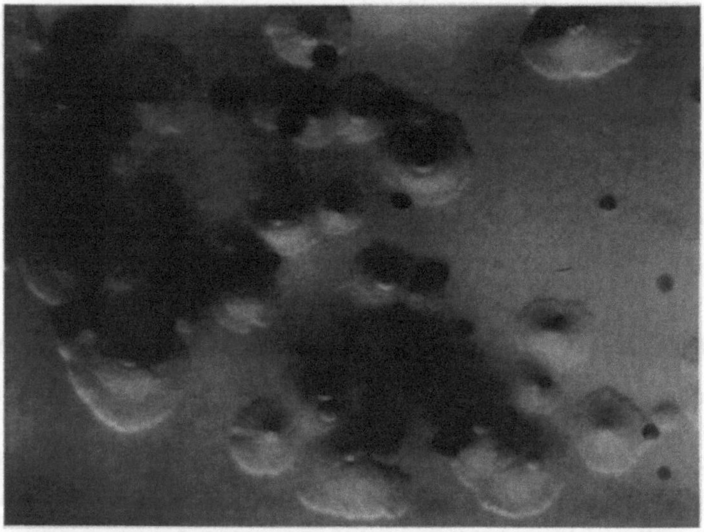

FIGURE 9.1. Culture of *Mycoplasma hominis* (fried-egg appearance) and *Ureaplasma urealyticum* (dark dots). Shephard A7 medium.

however, be a concomitant etiologic agent for NGU in male patients exhibiting urethral anatomic abnormalities or chronic inflammatory changes of the urethra [22].

Yeasts only rarely cause NGU. In yeast balanitis a nonspecific urethral inflammation may be observed [4].

## Other Causes

Anatomic abnormalities such as urethral strictures, phimosis, or changes after urethral traumatization may lead to secondary bacterial urethritis or abacterial dysuria. Particular sexual practices may also cause urethral discomfort with or without inflammatory signs.

## Epidemiology

NGU is the most common STD in men in the United States and in several European countries. Data from Great Britain show a tenfold increase in the frequency of NGU since 1951. More than 100,000 cases are reported annually [23]. For 1977 the Centers for Disease Control estimated 2.5 million cases of NGU in the United States and 1 million cases of gonorrhea [24]. NGU thus is more frequently observed than gonorrhea and comprises more than 70% of all acute cases of urethritis.

Epidemiologic data indicate that NGU patients, compared with gonorrhea patients, are more often white, are better educated, are members of a relatively higher socioeconomic status, are older at the age of first sexual experience, and have fewer sexual partners [4]. Homosexuals are reported to suffer less frequently from NGU than heterosexual men.

## Diagnosis

The diagnosis of NGU should be carried out as a two-step procedure:

1. Diagnosis of urethritis and exclusion of gonorrhea.
2. Diagnosis of the cause of the NGU as far as possible.

The diagnostic criteria for the definite demonstration of urethritis include [25]

Five or more PMN (polymorphonuclear leukocytes) in at least three fields of the Gram's stain examined with a magnification of ×1000.

No gonococci in the microscopic field or in culture (culture is necessary in a negative or doubtful Gram's stain and in all cases with possible forensic impact).

For a firm diagnosis, optimal examination is needed. In patients with no or only little discharge or with few or no PMNLs in the urethral smear, negative results should be confirmed by reexamination in the morning before the patient voids.

A search for *C. trachomatis* should be done routinely; it requires techniques with a high sensitivity and specificity (see also chap. 20). The immunofluorescence test with monoclonal antibodies is easy to perform, and a high concordance between the direct specimen test and culture technique is reported by many investigators [26,27].

The test for *U. urealyticum* on culture media should be performed in all NGU patients.

In men with primary HSV infection, the virus can be demonstrated from urethral swab or from first-voided urine by direct immunofluorescence technique or by culture methods.

## Management

Studies during the last 20 years have recognized the tetracyclines and erythromycin as the most effective drugs for treatment of NGU and as particularly active against *C. trachomatis*, the most common agent in NGU.

Although untreated NGU has been shown to regress spontaneously within 1 to 3 months in 50 to 70% of cases [28], most untreated disease remits with mild symptoms [29]. Furthermore, even in patients without symptoms, the microorganisms remain infectious and may lead to complications as well as to transmission to sexual partners. NGU therefore should be treated as early as possible.

### Tetracyclines

The standard antibiotic employed in NGU treatment is tetracycline hydrochloride or oxytetracycline, given as 500 mg every 6 hours for at least 7 days. The "second generation" tetracyclines (minocyline and doxycycline) are equally effective with only twice-daily administration of 200 mg for at least 7 days [30,31]. Side effects such as vestibular irritation (minocycline) or gastrointestinal symptoms (doxycycline) may occur.

### Erythromycin

Erythromycin is effective in the treatment of NGU and is preferred for patients who cannot tolerate tetracyclines as well as for pregnant women and children. The recommended dosage is four times 500 mg per day for 1 week. Because of tetracycline-resistant ureaplasmal isolates, erythromycin in future may become more important in NGU therapy. However, eradication of *C. trachomatis* infection may not always occur; a failure rate of about 30% was observed within 5 weeks after treatment with 250 mg of erythromycin four times daily for 7 days [32]. Better results were obtained when the drug was administered in a dosage of 500 mg twice daily for 2 weeks [33].

### Other

Antimicrobials such as sulfonamides and trimethoprim-sulfamethoxazole, as well as rifampicin, are not as useful in the treatment of NGU because of their lower efficacy against *U. urealyticum*.

### Partner Treatment

Concomitant treatment of sexual partners is mandatory in cases of NGU because it is known that *C. trachomatis* can be isolated from 30 to 60% of female partners of men with NGU [34,35].

Furthermore, chlamydial infection of the male and female genital tract is often symptomless and may last for months or years. It thus represents a reservoir for further *C. trachomatis* transmission.

### Recurrent or Persistent NGU

The cure rate for firmly diagnosed NGU is about 80%. Treatment of relapsing NGU represents one of the most difficult problems in genitourinary medicine. The causes for NGU recurrences are not fully understood and may include:

An unusual cause of NGU, unaffected by the therapy employed.
A persistent infectious agent, resistant to therapy.
Poor compliance by the patient.
No concomitant or concordantly performed partner treatment.
Sexual intercourse during therapy.
Reinfection.
Urethral foreign body or periurethral fistula, abscess, or strictural urethral disease.

Patients with recurrent or persistent NGU are most often observed 2 weeks after completing the first therapy schedule. Herpetic urethritis and infection with *T. vaginalis* should be considered.

## Prognosis

NGU is a self-limited disease and the clinical course usually is mild. However, 1 to 2% of patients develop epididymitis and conjunctivitis. Sexually acquired arthritis is described in 2% (see discussion of Reiter's disease following).

# Part 2. Reiter's Syndrome

In 1916, Hans Reiter described the clinical triad of purulent urethritis, conjunctivitis, and painful arthralgia that developed in a military officer, lasted for about 3 months, and was followed by a brief period of bloody diarrhea [36]. The clinical picture was referred to later as "conjunctivo-urethro-synovial syndrome," "arthritis urethritica," "non-gonococcal urethritis and conjunctivitis with arthritis," "post-dysenteric arthritis," "infectious uro-arthritis," and "venereal arthritis."

Reiter's syndrome (RS) is now characterized as a triad of arthritis, conjunctivitis, and urethritis, occurring together or sequentially with combinations of symptoms varying from case to case and from time to time [37]. The high frequency of RS and related conditions in certain families supports the hypothesis of hereditary predisposition. The frequency of rheumatic disorders is increased in family members of patients with RS, and most commonly acute polyarthritis following NGU, *Shigella*, and *Yersinia* infections is observed [38–40]. The family history therefore is a useful adjunct in the diagnosis of RS.

The pathogenesis of RS is poorly understood, and the etiologic role of a spirochete—as Reiter postulated—has not been confirmed. RS has been reported in two forms, postenteritic [39] and posturethritic [40] following genitourinary and gastrointestinal tract infections. In some patients with clinical features of RS there is no evidence of an infectious agent.

The incidence of RS in nontraumatic arthritis varies geographically and seems to be about 10%. Blacks are less susceptible than whites, possibly because of the lower prevalence of the HLA-B27 antigen in blacks.

## Trigger Mechanisms

RS seems to be of multifactorial origin and may represent the host response to different genital and intestinal infectious agents such as *C. trachomatis*, *N. gonorrhoeae*, *Shigella flexneri*, and *dysenteriae*, *Salmonella* species, *Y. enterocolitica*, and *Campylobacter* species.

One to three percent of patients with gut infections caused by *S. dysenteriae*, *Sh. flexneri*, and other intestinal pathogens develop reactive arthritis. Epidemiologic studies of dysentery epidemics during the World Wars, of seasonal nonspecific diarrhea, and of genital infections have shown that these conditions lead to a high incidence of RS.

Typical RS may also follow gonococcal urethritis. Even after successful treatment of gonorrhea, the so-called "postgonococcal arthritis" or typical RS may occur.

Among patients with NGU, arthritis develops in 1 to 2% and has been termed sexually acquired reactive arthritis (SARA) [41]. In 35% of cases of SARA (which may be understood as a monosymptomatic form of RS) the full clinical picture of RS can be observed.

Siboulet and Galistin [42] were the first to describe RS after chlamydial infection. Further investigations during the last 25 years have presented evidence that chlamydiae may play an etiologic role in the development of SARA and RS despite the fact that the isolation rate of chlamydiae from the urethra of men does not differ between those with SARA (35%) and those with uncomplicated NGU (40%) [43,44]. Some studies are the following:

1. Isolation of *C. trachomatis* from Synovial Tissue. Recently, Keat et al [45] were able to recover chlamydial elementary bodies in synovial membrane preparations or synovial fluid by the use of monoclonal antibodies. The microorganism could not be detected in any of the control specimens. These findings support those of other investigators, who reported electron microscopic evidence of chlamydia-like particles in the synovial membrane [46]. Though these observations provide evidence of an important role of *C. trachomatis* in arthritis, it is yet unclear if the presence of the microorganism within the joints may be interpreted as a widespread dissemination of genital infection or as a more specific intraarticular presence of chlamydial elementary bodies.
2. Immunologic Studies. In contrast to the titer in men with uncomplicated NGU (33%), high antichlamydial antibody titers have been found in a majority of male patients with SARA (87%), indicating dissemination of chlamydial antigen from the urethra to other organs [44,47,48]. In addition, an increase in lymphocyte transformation rate, with *C. trachomatis* used as antigen, was demonstrated in patients with RS.
3. Lymphogranuloma Venereum. Five percent of patients with chronic lymphogranuloma venereum develop aseptic polyarticular or oligoarticular arthritis.
4. Psittacosis. Polyarthralgia may occur during an infection with *C. psittaci*; the relationship between psittacosis and arthritis is, however, unclear. *C. psittaci* causes polyarthritis in cattle and sheep as one manifestation of severe systemic disease after oral infection, indicating that polyarthritis in animals may be the veterinary counterpart of RS in humans [49].
5. Animal Studies. After direct inoculation of *C. trachomatis* into joint spaces of macaque monkeys and rabbits, reinoculation of the recovered microorganisms induces arthritis [50]. In other experiments, arthritis developed in all mice inoculated with a human NGU strain into the knee joint [51]. These data indicate that chlamydial strains inducing NGU in humans lead to arthritis in certain animals (baboons, rhesus and macaque monkeys, chimpanzees).

Despite this evidence that *C. trachomatis* represents an important trigger factor for RS, many questions are still unanswered, for example, why not all of the genital chlamydial infections lead to arthritis. Possibly only particular serotypes of the organism cause SARA, or primary sensitization with the infectious agent and production of immune complexes are required to induce arthritis.

## Histocompatibility (HLA-) Antigen Association

There is a strong association between the HLA-B27 antigen located on the shorter arm of chromosome 6 and certain rheumatic diseases. HLA-B27 antigen is expressed in 70 to 80% of RS patients but in less than 10% of healthy controls [43,52,53]. For HLA-B27-positive persons, the risk for developing RS is approximately 100 times higher than for negative persons [54]. Among HLA-B27-negative but HLA-B7-, Bw22-, and Bw42-positive RS patients, about 70% show cross-reaction, indicating that these antigens may be present in linked genes, causing an abnormal immune response to certain infectious agents [55]. It may also be possible, however, that the HLA-B27 gene is not identical with but closely localized to a genome determining disease susceptibility.

The occurrence of RS in a given population depends on the incidence of HLA-B27 carriers. In the Finnish population, for example, 14% of the people are HLA-B27 positive. Two percent of the men develop SARA after NGU, compared with 0.8% in the British population, which exhibits a definitely lower percentage of HLA-B27 carriers [43].

Carriage of HLA-B27 antigen predisposes not only to RS but also to spondylitis, acute uveitis, and to a more severe development of other diseases, and therefore may be used as a prognostic parameter [56,57].

## Clinical Manifestations

RS is defined as a combination of articular, mucocutaneous, and ocular symptoms and often occurs after urethritis or enteritis. Not all of the clinical symptoms (acute arthritis, lower urogenital tract inflammation, conjunctivitis, and cutaneous lesions) may be observed at the same time. Some may be silent or can easily be overlooked by patient and/or physician (Table 9.3). The mean incubation period is about 4 weeks. RS occurs predominantly in young men, the mean age of onset being between 25 and 30 years. In women, RS exhibits the same clinical features and HLA haplotypes but may sometimes remain undiagnosed.

### Urogenital Inflammation

Urethritis is indistinguishable from uncomplicated NGU and occurs in up to 90% of male patients with RS. In sexually inactive children with postdysenteric RS, urethral inflammation may be interpreted as an immunologic reaction.

TABLE 9.3. Clinical manifestations of Reiter's syndrome.

| Manifestation | Form |
|---|---|
| Cutaneous lesions (12% of patients) | Pustular and hyperkeratotic lesions on skin of trunk, palms, soles, extremities |
| Oral lesions (10–15% of patients) | Ulcers or plaques on lips, cheeks, tongue, palate, tonsillar pillars |
| Ocular lesions (10–50% of patients) | Mild and transient conjunctivitis, acute anterior uveitis |
| Genital lesions (85–90% of patients) | Urethritis, circinate balanitis |
| Arthritis (86% of patients) | Polyarticular synovitis, polyarthritis (distal joints), fusiform dactylitis, sacroileitis |
| Rare systemic manifestations | Neurologic lesions, carditis (peri-, myo-, endo-), aortitis, amyloidosis, lymphadenopathy, pneumonitis, pleuritis, meningoencephalitis |

In women, the incidence of urogenital inflammation in RS is not exactly defined but is reported to occur in about 30% of cases.

## Arthritis

Articular symptoms show a wide range of asymmetric polyarthritis with involvement of four or more joints and fusiform dactylitis ("sausage digits"). In most cases arthritis starts in the distal weight-bearing joints, leading to knee effusions. Sacroileitis is most common in the posturethritis variant of RS and is also reported in association with other urogenital disorders such as prostatitis and salpingitis. Other spinal involvement is rare.

## Mucocutaneous Manifestations

Circinate balanitis represents a very frequent symptom of RS and appears as a painless serpiginous erosive dermatitis. In women, similar lesions in the vulvar region have been documented [58]. Skin lesions resemble those of psoriasis and are characterized by hyperkeratotic papules and plaques frequently involving the soles. Less commonly skin lesions appear as painless oral erosions and ulcers on the palate, tongue, lips, or pharynx. Nails are sometimes thickened and discolored (Fig. 9.2,9.3).

## Ocular Manifestations

In over half of RS patients, chronic ocular lesions (conjunctivitis, iritis, or rarely uveitis) can be observed.

## Other Manifestations

Transient cardiovascular involvement with benign electrocardiographic abnormalities, myocarditis, and pericarditis have rarely been observed. Neurologic complica-

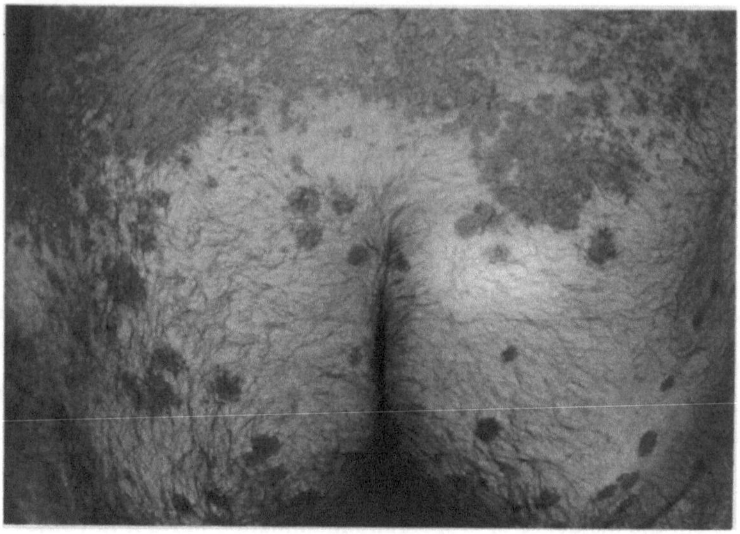

FIGURE 9.2. Reiter's syndrome: Papular and pustular lesions with psoriasiform scales.

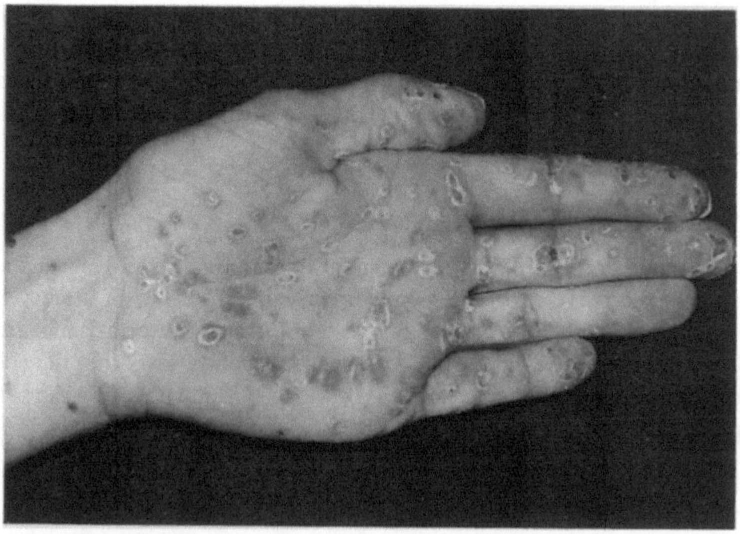

FIGURE 9.3. Psoriasiform lesions of Reiter's syndrome.

TABLE 9.4. Laboratory findings in Reiter's syndrome.

| |
|---|
| Erythrocyte sedimentation rate ↑ or normal |
| Normochromic or hypochromic anemia |
| Leukocytosis |
| Antinuclear antibodies positive |
| Rheumatoid factor positive |
| C-reactive protein ↑ |
| Circulating immune complexes positive |
| Serum α2 ↑ |
| Gammaglobulins ↑ |
| Complement factors C3, C4 ↑ or normal |
| HLA-B27 antigen 70–80% positive |
| Synovial fluid: |
| leukocyte count 500 to >50,000 mm³ |
| ≥90% neutrophils |
| Viscosity ↓ |
| Complement ↑ or normal |
| Proteins ↑ |
| Glucose normal |
| "Reiter cells" positive (nonspecific) |
| Evidence of nongonococcal urethritis 1–3% of patients |

tions (polyradiculitis, neuritis, and meningoencephalitis), generalized lymphadenopathy, thrombophlebitis, and amyloidosis have been reported (Table 9.3).

The acute stage of RS usually is self-limited. In about 18% of patients the condition becomes chronic with multiple recurrences [59]. At least two thirds of patients show disease activity even after 6 years. The clinical features of recurrences may be monosymptomatic or may present the full clinical picture of RS with different degrees of functional impairment. Death resulting from RS is very rare; it is due to aortitis, amyloidosis, or complications of treatment.

## Laboratory Findings

Specific laboratory features do not exist in RS (Table 9.4). The erythrocyte sedimentation rate usually is elevated, but there is no correlation with disease activity. Occasionally, leukocytosis, antinuclear antibodies, C-reactive protein, and circulating immune complexes are present. Macrophages containing leukocytes (so-called Reiter cells) are often observed in different kinds of arthritis, but are not diagnostic for RS.

A specific synovial mononuclear cell response to different microbiologic antigens has been described by Ford et al [60], demonstrating a distinct pattern in sexually transmitted and in enteric cases. Immunoproteins frequently are found in the synovium, indicating that immunologic mechanisms may play a role in the etiology of RS.

## Management

Specific antimicrobial treatment should be administered to patients with nongonococcal urogenital inflammation or infectious enteritis-associated RS; however, there is no evidence that antibiotic treatment has any effect on the course of arthritis or other symptoms of RS. Otherwise, early antibiotic therapy might influence the duration and extensity of the disease [61].

Most commonly, nonsteroidal antiinflammatory drugs are used for symptomatic treatment. Corticosteroids show little effect. In severe cases, methotrexate or immunosuppressive drugs such as azathioprine are used with good clinical response. Retinoids and photochemotherapy have been tried with excellent response for the treatment of mucocutaneous symptoms.

### References

1. Oriel JD, Reeve P, Powis P, et al: Isolation of chlamydia from patients with non-specific genital infection. *Br J Vener Dis* **48**:429–436, 1972.
2. Oriel JD, Reeve P, Wright JT, et al: Chlamydial infection of the male urethra. *Br J Vener Dis* **52**:46–51, 1976.
3. Richmond SJ, Hilton AL, Clarke SKR: Chlamydial infection. Role of Chlamydia Subgroup A in nongonococcal and postgonococcal urethritis. *Br J Vener Dis* **48**:437–444, 1972.
4. Holmes KK Handsfield HH, Wang SP, et al: Etiology of non-gonococcal urethritis. *N Engl J Med* **292**:1199–1206, 1975.
5. Dunlop EMC, Al Hussian MK, Garland JA, et al: Infection of the urethra by TRIC agent in men presenting because of non-specific urethritis. *Lancet* **1**:1125–1128, 1965.
6. Bowie WR, Wang S-P, Alexander ER, et al: Etiology of nongonococcal urethritis. Evidence for *Chlamydia trachomatis* and *Ureaplasma urealyticum*. *J Clin Invest* **59**:735–742, 1977.
7. Brown MB, Cassell GH, Taylor-Robinson D, et al: Measurement of antibody of *Ureaplasma urealyticum* by an enzyme-linked immunoassay and detection of antibody responses in patients with nongonococcal urethritis. *J Clin Microbiol* **17**:288–295, 1983.
8. Taylor-Robinson D, Evans RT, Coufalik ED, et al: *Ureaplasma urealyticum* and *Mykoplasma hominis* in chlamydial and non-chlamydial non-gonococcal urethritis. *Br J Vener Dis* **55**:30–35, 1979.
9. McCormack WM, Almeida PC, Bailey PE, et al: Sexual activity and vaginal colonization with genital mycoplasmas. *JAMA* **221**:1375–1377, 1972.
10. McCormack WM, Lee Y-H, Zinner SH: Sexual experience and urethral colonization with genital mycoplasmas: A study in normal men. *Ann Intern Med* **78**:696–698, 1973.
11. Lee Y-H, Tarr PI, Schumacher JR, et al: Reevaluation of the role of T-mycoplasmas in nongonococcal urethritis. *Sex Trans Dis* **3**:25–28, 1976.
12. Prentice MJ, Taylor-Robinson D, Csonka GW: Non-specific urethritis: A placebo-controlled trial of minocycline in conjunction with laboratory investigation. *Br J Vener Dis* **52**:269–275, 1976.
13. Coufalik ED, Taylor-Robinson D, Csonka GW: Treatment of nongonococcal urethritis with rifampicin as a means of defining the role of *Ureaplasma urealyticum*. *Br J Vener Dis* **55**:36–43, 1979.

14. Ford DK, Smith JR: Non-specific urethritis associated with a tetracycline-resistant T-mycoplasma. *Br J Vener Dis* **50**:373–374, 1974.
15. Taylor-Robinson D, Csonka GW, Prentice MJ, et al: Human intraurethral inoculation of ureaplasmas. *Quart J Med* **46**:309–326, 1977.
16. McCormack WM, Braun P, Lee Y-H, et al: The genital mycoplasmas. *N Engl J Med* **288**:78–79, 1973.
17. Bowie WR, Wang S-P, Alexander ER, et al: Etiology of non-gonococcal urethritis. In Hobson D, Holmes KK (Eds.): *Non-gonococcal urethritis and related infections*. Washington D.C.: American Society for Microbiology, 1977, pp. 19–29.
18. Braun P, Klein JO, Lee Y-H, et al: Methodologic investigations and prevalence of genital mycoplasmas in pregnancy. *J Infect Dis* **121**:391–400, 1970.
19. Swartz SL, Kraus SJ, Herrmann KL, et al: Diagnosis and etiology of nongonococcal urethritis. *J Infect Dis* **138**:445–454, 1978.
20. Hovelius B, Thelin I, Mardh P-A: *Staphylococcus saprophyticus* in the etiology of nongonococcal urethritis. *Br J Vener Dis* **55**:369–374, 1979.
21. Furness G, Evangelista AT, Kaminski Z: *Corynebacterium genitalium* (nonspecific urethritis *Corynebacterium*): Biologic reactions differentiating commensals of the urogenital tract from the pathogens responsible for urethritis. *Invest Urol* **15**:23–27, 1977.
22. Kuberski T: *Trichomonas vaginalis* associated with nongonococcal urethritis and prostatitis. *Sex Trans Dis* **7**:135–136, 1980.
23. Academic Department of Genitourinary Medicine of the Middlesex Hospital Medical School, the Communicable Surveillance Centre, and the Communicable Disease Unit: Sexually transmitted disease surveillance. *Br Med J* **2**:1375–1376, 1979.
24. Wiesner PJ: Selected aspects of the epidemiology of nongonococcal urethritis. In Hobson D, Holmes KK (Eds.): *Nongonococcal urethritis and related infections*. Washington, D.C.: American Society for Microbiology, 1977, pp. 9–14.
25. Oriel JD: Management of nongonococcal urethritis. *Drugs* **18**:398–402, 1979.
26. Stary A, Kopp W, Gebhart W, Söltz-Szöts J: Culture versus direct specimen test: A comparative study of *Chlamydia trachomatis* infections in Viennese prostitutes. *Genitourin Med* **61**:258–260, 1985.
27. Stamm WE, Harrison HR, Alexander ER, et al: Diagnosis of *C. trachomatis* infections by direct immunofluorescence staining of genital secretions: A multicenter trial. *Ann Intern Med* **101**:638–641, 1984.
28. Oriel JD: Treatment of nongonococcal urethritis. In Hobson D, Holmes KK (Eds.): *Nongonococcal urethritis and related infections*. Washington, D.C.: American Society for Microbiology, 1977, pp. 38–42.
29. Schachter J: Chlamydial infections. *N Engl J Med* **298**:428–435, 1978.
30. Jaffe HW: Nongonococcal urethritis: Treatment of men and their sexual partners. *Rev Infect Dis* **4**:772–777, 1982.
31. Bowie WR, Alexander ER, Stimson JB, et al: Therapy of nongonococcal urethritis. *Ann Intern Med* **95**:306–311, 1981.
32. Bowie WR: Treatment of chlamydial infections. In Mardh P-A, Holmes KK, Oriel JD, et al (Eds.): *Chlamydial infections*. New York: Elsevier Biomedical Press, 1982, pp. 231–244.
33. Oriel JD, Ridgway GL, Tchamouroff S: Comparison of erythromycin stearate and oxytetracycline in the treatment of nongonococcal urethritis: Their efficacy against *C. trachomatis*. *Scot Med J* **22**:375–379, 1977.
34. Arya OP, Alergant CD, Annels EH, et al: Management of nonspecific urethritis in men. *Br J Vener Dis* **54**:414–421, 1978.

35. Tait IA, Rees E, Hobson D, et al: Chlamydial infection of the cervix in contacts of men with nongonococcal urethritis. *Br J Vener Dis* **56**:37–45, 1980.
36. Reiter H: Ueber eine bisher unerkannte Spirochaeteninfektion (Spirochaetosis Arthritica). *Dtsch Med Wochenschr* **42**:1535–1536, 1916.
37. Lassus A, Lousa M: Reiter's disease. In Harris JRW (Ed): *Recent advances in sexually transmitted diseases*. Vol A. London: Churchill Livingstone, 1981, pp. 187–199.
38. Kousa M: Clinical observations on Reiter's disease with special reference to the venereal and nonvenereal etiology: A follow-up study. *Acta Derm Venereol* (Stockh) (Suppl 81), 58:1, 1978.
39. Paronen I: Reiter's disease: A study of 344 cases observed in Finland. *Acta Med Scand* Suppl 130, 1948.
40. Csonka GW: The cause of Reiter's syndrome. *Br Med J* **1**:1088–1090, 1958.
41. Keat AC, Maini RN, Nkwazi GC, et al: Role of *Chlamydia trachomatis* and HLA-B27 in sexually acquired reactive arthritis. *Br Med J* **1**:605–607, 1978.
42. Siboulet A, Galistin P: Arguments in favour of a virus aetiology of non-gonococcal urethritis illustrated by three cases of Reiter's disease. *Br J Vener Dis* **38**:209–211, 1962.
43. Kousa M, Saikku P, Richmond S, et al: Frequent association of chlamydial infection with Reiter's syndrome. *Sex Trans Dis* **5**:57–61, 1978.
44. Martin DH, Pollock A, Kou C-C, et al: *Chlamydia trachomatis* infections in men with Reiter's syndrome. *Ann Intern Med* **100**:207–213, 1984.
45. Keat A, Dixey J, Sonnex C, et al: *Chlamydia trachomatis* and reactive arthritis: The missing link. Lancet **1**:72–74, 1987.
46. Schumacher HR, Cherian PU, Sieck M, et al: Ultrastructural identification of chlamydial antigens in synovial membrane in acute Reiter's syndrome. *Arth Rheum* 29 suppl, abstr 115, 1986.
47. Vilppula AH, Yli-Kerttula VL, Ahlroos AK, et al: Chlamydial isolations and serology in Reiter's syndrome. *Scand J Rheum* **10**:181–185, 1981.
48. Thomas BJ, Reeve P, Oriel JD, et al: Simplified serologic test for antibodies to *Chlamydia trachomatis*. *J Clin Microbiol* **4**:6–10, 1976.
49. Storz J: Psittacosis agents as a cause of polyarthritis in cattle and sheep. *Vet Med Rev* **2/3**:125–139, 1967.
50. Smith DE, James PG, Schachter J, et al: Experimental bedsonial arthritis. *Arth Rheum* **16**:21–29, 1973.
51. Keat A, Thomas BJ, Taylor-Robinson, D: Chlamydial infection in the etiology of arthritis. *Br Med Bull* **39**:168–174, 1983.
52. Brewerton DA, Caffrey M, Nicholls A, et al: Reiter's disease and HLA-B27. *Lancet* **2**:996–998, 1973.
53. Friis J, Svejgaard A: Salmonella arthritis and HL-A27. *Lancet* **1**:1350, 1974.
54. Keat AC: HLA-linked disease susceptibility and reactive arthritis. *J Infect* **5**:227–239, 1982.
55. Arnett FC, McClusky OE, Schachter BZ, et al: Incomplete Reiter's syndrome: Discriminating features and HL-AW27 in diagnosis. *Ann Intern Med* **84**:8–12, 1976.
56. McCluskey OE, Lordon RE, Arnett FP: HL-A27 in Reiter's syndrome and psoriatic arthritis: A genetic factor in disease susceptibility and expression. *J Rheumatol* **1**:263–268, 1974.
57. Harris JR, Gelsthorpe K, Doughty RW, et al: HLA-27 and W10 in Reiter's syndrome and non-specific urethritis. *Acta Derm Venereol* (Stockh) **55**:127–130, 1975.

58. Thambar IV, Dunlop R, Thin RN, et al: Circinate vulvitis in Reiter's syndrome. *Br J Vener Dis* **53**:260–262, 1977.
59. Calin A: Reiter's syndrome. In: Kelly WN, et al (Eds.): *Textbook of Rheumatology.* Philadelphia: WB Saunders, 1981, p. 1033.
60. Ford DK, da Roza DM, Schulzer M: The specificity of synovial mononuclear cell responses to microbiological antigens in Reiter's syndrome. *J Rheumatol* **9**:561–567, 1982.
61. Keat AC, Maini PN, Pegrum GD, et al: The clinical features and HLA-associations of reactive arthritis associated with non-gonococcal urethritis. *Quart J Med* **48**:323–324, 1979.

CHAPTER 10

# Trichomoniasis

Larry E. Millikan

## Overview

A fairly frequent problem is infection by the urogenital protozoan *Trichomonas vaginalis*. It is perhaps the most common clinically recognized sexually transmitted disease in the United States, with about 2.5 million new cases occurring annually. Approximately 180 million new cases occur each year worldwide [1]. The infection has a continuous endemic source, for as many as half of the female carriers are totally asymptomatic. Newer treatments have greatly improved therapy for this disease, but diagnosis and the detection of carriers remain significant challenges. Symptomatic or asymptomatic urethritis or vaginitis due to *T. vaginalis* is the usual scenario. The spectrum of symptoms associated with this disease is wide. Ultimately, the diagnosis is established by identifying the causative organisms.

## Definition

Urethritis or vaginitis, with or without symptoms, and the finding of the protozoan *T. vaginalis* fulfill the criteria for diagnosis and definition.

## Clinical Findings

In women acute vaginitis is the most common syndrome in which the diagnosis of trichomoniasis is made. The infectious agent primarily involves the stratified squamous epithelium of the lower urogenital tract; it spares the columnar cells. Involvement of the endocervix is quite rare, so that specimens for diagnosis should be taken from the exterior cervix or vaginal area. The urethra and Skene's glands are involved much of the time [2].

In reviewing the history, the focus should be on symptoms of pruritus, discharge, odor, and any urinary tract symptoms. Involvement of the vulva is very important. In the differential consideration of acute vaginitis or lower genital symptoms (discharge, urinary frequency or dysuria, abnormal bleeding, itching, and/or foul odor),

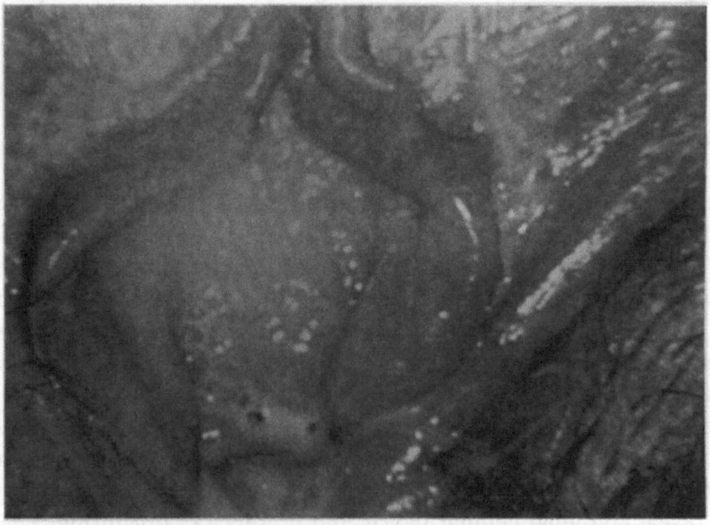

FIGURE 10.1. *Trichomonas* infection. Note the copious, frothy, yellow-white discharge. (Courtesy of Burroughs Wellcome Co., Research Triangle Park, NC)

one can often separate out the various etiologies by compartmentalization of symptoms: (a) primarily urethritis, (b) primarily cystitis, (c) primarily vaginitis, or lastly (d) vulvitis [3] (see Differential Diagnosis below). However, a significant percentage of women are asymptomatic. (While we generally do not consider trichomoniasis a problem in premenarchal women, the infection has been described as an initial sign of sexual abuse [4].)

The primary symptom causing the patient to seek medical attention is usually vaginal discharge (Fig. 10.1), (present in half to three quarters of patients) [5]. It is malodorous in a small number of patients. Pruritus, dyspareunia, and dysuria are equally infrequently reported. In a few patients there may be lower abdominal pains and tender inguinal adenopathy. Urinary frequency can be noted. In acute infection, signs and symptoms range from nil to extensive. At the latter extreme there may be marked erythema and edema of the labia and a profuse vaginal discharge. The typical or classic discharge is frothy, bubbly, and sometimes described as yellow-green. This, however, is also seen in nonspecific forms of vaginitis. Punctate hemorrhages of the cervix have also been described; they result in a strawberry appearance [3]. It is obvious from the broad range of signs and symptoms and a significant asymptomatic carrier group that diagnosis often rests on a very high index of suspicion in the female patient.

The diagnosis of trichomoniasis in men is, on the basis of clinical symptoms, often very difficult. Indeed, the diagnosis is established by association with an infected female sexual partner. In florid cases, differentiation from nonspecific urethritis often is accomplished by therapeutic trials. Exact clinical differentiation is often not possible. Therefore, careful history, especially of sexual contacts, and subsequent tests (see below) are appropriate.

## Histopathology

The traditional literature emphasizes the specificity of parasitization of the *Trichomonas*. This theory has also been used to explain the older range of infection (with the exception of the previously mentioned infection in the child after sexual abuse). Estrogen use seems to affect susceptibility by altering the vaginal environment, encouraging the growth and parasitism of *Trichomonas*. It has always been assumed that the primary site or residence of the organism is on stratified squamous epithelium.

Because of the superficial and often transient and mild nature of infections, biopsy for diagnosis is not a standard technique. Hence there is limited information on the histopathology of the pathologic process in the urethra and vagina. Scrapings for diagnosis reveal epithelial cellular debris and presence of organisms. The binding characteristics that limit the organism's association to the squamous epithelium have been studied [6].

Alderete and Guillermo looked at *T. vaginalis* and its attachment in cell culture. Interestingly, the pathogen was found to adhere more strongly to epithelial lines than to human fibroblast cell lines. This supports the previous concept of preferential parasitism to the epithelium. Of equal interest is the fact that the avirulent trichomonad *T. tenax* was not found to adhere to the cell monolayers. *T. tenax* is a common trichomonad in other parts of the body. Also these investigators noted cell damage when *T. vaginalis* attached to the cells, while *T. tenax* did not cause the same degree of cell destruction or inflammation. They concluded that the pathogen adheres to the host cells through surface proteins in a specific receptor-ligand fashion. Additionally, their studies give some insight into the mechanism of actions of some of the therapeutic agents [6].

Histopathologic studies of other parts of the urogenital tract are lacking; however, a recent report by Gardner and fellow investigators have demonstrated *T. vaginalis* in the prostate gland [7]. Previously, solid evidence for this had been lacking. Gardner et al provided convincing evidence of *T. vaginalis*-like organisms in lumina, intraepithelial vacuoles, and subepithelial stroma. They confirmed these findings with specific immunostaining for the organism. The immunostaining was necessary because in many of these cases the specimen was poorly preserved because it was obtained up to 24 hours postmortem. Reasonable confirmation through special immunoperoxidase stains for specific organelles was thus necessary. These findings strongly suggest widespread involvement in the prostate gland by *T. vaginalis* and question the previous dogma about specificity for epithelial structures.

In contrast to tissue histopathology, cytology of *T. vaginalis* is fairly well developed. The organism is ovoid, 10 to 20 μ wide, and characteristically very motile [8]. Ultrastructural studies have shown four free anterior flagella and a recurrent flagellum in the membrane, which extends for about two thirds the length of the cell. These four or five flagella are the primary means of locomotion. Ultrastructurally these organisms contain a large nucleus with scattered chromatin typical of eucaryotic cells and a Golgi apparatus–skeletal organelles centered around a microtubular, oriented axostyle. The axostyle projects from the posterior end as a slender spike. The organism absorbs soluble nutrients through the cell membrane and particulate material by endocytosis. This process involves the standard steps–lysosomal fusion, digestion, and ulturate end vacuole formation.

It is presumed that *T. vaginalis* exists only in this squamous form, for attempts to identify cyst or vegetative forms or other unusual long-lasting states of the parasite have not been successful. Special stains have been very useful in the identification of the organism. Traditionally histochemistry has been used, including periodic acid Schiff reaction and methenamine silver stain. The use of Giemsa's and acridine orange stains has also been proposed, but apparently none of these on fresh tissue have an advantage over wet mounts.

Because use of wet mounts and special stains of a more traditional nature seems to miss the diagnosis in one quarter to one third of patients, monoclonal technology has now been focused on this infection [9,10]. The result is a direct specimen test (Trichomonas Direct Specimen Test, Integrated Diagnostics, Inc., 1440 4th St., Berkeley, CA 94710). This test involves the mixture of three monoclonal antibodies that provide immunofluorescence staining of the membrane, cytoplasm, flagella, and nuclei of *T. vaginalis* and *Tritrichomonas foetus*. This test seems very promising. The test kit involves a positive control slide, a negative control slide, and the test material. Positive diagnosis is made when three or more organisms are identified within a 10-mm scan area. The limitations are the usual ones, importantly a concentration of organisms below 300/ml in the vaginal urethral discharge. This seems to be the cutoff in sensitivity. There is cross-reaction with *T. hominis* and *T. foetus*, but these are not usual inhabitants of the human urogenital tract. This may be a very important diagnostic tool in the future for confirmation of diagnosis.

## Natural History

The exact natural history of trichomoniasis is not entirely clear, for in most countries it is not a reportable disease. Presumably there are a large number of asymptomatic cases in both sexes. The infection has been diagnosed in up to 4% of men attending sexually transmitted disease clinics for other complaints [11]. The previously mentioned changes in the vaginal epithelium largely preclude infection in premenarchal patients. As previously mentioned, it seems that the peak incidence of the infection is usually in middle-aged men and women. Studies have suggested that in symptomatic men with nongonococcal or nonspecific urethritis, 5 to 15% have trichomoniasis [12]. From these data, one can synthesize some aspects of the natural history of the infection. Women who have never had intercourse are never affected [13]. With sexual development in the male and female, the environment becomes appropriate for parasitization by the protozoan on the epithelium of the lower urogenital tract. Sexual activity with an asymptomatic carrier allows maintenance of the infection and ease of spread. The correlation of the infection with the level of sexual activity is rather direct, as might be expected. The rate of infectivity also seems very high, with 70 to 80% of persons acquiring the infection after intercourse with an infected partner. It would seem that the main reservoir is the asymptomatic individual; the large number of them assures prolonged persistence of this infection, in spite of advances in therapy.

## Complications

As mentioned, a significant percentage of the population is asymptomatic. This would suggest that severe infections and complications are quite rare. There is very little evidence to suggest that *Trichomonas* infection leads to complications of an early or a late nature.

## Differential Diagnosis

The primary presenting symptoms in men are those of urethritis and in women those of inflammation of the lower urogenital tract.

In women, symptoms suggesting cystitis, urethritis, and vulvovaginitis all remotely may be related to trichomoniasis. Cystitis and urethritis, however, are more likely to be caused by *Chlamydia*, *Neisseria*, or herpes simplex virus. The differential diagnosis for these three infections is usually straightforward, and appropriate confirmatory tests are now routinely available. Ancillary tests including examination, Tzanck smear of the vesicles in herpes simplex, and specific stains of urethral discharge also are important in establishing the diagnosis. Appropriate tests for trichomoniasis, already mentioned, are also part of this evaluation.

Vulvovaginitis is generally secondary to *Trichomonas*, *Candida*, or *Gardnerella* infection. A few discriminating findings allow differentiation. It has been claimed [3] that a major sign of trichomoniasis is the "strawberry cervix": a cervix covered with petechial lesions. This sign is seen in 25 to 30% of patients.[3] Motile trichomonads in a saline suspension of discharge is usually helpful. With candidosis, the usual clumpy discharge, which can be strongly positive on KOH exam, is usually quite straightforward. Culture can be used to confirm the diagnosis. The use of oral contraceptives or the presence of diabetes mellitus is often an important predisposing factor and a clue to the diagnosis. Nonspecific vaginosis can be caused by several organisms.

*Gardnerella vaginalis* (previously *Haemophilus vaginalis*) is a third cause of acute vaginitis. It presents with an extensive foul-smelling discharge that has very few white cells and a higher than usual pH (above 4.5). Sweet [3] claimed that the clue cell is an important finding for establishing the diagnosis. In some instances, a heavy malodorous discharge that appears to be acute vaginitis can be associated with a fulminant *Neisseria* infection.

## Therapy

At present there remains one therapeutic agent of choice for *Trichomonas* infections. Metronidazole was introduced in 1960. It is one of a number of imidazoles that have a fairly broad spectrum of activity against mycoses, parasites, protozoans, and gram-positive bacteria. It is currently available in the United States as a liquid, as 250-mg tablets, and as 500-mg tablets. The drug should be taken orally on an empty stomach. Administration with or after meals results in delayed absorption and lower blood levels. Lossick [14] has summarized most of the studies done since 1962. They show remarkable cure rates, generally between 98 and 100%. Only a few studies had a cure rate below 85%; the lowest in Lossick's tabulation was the 1-g single-dose treatment, which in one study had a 100% cure rate and in another a 55% cure rate.

Several principles of therapy seem appropriate: Treatment of asymptomatic patients would be desirable and is increasingly recommended. The most common treatment regimens for all patients are the 2-g single dose and the 250-mg three times per day for 7 days dosage. Treatment of the regular sexual partner of the infected patient seems appropriate. The high rate of infection is reason enough for prophylactic treatment.

The recurring question in the treatment of trichomoniasis with metronidazole is that of long-term carcinogensis. Lossick [14] concluded that by current standards metronidazole seems to be a potential weak human carcinogen and probably not of clinical concern. In more than two decades, studies to adequately evaluate this issue have yet to be done. Some studies suggest an increased incidence of carcinoma of the cervix in patients with *Trichomonas* infection, but before the use of metronidazole, these patients were also at increased risk. Whether this relates to infection, promiscuity, or infection with other agents such as herpes still has not been clarified. It would seem judicious to treat with the lowest possible dose that achieves a cure, to minimize unnecessary exposure to the drug. In 1985 treatment guidelines from the U.S. Department of Health and Human Services [15] recommended the 2-g single dose with the 250-mg tid for 7 days dosage an alternative. Because of the questions of carcinogenicity, metronidazole is contraindicated early in pregnancy and alternative therapy (see below) should be used. Neonatal infections should be treated with 10 to 30 mg/kg of body weight daily for 5 to 8 days [15].

## Alternative Therapy

In the United States, clotrimazole is the recommended treatment modality for trichomoniasis in pregnancy. The intravaginal preparation has shown reasonable success.

Other agents have been used outside the United States. Many of these are related to metronidazole; they include tinidazole and nimorazole. Because this is an area of active pharmacologic research, other drugs undoubtedly will be found to be effective therapy. Alderete and Guillermo's study [6] of the parasitism of *Trichomonas* in tissue culture provides an intriguing potential for the screening of new drugs. Iodoacetate and metronidazole both interfered with parasite attachment. Similarly when this drug was added to tissue culture, the parasites were released from the cells. This may ultimately be an important way to determine new drugs.

## Prognosis

With newer forms of therapy, prognosis seems excellent. The only caveat might be the fact that there is an obvious large reservoir of asymptomatic carriers. Perhaps an aggressive public health stand in this area in the future may markedly decrease the incidence of disease.

### References

1. Krieger JN, Holmes KK, Spence MR, et al: Geographic variation among isolates of *Trichomonas vaginalis*: Demonstration of antigenic heterogenicity by using monoclonal antibodies and the indirect immunofluorescence technique. *J Infect Dis* **152**(5):979–984, 1985.
2. Wisdom R, Dunlop EMC: Trichomoniasis: Study of the disease and its treatment in women and men. *Br J Vener Dis* **41**:90–95, 1965.
3. Sweet RL: Importance of differential diagnosis in acute vaginitis. *Am J Obstet Gynecol* **152**:7:921–923; 1985.
4. Jones JG, Yamauchi T, Lambert B: *Trichomonas vaginalis* infestation in sexually abused girls. AJDC **139**:846–847, 1985.
5. Fouts AC, Kraus SJ: *Trichomonas vaginalis*: Reevaluation of its clinical presentation and laboratory diagnosis. *J Infect Dis* **141**:137–142, 1980.
6. Alderete JF, Guillermo EG: Specific nature of *Trichomonas vaginalis* parasitism of host cell surfaces. *Infect Immunol* **50**:701–703, 1985.
7. Gardner WA, Culberson DE, Bennett BD: *Trichomonas vaginalis* in the prostate gland. *Arch Pathol Lab Med* **110**:430–432, 1986.
8. Wherton A, Honigberg BM: Structure of trichomonads as revealed by scanning electron microscopy. *J Protozool* **26**:56–62, 1979.
9. Chang TH, Tsing SY, Tzeng S: Monoclonal antibodies against *Trichomonas vaginalis*. *Hybridoma* **5**:43–51, 1986.
10. Connelly RJ, Torian BE, Stibbs HH: Identification of a surface antigen of *Trichomonas vaginalis*. *Infect Immunol* **49**:270–274, 1985.
11. Wright RA, Judson FN: Relative and seasonal incidences of the sexually transmitted diseases: A two year statistical review. *Br J Vener Dis* **54**:433–439, 1978.
12. Krieger JN: Urologic aspects of trichomoniasis. *Invest Urol* **18**:411–418, 1981.
13. Dunlop EMC, Wisdom AR: Diagnosis and management of trichomoniasis in men and women. *Br J Vener Dis* **41**:85–90, 1965.
14. Lossick JG: Treatment of *Trichomonas vaginalis* infections. *Infect Dis* **4**(Suppl.):801–818, 1987.
15. U.S. Department of Health and Human Services: *STD Treatment Guidelines 1985*. Washington, D.C.: U.S. Government Printing Office, 1985.

CHAPTER 11

# Genital Candidosis

Tomasz F. Mroczkowski

## Overview

Genital candidosis results from infections by *Candida* species, yeastlike organisms that belong to the family Cryptococcaceae, Fungi Imperfecti. At least seven species of *Candida* and two of *Torulopsis* are of medical importance. Two of them are of significance as sexually transmitted agents – *C. albicans* and *T. glabrata* – of which *C. albicans* is overwhelmingly the most frequent genital yeast pathogen [1–3].

The yeasts have a predilection for mucous membranes and moist skin surfaces and have frequently been isolated from mouth, throat, large intestine, vagina, and skin in healthy individuals [1]. The question of whether *C. albicans* can be a genital commensal in some cases, that is, present without producing symptoms, or whether it should always be considered a pathogen still remains unanswered. More and more investigators agree that detection of *C. albicans* on the genitalia indicates a disease-like state that should be treated [4].

*C. albicans* has been identified as the cause of several diseases, of which candidal vaginitis and vulvovaginitis in women and balanitis or balanoposthitis in men may be considered in the category of sexually acquired infections.

Generally, a genital yeast infection is a minor condition in both sexes, but its high incidence and frequent recurrences, especially in women, along with the discomfort experienced by the infected patient make the disease of special concern.

## Synonyms

Synonyms for genital candidosis are genital candidiasis and moniliasis.

## Epidemiology

According to gynecologists, *C. albicans* is currently the most common actual or potential pathogen in the female genital tract [5]. Among women attending family planning clinics, the incidence of vaginal candidosis was 21% [6], as opposed to 37%

found at sexually transmitted disease clinics [3]. Other studies have reported similar isolation rates in STD and non-STD clinic populations [7,8].

It is estimated that about half a million women attending clinics for sexually transmitted disease in the United States have vaginal candidosis [9]. The peak incidence of genital candidosis in women occurs between ages 16 and 30, corresponding to the ages of high sexual activity [4]. Strictly speaking, genital candidosis is probably not a sexually transmitted disease. Sexual acquisition of candidosis by women is probably rare, whereas men commonly acquire it from a woman with vaginal candidosis [10,11]. Male contacts of infected women often have positive urine culture and/or urethritis, and about 10% may have symptoms of balanoposthitis [3,12]. Some authors have presented evidence that yeast infections are spread sexually in up to 40% of genital candidosis [13]. A relationship between oral sex and genital candidosis has also been reported [14–16]. The latter route of infection is supported by isolation of the same strain of *C. albicans* from the oral cavities of women and from the genitalia of their sexual partners [14]. Infants born to mothers with genital candidosis are at risk of acquiring oral thrush. The incidence of neonatal oral candidosis is several times higher among babies born to women with genital candidosis than among those born to uninfected mothers [17,18].

Vaginal candidosis has also been observed in sexually inactive women. The intestinal tract is a possible source of infection for these patients, as genital infection is often associated with the presence of the same strain of yeast in the digestive tract [14,19,20].

## Pathogenesis and Predisposing Factors

The mechanism by which *C. albicans* and other yeasts cause genital infection is rather poorly understood. There is little doubt that *Candida* may remain in some individuals without causing recognizable symptoms or signs. In others periods of asymptomatic colonization follow episodes of mild to acute exacerbations. In some patients candidosis is a chronic, unremitting disease. It seems that the basis for these differences is very complex, since a great number of factors may play a role. Among these are microbial virulence expressed both by the ability of the yeast to multiply and to produce toxic metabolites, hydrolytic enzymes, and so on, and by host resistance, which can be reduced by the so-called predisposing factors commonly observed among patients with genital candidosis (Table 11.1).

Predisposing host factors that count in genital (and other) candidosis include endocrine disorders (of which diabetes mellitus seems to be the most important), certain malignancies, AIDS, and other diseases. Pregnancy and menstruation seem to aggravate candidosis, as does prolonged use of antibiotics, steroids, or immunosuppressive drugs. The role of oral contraceptives is not entirely clear, although the overwhelming majority of studies point out an increased risk of genital candidosis in women using them. Among environmental factors, increased warmth and moisture attributed to the wearing of synthetic fiber undergarments have been implicated [21]. Moreover, any trauma, skin breaks, or mucous membrane abra-

TABLE 11.1. Factors predisposing to genital candidosis.

| | |
|---|---|
| Pregnancy | Endocrine disorders |
| Menstruation | Diabetes mellitus |
| | Hypothyroidism |
| Medications | Hypoparathyroidism |
| Broad-spectrum antibiotics | Hypoadrenalism |
| Immunosuppressants | |
| Corticosteroids | Malignancies |
| Oral contraceptives | Lymphosarcoma |
| Metronidazole | Hodgkin's disease |
| Environmental | Other diseases |
| Poor hygiene | AIDS |
| Excessive warmth and moisture due to wearing of synthetic-fiber undergarments | Severe anemia<br>Agammaglobulinemia<br>Malnutrition<br>Pancreatitis |
| Trauma, abrasion, and breaks in the skin and mucous membranes | Obesity |

sions disturbing the mechanical barriers provided by the skin and ciliated epithelial surfaces provide an opportunity for *Candida* to invade the tissue [22].

The pathogenic mechanisms through which predisposing factors contribute to development or exacerbation of the disease are again complex and not completely understood. There is little doubt, however, that humoral and cell-mediated immunity plays a very important role [1,23–25]. The increased prevalence of oral and vaginal thrush in women, and of oral and penile thrush in male patients with AIDS, points out the role of T helper lymphocytes in the pathogenesis of candidosis. It is probable that the same mechanism plays a role in lymphosarcoma and Hodgkin's disease. Frequent candidal infections in malnourished patients and in persons with agammaglobulinemia may suggest a role of gammaglobulins in candidosis.

The high incidence of vaginal candidosis in pregnancy can be explained by (a) changes in the hormonal status of pregnant women, which results in an increase in glycogen stores in the vaginal epithelium, and by (b) the depressed cellular immunity observed in pregnancy [26]. The incidence increases during the course of gestation. Symptomatic candidal vulvovaginitis was observed in about 10% of pregnant women during the first trimester and in 23 to 55% of women during the third trimester [17,27–29]. An even high incidence of candidal vulvovaginitis (up to 90%) was observed in pregnant women who had been vaginal carriers of *C. albicans* [1,2,8,29].

It is generally accepted that candidal infections (including genital) are more prevalent in diabetics than in the general population [30–33], and recurrent episodes of genital candidosis may sometimes be the first noticeable manifestation of this serious disease. Even so, some authors claim that the incidence of candidosis in diabetics is not increased when the disease is well controlled [32,33]. Vulvovaginal candidosis is common in girls suffering from diabetes, and in 77% of them cultured for *C. albicans* results are positive [31]. Almost 100% of cultures taken from girls with symptoms and signs of vulvovaginitis grew *C. albicans* [31]. In two thirds of the patients, the same yeast flora was cultured from the anus as well as the vulva [31]. It has been observed that a decrease in glycosuria is associated with remission of signs and cessation of symptoms [32].

The role of oral contraceptives in genital candidosis is controversial. It has been suggested that birth control pills encourage yeast growth, on the basis of findings that a significantly higher percentage of infected than uninfected women use oral contraceptives [34]. Other reports, however, have claimed that the incidence of candidosis in women using birth control pills is no higher than in women using other forms of contraception [5,12]. It is probable that oral contraceptives may predispose to vaginal carriage but that other factors may be necessary for the development of vulvovaginitis.

Many patients develop genital candidosis during the course of treatment with broad-spectrum antimicrobials [35,36]. Bisschop et al [37] demonstrated that vaginal fluid aspirated from randomly selected healthy women could serve as a culture medium for *C. albicans*, but the addition of broad-spectrum antibiotics significantly enhanced its growth-promoting activity. This might at least partly explain the phenomenon of frequent development of genital candidosis in patients treated with antibiotics.

## Clinical Findings

### Women

About 30% of women with genital candidosis may be asymptomatic [6]. Others may complain of minimal to severe symptoms. Symptoms of vulvovaginal candidosis are of abrupt onset, usually prior to menstruation. The most common manifestation is vulvar pruritus, present in 81 to 90% of symptomatic women [38,39]. About three fourths of female patients complain of vulvar soreness [33]. Some complain of burning, especially during and after intercourse, and of pruritus and burning around the anus. Dysuria may also occur if the urine comes in contact with the inflamed vulva.

Physical examination reveals an erythematous, somewhat edematous vulva, frequently with excoriations, although none of these findings are constant. In one prospective study, vulvar redness was observed in 54.5% of patients with symptomatic candidosis [38]. The vagina may be erythematous and may contain a thick, cottage-cheese-like discharge, which adheres to the vaginal wall and forms white, curdy patches (Fig. 11.1). These patches are more common in pregnant women [22]. On rare occasions the discharge may be thin and watery, producing a white sheen on the vagina and vulva. Vulvar candidosis may extend to the adjacent skin (Fig. 11.3) and concomitant perianal involvement as a papulopustular dermatitis may accompany vaginal lesions. Remote satellite lesions may be seen on the labia, inner thighs, or perineum. As in healthy women, the pH of vaginal secretion is less than 4.5, and the odor of vaginal fluid mixed with KOH is normal.

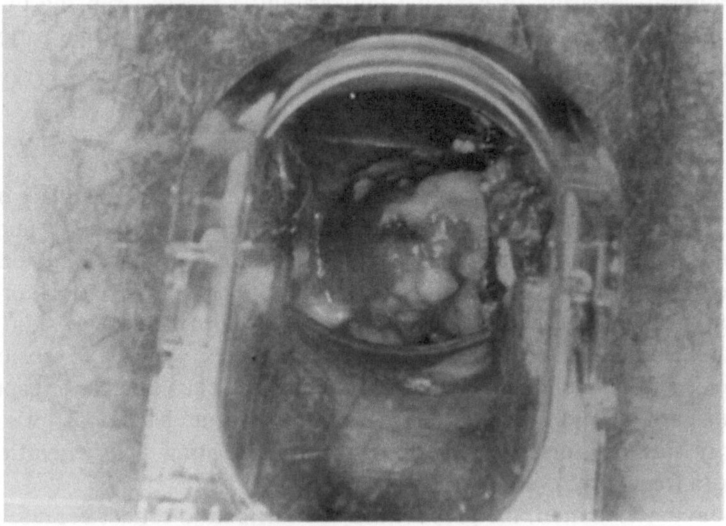

FIGURE 11.1. Vaginal candidosis: white cottage-cheese-like discharge adhered to the vaginal wall and cervix.

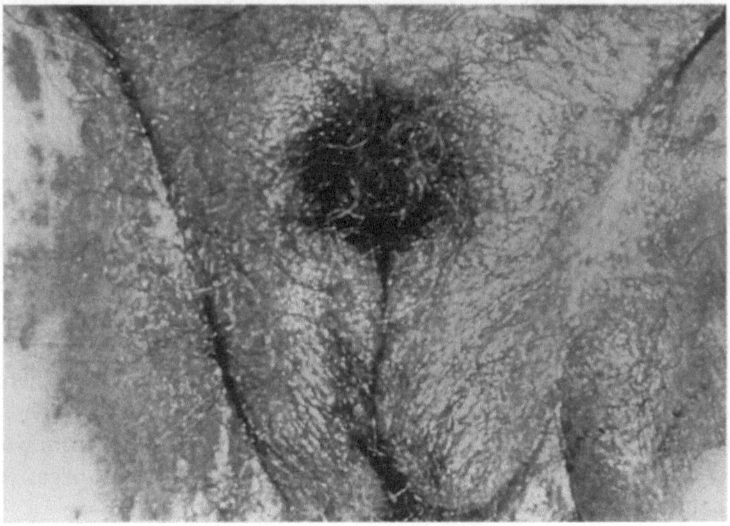

FIGURE 11.2. Vulvar candidosis extending to the adjacent skin.

The clinical spectrum of candidal vulvovaginitis ranges from the typical presentation just described to minimal pruritus experienced by some patients prior to menstruation.

### Men

Men with genital candidosis may have no symptoms or may complain of various degrees of itching, burning, or irritation. This symptom may occur immediately after coitus or a few days following. Symptomatic disease is more common in uncircumcised men [40] but is not confined to them. The manifestations of candidal infection of the penis usually include erythema appearing as "glazed skin" [41], but may also include small, scattered erythematous papules, vesicles, or erosions on the glans penis and/or on the inner aspect of the prepuce. The vesicular or papulopustular lesions are more characteristic for early, more acute balanoposthitis, while in chronic or subsiding disease, mild desquamation, crusting, and lichenification are seen more frequently.

In uncircumcised men, the prepuce may be difficult to retract because of edema and fissuring. A white discharge may be present, or adherent white patches resembling smegma may be seen (Fig. 11.2). Occasionally the scrotal skin may be involved, with scaling, pruritic lesions present. Intertriginous candidiasis may be seen on opposing surfaces of the scrotum or in the crural region. Perianal lesions may be present in homosexual men. Candidal urethritis has been reported as well, but uncommonly [42].

### Complications

A rare complication in men with candidal balanoposthitis is phimosis, while in women frequent recurrences of vulvovaginitis causing dyspareunia may result in sexual neurosis. In immunocompromised patients, disseminated candidosis may occur. The clinical triad of fever, an erythematous eruption, and muscle tenderness in immunocompromised patients receiving broad-spectrum antibiotics should alert the physician to possible disseminated candidosis. Immediate antifungal therapy should be considered, since the complication is frequently fatal [43]. There is a possibility that *C. albicans* may inhibit *Neisseria gonorrhoeae*, impairing detection and confirmation of gonorrhea [44,45]. Failure to culture gonococci from women suspected of having gonorrhea should be considered a possible false-negative result if genital candidosis is present.

## Diagnosis

Diagnosis of genital candidosis is established by clinical findings, laboratory tests, and exclusion of other causes of vulvovaginitis or balanoposthitis. Even though the clinical picture may be very suggestive for candidosis, diagnosis on clinical grounds alone is generally unreliable and should be confirmed by demonstration of the pathogenic microorganism by laboratory tests.

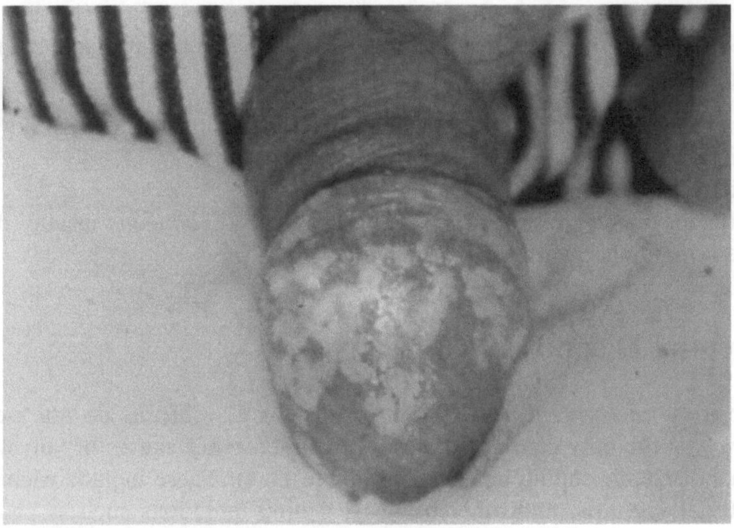

FIGURE 11.3. Candidal balanitis: white adherent patches on the glans of the penis.

## MICROSCOPIC EXAMINATION

### Potassium Hydroxide Preparation

Microscopic examination of vaginal or subpreputial discharge in wet mounts with 10% KOH allows the visualization of yeast forms and pseudohyphae. Potassium hydroxide dissolves epithelial and inflammatory cells, leaving behind fungal elements and making them easy to observe. The KOH solution destroys other elements, and thus cannot be used for the diagnosis of conditions other than fungal.

### Gram-stained smears

In Gram's stain *Candida* appear as dense, gram-positive, ovoid bodies. Pseudohyphae are long tubes of the same diameter as the spores; they may appear clear with gram-positive dots. The sensitivity of Gram's stain is probably higher than that of a wet mount, but the latter method is more popular, especially among gynecologists, for rapid diagnosis of vaginal candidosis in the office. Gram-stained smears may also serve to detect "clue cells" and *N. gonorrhoeae*, but are not useful for detection of another frequent case of vulvovaginitis, *Trichomonas vaginalis*.

## CULTURE

Culture is the most sensitive and reliable method for identification of *C. albicans* both in symptomatic and asymptomatic patients. It has been suggested that 40 to 60% of yeast infections in women would be missed if diagnosis depended only on microscopic examinations [46,47]. The most reliable identification and differentiation of *Candida* species are provided by Sabouraud's and Neckerson media [48].

Culture does, however, have disadvantages: it is relatively expensive and several days are needed to obtain the results. Other methods that are available but not routinely applied are

Fluorescent antibody stains and enzyme-linked immunoabsorbent assay (ELISA) techniques
Serologic tests
Biopsy (taken mainly for scientific purposes, since *C. albicans* usually does not invade layers underneath the epithelium

## Differential Diagnosis

Even positive microscopic and culture results for *C. albicans* do not mean that *C. albicans* is the only cause of disease. In women other causes of vulvovaginitis or vaginal discharge should be ruled out (Table 11.2). These include trichomoniasis, bacterial vaginitis, and other bacterial genital infections such as gonococcal or chlamydial cervicitis. Secondary syphilis, genital herpes, and genital warts may be the cause of vaginal discharge or vulvitis as well. Other conditions that should be considered in the differential diagnosis in women include postmenopausal vaginitis and vaginal discharge due to foreign bodies, chemical irritants, douches, or deodorants.

In men, the differential diagnosis should include balanitis or balanoposthitis caused by other microorganisms. Other sexually transmitted diseases to consider are syphilis (primary and secondary), genital herpes, genital warts, gonorrhea, Reiter's syndrome, and scabies. Among noninfectious causes, seborrheic dermatitis and contact dermatitis, lichen planus, psoriasis and erythema multiforme, and hypersensitivity reactions to contraceptives, creams, antiseptics, and condoms should be mentioned.

## Management

Genital candidal infection may be treated with a number of topical antifungals. As an initial step, the vulva or glans penis (after retraction of the prepuce) should be gently cleaned with mild soap and water, rinsed, and dried.

Topical creams are applied to external skin and mucous membrane lesions. Vaginal lesions are treated with vaginal tablets, creams, or suppositories inserted with an applicator.

### Candidal Vulvovaginitis

The following are possible regimens:

Miconazole nitrate, 2% vaginal cream or 100-mg suppositories, intravaginally, once daily at bedtime for 7 days

TABLE 11.2. Helpful diagnostic features in the differential diagnosis of vaginal discharge.

| Feature | *Candida* | *Trichomonas* | Bacterial | Other: *N. gonorrhoeae*; *C. trachomatis* |
|---|---|---|---|---|
| Itching | ++++* | +/− | +/− | +/− |
| Vulvar sore, vaginal discomfort | +++ | ++++ | ++ | + |
| Odor | + | ++ | ++++ | + |
| Dyspareunia | +++ | ++++ | + | +/− |
| Relationship to menstrual cycle | ++++ | − | − | − |
| Recent new sex partner | + | +/− | − | ++++ |
| Onset of symptoms related to systemic antibiotic use | ++++ | − | − | − |

*(+) occasionally to (++++) nearly always; (−) no symptoms.

Miconazole nitrate, 200-mg suppositories, intravaginally, once daily at bedtime for 3 days
Clotrimazole, 1% vaginal cream or 100-mg tablets, intravaginally, once daily at bedtime for 7 to 14 days
Clotrimazole, 2% vaginal cream or 200-mg tablets, intravaginally, once daily at bedtime for 3 days
Clotrimazole, 500-mg tablets, intravaginally as a single dose
Nystatin cream, tablets or suppositories, 100,000 units intravaginally, once daily for 14 days
Ketoconazole, 200-mg tablet, orally, once daily for 7 to 14 days or other regimens [49–51].

Recurrences have been frequently observed in apparently adequately treated women. In these cases elimination of predisposing factors (control of diabetes mellitus, discontinuation of oral contraceptives, etc.) [32,52] should be considered. Some authors recommend simultaneous treatment of male sexual partners [4] or oral administration of antifungals to prevent reinfection from the gastrointestinal tract [52].

## CANDIDAL BALANITIS OR BALANOPOSTHITIS

Men with genital candidosis should be treated by cleansing the affected site, drying thoroughly, and applying miconazole or clotrimazole cream twice daily for 7 to 14 days. Hydrocortisone creams plus 1 to 3% vioform, local applications of 1% aqueous solution of gentian violet, or frequently changed saline compresses are also helpful.

As is the case in treatment of women's genital candidosis, elimination of predisposing factors or treatment of sexual partners is recommended.

In intractable cases, oral ketoconazole, 200-mg tablets one to two times daily for 7 to 14 days, may be used. The infrequent reports of hepatotoxicity require careful use of this agent.

## References


1. Odds FC: *Candida* and *Candidosis*. Baltimore: University Park Press, 1979.
2. Hurley R, Leask B, Faktor JA, et al: Incidence and distribution of yeast species and of *Trichomonas vaginalis* in the vagina of pregnant women. *J Obstet Gynaecol Br Com W* **80**:252–257, 1973.
3. Willmott FE: Genital yeasts in female patients attending a VD clinic. *Br J Vener Dis* **51**:119–122, 1975.
4. Oriel JD, Patridge BM, Denny MJ, et al: Genital yeast infections. *Br Med J* **4**:761–764, 1972.
5. Merkus JM, Bisschop MP, Stolte LAM: The proper nature of vaginal candidosis and the problem of recurrence. *Obstet Gynecol Surv* **40**:493–504, 1985.
6. Goldacre MJ, Watt B, Loudon N, et al: Vaginal microbial flora in normal young women. *Br Med J* **1**:1450–1453, 1979.
7. Thin RN, Rendell P, Wadsworth J: How often are gonorrhea and genital yeast infection sexually transmitted? *Br J Vener Dis* **55**:278–280, 1979.
8. Persson K, Persson K, Hansson H, et al: Prevalence of nine different microorganisms in the female genital tract: A comparison between women from a venereal disease clinic and from a health control department. *Br J Vener Dis* **55**:429–433, 1979.
9. NIAID Study Group: Sexually Transmitted Diseases: 1980 Status Report. Washington, D.C.: U.S. Government Printing Office, 1981, pp. 181–193, 249–254.
10. Masteron G. Sengupta SM, Schofield CBS: Natamycin in genital candidosis in men. *Br J Vener Dis* **51**:210–212, 1975.
11. Rodin P, Kolator B: Carriage of yeasts on the penis. *Br Med J* **1**:1123–1124, 1976.
12. Diddle AW, Gardner WH, Williamson PJ, et al: Oral contraceptives medications and vulvovaginal candidiasis. *Obstet Gynecol* **34**:373–377, 1969.
13. Thin RN, Leighton M, Dixon MJ: How often is genital yeast infection sexually transmitted? *Br Med J* **2**:93–94, 1977.
14. Warnock DW, Speller DCE, Milne JD: Epidemiological investigation of patients with vulvovaginal candidiasis. *Br J Vener Dis* **55**:357–361, 1979.
15. White W, Spencer-Phillips PJ: Recurrent vaginitis and oral sex. *Lancet* **1**:621, 1979.
16. Oates JK: Recurrent vaginitis and oral sex. *Lancet* **1**:785, 1979.
17. Morton RS, Rashid S: Candidal vaginitis: Natural history, predisposing factors and prevention. *Proc Roy Soc Med* **70**(Suppl 4):3–13, 1977.
18. Hurley R, deLouvois J: *Candida* vaginitis. *Postgrad Med J* **55**:645–647, 1970.
19. Miles RM, Olsen L, Rogers A: Recurrent vaginal candidiasis: Importance of an intestinal reservoir. *JAMA* **238**:1036–1037, 1977.
20. Hilton AL, Warnock DW: Vaginal candidiasis and the role of the digestive tract as a source of infection. *Br J Obstet Gynecol* **82**:922–926, 1975.
21. Elegbe IA, Botu M: A preliminary study on dressing patterns and incidence of candidiasis. *Am J Public Health* **72**:176–177, 1982.
22. Felman YM, Nikitas JA: Genital candidiasis. *Cutis* **31**:369–382, 1983.
23. Dwyer JM: Chronic mucocutaneous candidiasis. *Ann Rev Med* **32**:491–497, 1981.
24. Syverson RE, Buckley H, Gibian J, et al: Cellular and humoral immune status in women with chronic *candida* vaginitis, *Am J Obstet Gynecol* **134**:624–627, 1979.
25. Mathur SM, Virella G, Koistinen J, et al: Humoral immunity in vaginal candidiasis. *Infect Immunol* **15**:287–294, 1980.

26. Brunham RC, Martin DH, Hubbard TW, et al: Depression of the lymphocyte transformation response to microbial antigens and to phytohemagglutinin during pregnancy. *J Clin Invest* **72**:1629–1638, 1983.
27. Paavonen J, Heinonen PK, Aine R, et al: Prevalence of nonspecific vaginitis and other cervicovaginal infections during the third trimester of pregnancy. *Sex Trans Dis* **12**:5–8, 1986.
28. Carrol CJ, Hurley R, Stanley VC: Criteria for diagnosis of *candida* vulvovaginitis in pregnant women. *J Obstet Gynaecol Br Com* **80**:258–263, 1973.
29. Hopsu-Havu VK, Gronroos M, Punnonen R: Vaginal yeasts in parturients and infestation of the newborns. *Acta Obstet Gynecol Scand* **59**:73–77, 1980.
30. Gilgor RS: Cutaneous infections in diabetes mellitus. JE Jelinek (Ed): *The Skin in Diabetes*. Philadelphia: Lea & Febiger, 1986, pp. 111–132.
31. Sonck CE, Somersalo O: The yeast flora of the anogenital region in diabetic girls. *Arch Dermatol* **88**:846–852, 1963.
32. Vallance-Owen J, Diabetes mellitus. *Br J Dermatol* **81**(Suppl 2):9–13, 1969.
33. Bagdade JD, Infection in diabetes. *Postgrad Med* **59**(1):160–164, 1976.
34. Bramley M, Kinghorn G: Do oral contraceptives inhibit *Trichomonas vaginalis*? *Sex Trans Dis* **6**:261–263, 1979.
35. Oriel JD, Waterwarth PM: Effect of minocycline and tetracycline on the vaginal yeast flora. *J Clin Pathol* **218**:403–406, 1975.
36. Caruso LJ: Vaginal moniliasis after tetracycline therapy. *Am J Obstet Gynecol* **90**:374–378, 1964.
37. Bisschop MP, Merkus JM, Van Cutsem J: The influence of antibiotics on the growth of *Candida albicans* in the vagina: An experiment with vaginal fluid. *Eur J Obstet Gynecol Reprod Biol* **20**:113–119, 1985.
38. Gough PM, Warnock DW, Turner A, et al: Candidosis in the genital tract in non-pregnant women. *Eur J Obstet Gynecol Reprod Biol* **19**:237–246, 1985.
39. Gardner HL, Kaufman RH: *Benign Diseases of the Vulva and Vagina*. Chap. 12, Candidiasis. Boston: G.K. Hall Medical Publishers, 1981.
40. Davidson F: Yeasts and circumcision in the male. *Br J Vener Dis* **53**:121–122, 1977.
41. Waugh MA, Evans EGV, Nayyar KC, et al: Clotrimazole (Canesten) in the treatment of candidal balanitis in men with incidental observations on diabetic candidal balanoposthitis. *Br J Vener Dis* **54**:184–186, 1978.
42. Mroczkowski TF: Post-gonococcal urethritis in men. Part II. Etiology and treatment. *Przegl Derm* **63**:173–179, 1976.
43. Jacobs MI, Magid MS, Jarowski CI: Disseminated candidiasis. *Arch Dermatol* **116**:1277–1279, 1980.
44. Hipp SS, Lawton WD, Chen NC, et al: Inhibition of *Neisseria gonorrhoeae* by factor produced by *Candida albicans. Appl Microbiol* **27**:192–196, 1974.
45. Wallin J, Gnarpe H: Possible inhibition of *N. gonorrhoeae* by *C. albicans*. *Br J Vener Dis* **51**:174–175, 1975.
46. Burgess SG, Manusco PG, Kalish PE, et al: Clinical and laboratory study on vaginitis. Evaluation of diagnostic methods and results of treatment. *NY J Med* **70**:2086–2091, 1970.
47. O'Connor BH, Adler MW: Current approaches to the diagnosis, treatment and reporting of trichomoniasis and candidiasis. *Br J Vener Dis* **55**:52–57, 1979.
48. Martius J, Hartman AA: Untersuchungen zur Nachweissicherheit und Haufigkeit genitaler Mykosen bei Schwangeren. *Z Geburts Perinatol* **187**:121–123, 1983.

49. Fregoso-Duenas F: Ketoconazole in vulvovaginal candidosis. *Rev Infect Dis* **2**:620–622, 1980.
50. Sobel JD: Management of recurrent vulvovaginal candidiasis with intermittent ketoconazole prophylaxis. *Obstet Gynecol* **65**:435–440, 1985.
51. Ledger WJ: Infection in the Female. Chap. 8, Community-acquired gynecologic infections. Philadelphia: Lea & Febiger, 1986, p. 127.

CHAPTER 12

# Scabies and Pediculosis

Lawrence Charles Parish and Joseph A. Witkowski

## Part 1. Scabies

### Overview

Scabies has been known since antiquity. It was among the first diseases to be correlated with a parasitic agent. Although treatment is simple and straightforward, the word scabies often creates pandemonium [1].

### Synonyms

A synonym for scabies is "the itch."

### Definition

Scabies is a parasitic disease caused by *Sarcoptes scabiei* var *hominis*, a mite that can barely be seen by the naked eye. It measures 270 to 380 μm, with the ova being 100 × 150 μm. The mite is transmitted only by close contact, for it can barely survive off the human body for more than several minutes, probably due to its temperature requirements [2].

The sexual transmission of scabies was demonstrated very eloquently by Mellanby [3]. During World War II he subjected conscientious objectors in England to a series of experiments to prove the contagiousness of the mite. The subjects exchanged underwear, slept in the same bed, and cohabitated. He proved conclusively that intimate contact is necessary for transmission. There is even a direct ratio of the number of mites to which a subject is exposed, the length of exposure, and the chance of infestation.

### Clinical Findings

Scabies infests all parts of the body save the face, except in infants and immunocompromised patients. Characteristic signs are the burrow, inflammatory vesicles, urticarial papules, excoriations, dermatitis, and pyoderma.

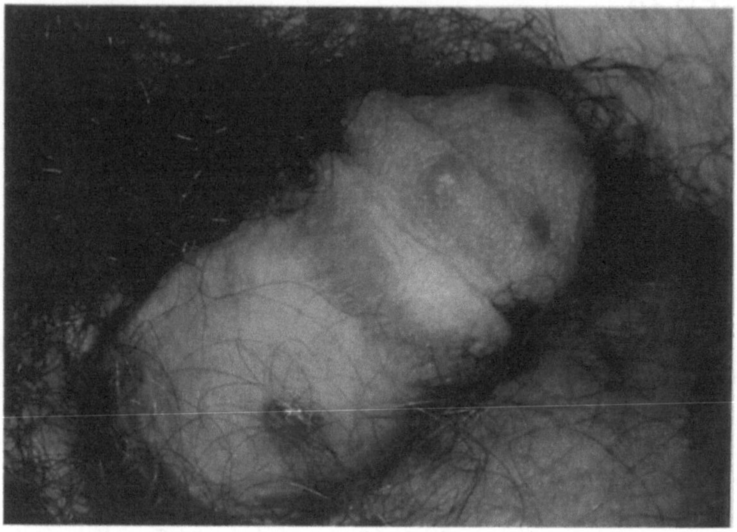

FIGURE 12.1. A 30-year-old man had pruritus of the penis, which he attributed to detergent remaining in his underpants. Clinical inspection revealed scabies, which was confirmed on microscopic examination.

The burrow is pathognomonic. It is a short 2- to 4-mm irregular line, often with a vesicle at the end. This represents the movement of the pregnant female mite. When the host reacts, an allergic response occurs, this being the red papule or vesicle. Because the developing pruritus is so marked, the patient digs into the skin. This leads to oozing, weeping, redness, and resultant secondary infection.

When the infestation has been present for some time, nodules can be found, particularly on the penis. These are frequently recalcitrant to scabicidal therapy.

Scabetic lesions are located on the cooler parts of the body. This makes the penis (Fig. 12.1) and the breast (Fig. 12.2) ideal areas for the mite to breed. The finger webs, waist, periaxillary areas, buttocks, and ankles are also good locations. The mite can flourish under the fingernails very nicely.

The diagnosis can be made by scraping the burrow with a scalpel blade. Often, the area that is itching the most will contain a mite (Fig. 12.3) and perhaps some ova. These can be examined microscopically under oil immersion. KOH digestation is used by some workers to dissolve the accompanying stratum corneum.

## Histopathology

The usual picture shows an inflammatory response with eosinophils in the dermis and spongiosis, exocytosis, and parakeratosis of the epidermis. Sometimes the mite can be observed in the stratum corneum.

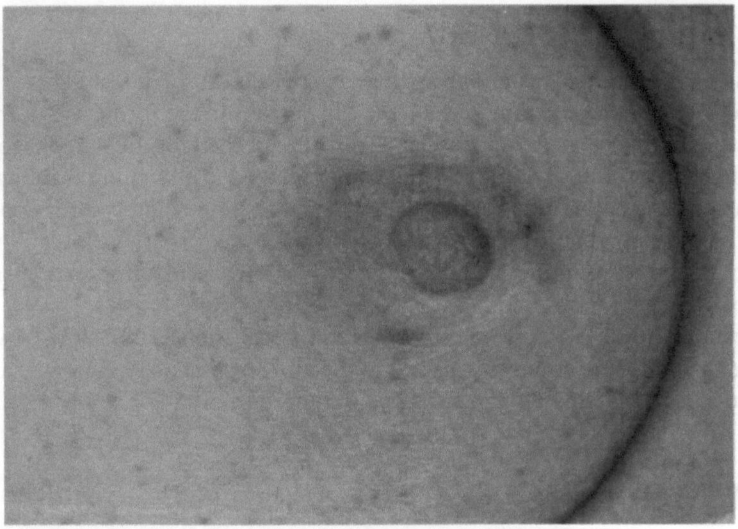

FIGURE 12.2. Four weeks after sexual contact with a new partner, this woman began to itch on her breasts. The papules on the areolae and those on the abdomen proved to be due to the scabies mite.

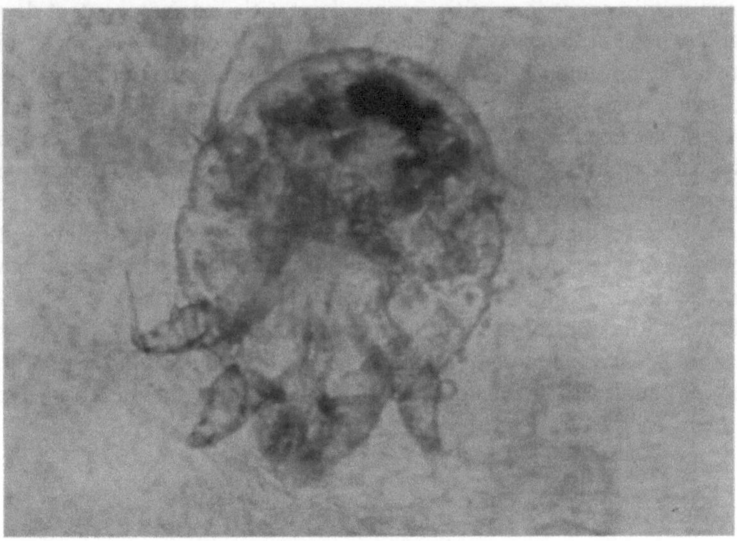

FIGURE 12.3. Although the scabies mite can be seen by some observers with the naked eye, visualization is much easier under the light microscope.

## Natural History

The first signs of scabies occur approximately 4 weeks after contact. This is because the life cycle is 19 days. From the time the egg hatches to the formation of the larval stage may be 3 to 4 days. An additional 12 days are needed for the nymphs to mature to adulthood, at which time the female is impregnated. The itching is thought to be due to her movement under the skin, as the male dies immediately after copulation, and to the development of hypersensitivity to the mite.

The pruritus, worse at night, makes the host scratch. This process transmits the mites to other parts of the body, where infestation occurs.

Untreated, the disease may last for several years; hence the term "seven-year itch." As the patient becomes sensitized to the antigen, itch may increase, and reinfestation can cause clinical signs to develop more rapidly [4].

## Complications

Scabies can lead to secondary bacterial infection. More serious effects are conceivable but unlikely.

## Differential Diagnosis

Scabies can mimic neurodermatitis, atopic dermatitis, or even contact dermatitis, particularly when the burrow is not present. This is due to the nonspecific red patches that may develop. When these coalesce or become plaquelike or dotted with vesicles, lichen planus and dermatitis herpetiformis may even be confused.

Two other ectoparasites need to be considered. Canine scabies occurs from close contact with a pet that is infested with *S. scabiei* var *canis*. The mite causes crusting on the animal's ears and abdomen. When the pet is cuddled, the mite transfers to the person, creating a red papular eruption, usually on the abdomen. Rarely does the mite penetrate the human stratum corneum, so that treatment is symptomatic [5].

*Cheyletiella* is a mite, most commonly found on rabbits and cats. When the animal is petted, the mite is transmitted to the human host, where it can feed. Often, the mite does not survive. Lesions may mimic those of scabies, but there are no burrows. The red papules are in clusters, which can develop central necrosis. Treatment is the same as for scabies [6].

## Management

The treatment of scabies is quite simple. Lindane 1% lotion or cream is applied to the body from the neck to the toes and allowed to remain for 12 hours. It can then be washed off. Bathing before, or for that matter after, the application of the miticide is unnecessary. Six hours is probably sufficient to kill the mites; however, the 12 hours is a reasonable compromise over the once-recommended 24 hours. No resistance to lindane is known. When a seeming therapeutic failure occurs, it most likely represents reinfestation [7].

Alternate regimens include a crotamiton lotion and 5% precipitated sulfur in petrolatum.

Contacts, both sexual and in the same domicile, should also be treated to prevent reinfestation. Care should be given to applying the medicaments to the nails, as the mite can be harbored under the nails [8]. Clothing need not be boiled or fumigated, as the mite cannot live off the body for more than a short time.

Within 24 hours of therapy, the itching should be reduced by half. Topical steroids can then be employed to further reduce the pruritus, which can last for several weeks. The nodules, particularly on the penis, may require intralesional steroids to resolve them. Sometimes, 5% crude coal tar in petrolatum can alleviate the itching.

## Prognosis

Scabies can be easily eradicated by proper treatment.

# Part 2. Pediculosis

## Overview

Three members of the Anaplora family can afflict humans: *Pediculus capitis* (head louse), *P. corporis* (body louse), and *Pthirus pubis* (crab louse). Since the head louse is usually troublesome to children only and the body louse lives on clothing rather than on the host, this discussion will be limited to the crab louse, which can cause severe itching [9].

## Synonyms

Synonyms for pediculosis are lice and crabs.

## Definition

The crab louse likes the pubic region, where it resides on the pubic hair and feeds on the adjacent skin. It and its nits can be found elsewhere on the body, wherever there is hair.

## Clinical Findings

Phthiriasis can occur in anyone who has contacted *P. pubis*. The louse is less than 2 mm in length (female 1.75 mm; male 1.25 mm) with the egg being 0.8 × 0.3 mm. *P. pubis* is less hardy than the other two types of lice, despite its crablike claws. It

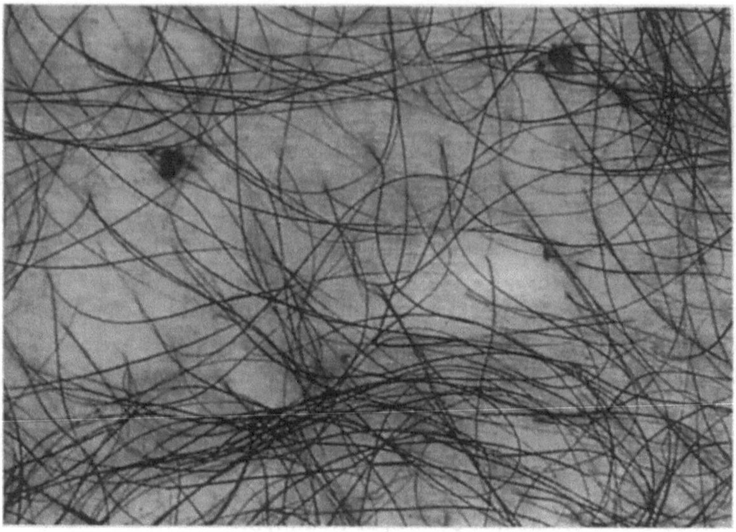

FIGURE 12.4. Although the itching caused by the crab louse is intense, the clinical picture often shows very little, as depicted here.

has a life cycle of about 30 days. It can live off the body for a few days, but is dead within 7 days unless it has had a blood meal. On the other hand, the nits can survive for several weeks [10].

The patient usually presents with itching on the groin. Rarely can more than one or two lice be seen, but the puncture marks are usually present. Secondary excoriation or dermatitis may be seen, and only rarely will maculae ceruleae, the slate-gray macules, be visualized (Fig. 12.4). *P. pubis* can be found on the eyelashes (pediculosis ciliaris) (Fig. 12.5) or on the chest, axillae, legs, or even the scalp (extrapubic pediculosis) [11].

## Histopathology

A nonspecific dermatitis may be found.

## Natural History

Pediculosis pubis may smolder for several months, as the nits may remain protected. Transmission is generally by intimate contact, although it is conceivable that the parasite is passed on by the exchange of clothes. The louse is sensitive to temperature, so that a temperature above 32°C or below 28°C may lead to its demise.

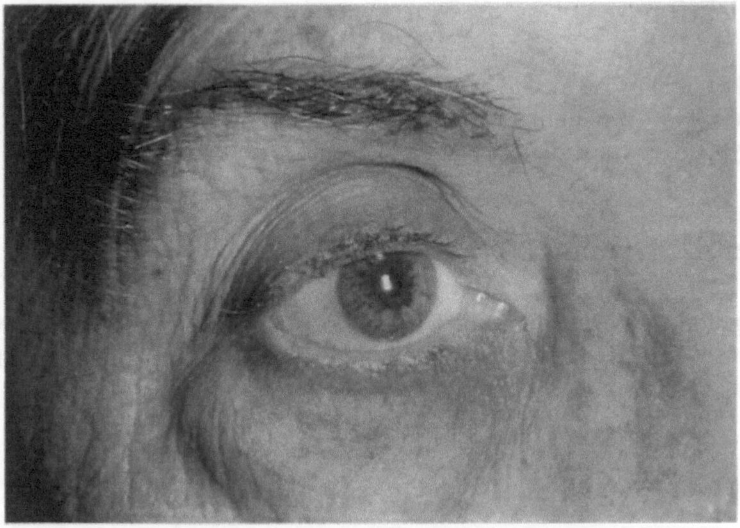

FIGURE 12.5. Pediculosis ciliaris may be transmitted indirectly. This 70-year-old woman contracted the nits on her eyelashes from her 44-year-old son who had many sexual contacts.

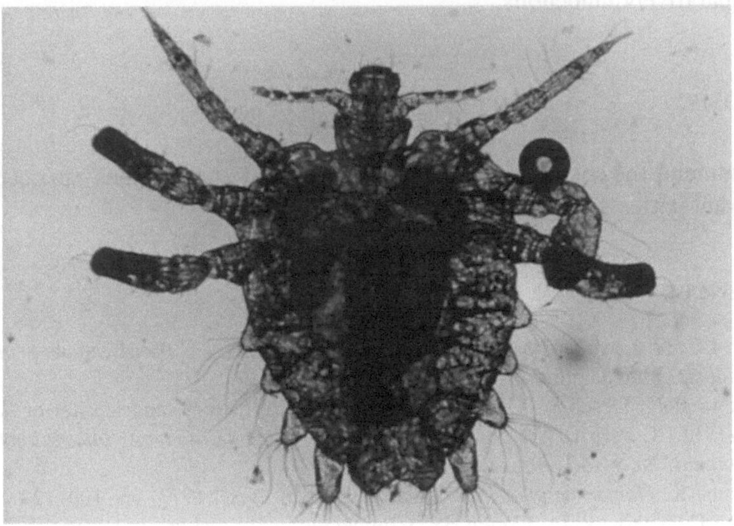

FIGURE 12.6. The crab louse can be visualized without the aid of a microscope.

## Complications

The marked itching can lead to excoriations and secondary bacterial infection. The pubic louse (Fig. 12.6) unlike the body louse which may transmit epidemic typhus, murine typhus, or epidemic relapsing fever, causes no known disease.

## Differential Diagnosis

A finding of the louse and nits, which can give a grainy feeling to the hair, confirms the diagnosis. Contact dermatitis or even a dermatophytosis may be suggested in the earliest stages [12].

## Management

Shampooing the entire body with lindane 1% shampoo for 4 minutes now and again in 7 days should eradicate the condition. The nits may remain for several weeks, unless combed out or cut off. There is no known resistance to lindane. Alternate treatment includes copper oleate cream or pyrethrin cream or shampoo [13,14].

All contacts and household members should be treated, as the therapy is so simple and comparatively innocuous.

## Prognosis

With treatment, the condition is immediately cured. Reinfestations can occur, even in observant patients.

### References


1. Parish LC: *History of scabies*. In M Orkin, HI Maibach, LC Parish, et al: *Scabies and Pediculosis*. Philadelphia: JB Lippincott, 1977, pp. 1–7.
2. Andrews JRH, Desch Jr. CE: The morphology, life history, and habitat of *Sarcoptes scabiei*. In LC Parish, WB Nutting, RM Schwartzman: *Cutaneous Infestations of Man and Animal*. New York: Praeger, 1983, pp. 53–69.
3. Mellanby K: *Human Guinea-Pigs*. London: Merlin Press, 1973, pp. 109–123.
4. Parish LC, Witkowski JA, Cohen HB: Clinical picture of scabies. In LC Parish, WB Nutting, RM Schwartzman: *Cutaneous Infestations of Man and Animal*. New York, Praeger, 1983, pp. 70–78.
5. Schartzman RM: Scabies in animals. In LC Parish, WB Nutting, RM Schwartzman: *Cutaneous Infestations of Man and Animal*. New York: Praeger, 1983, pp. 90–99.
6. Miller WH: Cheyletiella infestation. In LC Parish, WB Nutting, RM Schwartzman: *Cutaneous Infestations of Man and Animal*. New York: Praeger, 1983, pp. 255–260.

7. Lomholt G, Parish LC: Scabies. In A Rook, LC Parish, JM Beare: *Practical Management of the Dermatologic Patient*. Philadelphia: JB Lippincott, 1986, pp. 187–189.
8. Witkowski JA, Parish LC: Scabies: Subungual area harbor mites. *JAMA* **252**:318–319, 1984.
9. Busvine JR: *Insects, Hygiene and History.* London: Athlone Press, 1976, pp. 1–262.
10. Kim KC, Pratt HD, Stojanovich CJ: *The Sucking Lice of North America*. University Park, Pa.: Pennsylvania State University Press, 1986, pp. 209–211.
11. Ackerman AB: Crabs: The resurgence of *Phthirius* (sic) *pubis*. *N Engl J Med* **278**:950–951, 1968.
12. Witkowski, JA, Parish LC: The usual and not so usual forms of pediculosis. In LC Parish, WB Nutting, RM Schwartzman: *Cutaneous Infestations of Man and Animal*. New York: Praeger, 1983, pp. 125–137.
13. Rasmussen JE: Pediculosis: Treatment and resistance. In JP Callen, MV Dahl, LE Golitz: *Advances in Dermatology.* Chicago Year Book Medical Publishers, 1986, Vol. 1, pp. 109–123.
14. Parish LC, Lomholt G: Pediculosis. In A Rook, LC Parish, JM Beare: *Practical Management of the Dermatologic Patient*. Philadelphia: JB Lippincott, 1986, pp. 150–152.

CHAPTER 13

# Herpes Progenitalis

Michihito Niimura and Steven Emmet

## Overview

The word *herpes* comes from the Greek word *herpein*, meaning "to creep." It has been used to describe a wide variety of diseases [1]. The following is a capsule summary of some of the more important sources [2]:

100 A.D.: Herodotus described "an eruption which appears about the mouth at the crises of simple fevers."
1694: Richard Morton was the first to use the word *herpes* to describe facial herpes with fever.
1736: Astruc described herpes of the genitals in both men and women.
1876: Piffard grouped both oral and genital herpes together and separated them from herpes zoster.
1905: Cushing noted that herpes facialis commonly occurred after trigeminal ganglion surgery for "tic dolouroux."
1912: Grueter transmitted a patient's herpetic keratitis to a rabbit's eye and back to the cornea of a blind man.
1921: Lipshutz maintained that herpes febrilis and herpes genitalis were different but related.
1921: Lauda established the filterability of the organism, implying a viral nature.
1923: Levaditi and Nicolau described the genital transmission of herpes from a female to a male rabbit.
1930s: Andrews and Carmichael noted that herpes simplex could recur despite serum antibodies to the virus.
1944: Tzanck described multinuclear giant cells after staining of material scraped from the base of a herpetic vesicle.
1957: Huang Zi Shang was the first to serologically differentiate between herpes simplex virus 1 and 2.
1961: Roizman discussed latency and the dynamic versus the nonreplicating state.
1971: Steven and Cook showed that 2 weeks after a foot pad infection in the mouse, explanted mice spinal ganglia would release herpes simplex virus.

## Synonyms

Synonyms for herpes progenitalis are herpes genitalis and genital herpes simplex.

## Etiologic Agent

The *Herpesvirus* family contains about 80 members, of which 5, now grouped in the Alpha herpes viriniae subfamily, Epstein-Barr virus, cytomegalovirus, varicella-zoster virus, Herpes simplex virus (HSV) types 1 and 2, are pathogenic for humans [3]. HSV is a double-stranded DNA virus surrounded by a lipid envelope which is derived from the cellular nuclear membrane. The core is about 85 to 110 nm and the total diameter is from 150 to 200 nm. The DNA, which is wrapped in a fibrillar spool, is of two types, a long one (82%) and a short one (12%). The ends of the DNA are anchored to the underside of the capsid shell, and there is enough DNA material to code for about 80 to 100 proteins. Only about 50 are known to exist; 30 are structural and the rest play a role in inducing such enzymes as thymidine kinase, DNA polymerase, and DNase. About 50% of the DNA of types 1 and 2 is homologous. In the latent stage the viral genome assumes a circular or concatameric shape. The tegument is filled with a fibrillar material of an unknown nature. The capsid is composed of 162 capsomeres, 150 of which are hexameric and 12 pentameric. The lipid envelope contains five viral glycoproteins, gB through gF; gB plays a role in penetration and fusion, gD in attachment. IgG Fc attaches to gE. gD also stimulates virus neutralization activity [4]. At the cellular level, viral infection takes place in the following sequence: adsorption, penetration, eclipse, DNA replication, nucleocapsid encapsulation, and release. Recent data indicate that HSV types 1 and 2 may bind to different sites on the cell, and that after DNA replication two types of bodies are left in the nucleus, a type A basophilic Feulgen-positive body with viral DNA in it and an eosinophilic inclusion body devoid of both protein and DNA. Each cell makes from 500,000 to 200,000 virions, but not all are complete viral particles [5].

The herpesvirus does not survive well outside of its normal host, humans, and it is readily inactivated by a low pH, ultraviolet light, ether, chloroform, merthiolate, and $AgNo_3$. It will survive 24 hours in distilled water, 4 hours in tap water, and not at all in spa water. In an investigation of the many claims that it is transmitted on a toilet seat, it was found that the virus will survive for 4.5 hours on a plastic surface, if the temperature is 37° to 40°C and the ambient humidity is high [6].

## Epidemiology

HSV has humans as its only natural reservoir. It is found throughout the world, in both primitive and advanced societies. One-hundred percent of the Bantu and 77% of the citizens of Uganda have antibodies to it, as do 100% of the Tiriyo tribe in Brazil. Women may have a slightly greater incidence of antibodies. Crowding seems to promote spreading, so while epidemics do not occur, there have been outbreaks in nurseries, orphanages, and children's homes. Reporting is not mandatory, but several studies suggest there may be 100 million episodes of oral herpes per year in the United States and 5 to 20 million episodes of genital herpes. Approximately 500,000 new cases of genital herpes occur yearly, which represents a ninefold increase between 1966 and 1981. Most newly affected women are between 20 and 24 years of age, most men between 25 and 29.

In serologic studies for antibodies to the herpesvirus, (both types 1 and 2), among the lower socioeconomic classes (probably secondary to crowding) 50% of children from 1 to 5 years of age and 100% of adults are positive. In the higher classes and in graduate school populations, 30 to 40% have antiherpes antibodies. When tests were performed specifically for type 2, or genital herpes, the following positive results were noted [5]: nuns, 3%; middle class 25%; heterosexuals at a VD clinic, 26%; homosexuals, 46%; lower classes 46 to 60%; and prostitutes, 70 to 80% [7].

The presence of antibodies does not denote an infectious state: in an actual study of oral viral shedding, 20%of asymptomatic children from 7 months to 2 years of age, 9% from 3 to 14 years, and 2.4% of adults shed HSV type 1. In other studies, from about 1 to 8% of children and from 0.75 to 9% of asymptomatic adults shed virus in the oral cavity. In one longitudinal study, oral herpes could periodically be recovered from 32% of asymptomatic children [8].

Pap smears can be used to detect genital herpes in women; from 0.03 to 6 to 9% of asymptomatic women have positive smears. In actual cultures of asymptomatic women, 0.25 to 1.5% of private gynecologic patients, 1.6 to 8% of VD clinic patients, and 12% of young prostitutes were positive for HSV type 2.

Interestingly enough, only 2.8% of female prostitutes over age 30 had positive HSV type 2 cultures. When male VD clinic patients had material from the epididymis, prostate, and urethra cultured, 0.3 to 15% of patients were positive for HSV type 2. When unselected cadavers were examined via explant culture, 55% had latent herpesvirus type 1 in the trigeminal ganglion and 20% had latent herpesvirus type 2 in the sacral ganglia.

## Clinical Findings

The clinical picture of HSV infections depends on the age of the patient, prior antibody and present immune status, and the site affected [9]. About 10% of children develop an acute gingivostomatitis characterized by painful blisters and erosions coalescing to form crusted yellow plaques on the lips and ulcerations on the tongue, gums, and palate. The regional lymph nodes are enlarged, and there is fever, malaise, and an inability to eat and occasionally to drink. Hospitalization is rarely necessary and resolution usually takes 2 to 3 weeks. Eleven percent of college students with pharyngitis have herpes simplex as an etiology, with individual and then confluent ulcers on the lips, gums, hard palate, tonsils, and posterior pharynx and accompanying fever, malaise, and regional adenopathy. Spontaneous resolution takes 2 to 3 weeks.

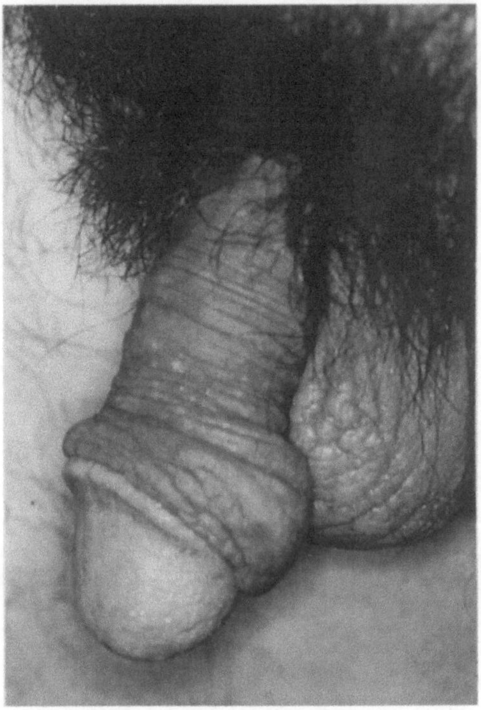

FIGURE 13.1. Primary genital herpes in a man.

## PRIMARY GENITAL HERPES

Adults without protective antibodies develop primary herpes after a 2- to 20- (average 6)day incubation period. Scattered vesicles with red areolae form at the site of inoculation, and then coalesce to form ulcers that either remain moist or develop a crust, depending on whether they are on mucous membranes or epidermal surfaces. As old areas heal, new areas form. Regional lymphadenopathy is associated with fever and malaise. Even in patients with protective antibodies, untreated primary herpes may last 2 to 6 weeks.

In almost all cases, HSV 1 is the cause of oral lesions, though HSV type 2 is also seen. Scattered perioral lesions are seen in conjunction with ulcerations of the lips, tongue, buccal areas, and posterior pharynx. Genital herpes, almost always caused by HSV type 2 (though type 1 genital cases have been documented), in men occurs on the glans, prepuce, shaft, and sulcus. Mechanical flow studies predict that secretions and bacterial and viral organisms should concentrate in the sulcus, and indeed many venereal diseases do concentrate in that area. Scattered lesions may be seen on the scrotum, thigh, and buttocks (Fig. 13.1). In women, primary herpetic lesions are seen on the labia majora and minora and often spread to the perineum and inner thighs (Fig. 13.2). Both vaginal discharge and cervicitis are often present, and the cervix is tender and bleeds easily. Pelvic lymphadenopathy may be associated with deep pelvic pain, and dysuria may be present [10]. Genital herpes in both sexes

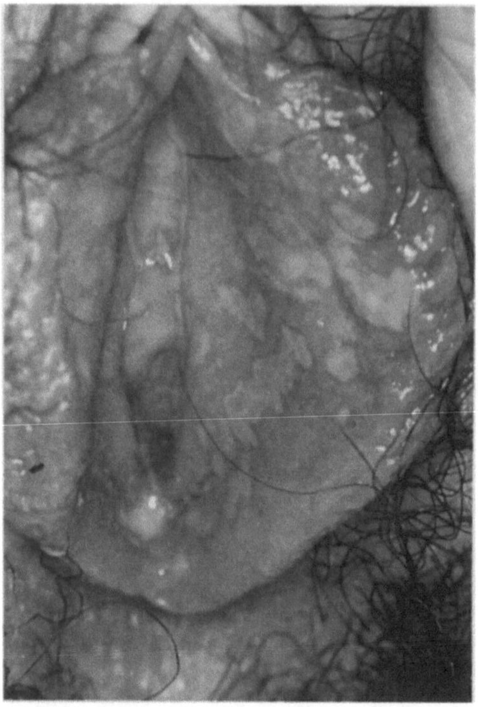

FIGURE 13.2. Primary genital herpes in a woman.

may have a concurrent meningitis, characterized by headache, fever, nuchal rigidity, cerebrospinal fluid (CSF) pleocytosis (with normal sugar content), and a positive viral CSF culture.

Historically initial attacks are often seen in patients who already have protective antibodies, probably secondary to herpetic pharyngitis as children. These attacks are far milder and heal more quickly with fewer days of viral shedding.

## Recurrent Genital Herpes

Recurrent lesions are the hallmark of herpes simplex infections. From 14 to 55% of patients with HSV type 1, and 50 to 80% of patients with HSV type 2 infections, will have recurrences in 1 year. HSV type 2 rarely recurs periorally and HSV type 1 rarely recurs genitally. In one unselected professional group, 2% had a monthly outbreak of herpes, 13% had one outbreak every 2 to 11 months, and 24% had attacks yearly or less often. In our experience, both the frequency and severity of the attacks diminish with time. Some of the alleged inducers of oral herpes include cold, colds, fever, wind, local irritation, menses, stress, and sun. Recurrences of genital herpes are said to be related to menses, sex, and stress. Incidentally, HSV type 2 is quite heat labile, which may explain why fever rarely causes its recurrence. Most if not all of the above have been shown to be associated with an increase in prostaglandin E, which facilitates viral growth in culture. Sunlight, thought to provoke recurrence, does cause a demonstrable decrease in cellular immunity.

Eighty percent of patients with recurrent type 1 and 50 to 70% of patients with recurrent type 2 herpes have prodromes 1 to 2 days prior to a clinical outbreak. These consist of itching, burning, and neuralgia. Biopsy with culture studies have shown that virus is present in the affected areas even before clinical lesions occur, so these patients are infectious even in the prodromal phase. Usually only one to four lesions occur, last an average of 8 days, and show maximal viral shedding during the first 4 days. Oral lesions remain on the vermillion border and skin, rarely involving mucous membranes. Recurrent genital lesions are also mostly on the labia majora and minora or penile shaft; rarely is there a vaginal discharge or cervical involvement. Oddly enough, higher HSV type 2 antibody levels are associated with a higher rate of recurrence [11]. Patients usually have recurrences of the same strains, but multiple strain recurrences have been documented, especially in immunosuppressed patients.

### Rectal Herpes

Rectal herpes, often seen in homosexuals, is commonly due to HSV type 1, either because of digital or oral contact. Tenesmus, anal pain, proctitis, discharge, and ulcerations as far as 10 cm into the anal canal may be seen. Dysuria may also develop, probably secondary to spinal ganglia involvement [12].

## Histopathology

During performance of a biopsy for routine hematoxylin and eosin examination, the use of Bouin's fixative (rather than formalin) will enhance the demonstration of intranuclear inclusion bodies and giant cells. On biopsy, one sees ballooning and reticular epidermal degeneration leading to acanthosis and intraepidermal vesicles. The swollen balloon cells have an eosinophilic cytoplasm and one or more nuclei. Coalescence of cells that have undergone reticular degeneration and rupturing of cell walls leads to multilocular vesicles. This is seen primarily in the upper and peripheral areas of the lesion (Fig. 13.3). Balloon cells may have eosinophilic bodies with clear halos in the nucleus. The upper dermis usually has an inflammatory infiltrate of neutrophils; they may be both in and around capillary walls [13]. ELISA (enzyme-linked immunoabsorbent assay) examination of biopsy specimens is also possible. Laboratory-developed antibodies to herpesvirus are linked to a horseradish immunoperoxidase, and the treated specimen is then immersed in 3,3'-diaminobenzidine with $H_2O_2$; herpetically infected cells turn brown. As with the immunofluorescent stain, the best results are seen in early lesions with higher viral counts.

Electron microscopy offers a rapid (several hours) method of detecting herpesvirus in tissue specimens. The classic picture of an 80- to 100-nm electron-dense core, capsomeres in an icosahedral shape with cubic symmetry, in a virus with a

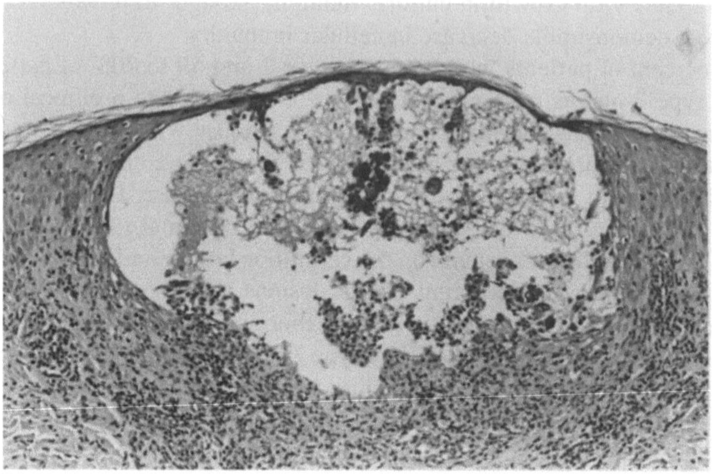

FIGURE 13.3. Ballooning and reticular epidermal degeneration of vesicle in herpesvirus infection.

total diameter of approximately 150 nm is diagnostic of the herpes group. More specific typing is not possible [14].

## Natural History

The virus is spread by close physical contact, so HSV type 1 is associated with kissing and sharing of eating utensils and HSV type 2 is spread by sexual contact or contact with genital secretions. Many patients may not even be aware of initial genital lesions. In one study, only 3% of pregnant patients were aware that they had had genital herpes, but 57% had type 2 antibodies. Only 6% of their spouses had positive histories, but 40% had type 2 antibodies.

In mice, virus can be recovered from the dorsal root ganglia as early as 2 weeks after an initial infection. Presumably in humans, the virus also travels via sensory axons to the dorsal root ganglia and enters a latent phase. Roizman (1961) initially raised the possibilities of either continuous production and destruction or a non-replicating state for the latent virus; apparently the latter is correct. The HSV genome is integrated into the host DNA and is not visible even with electron microscopy. With the exception of virus inoculated directly into the eye or CNS, latency seems to be proportional to viral thymidine kinase (TK) production. TK production may range from 0 to 100%, and TK-negative viruses rarely, if ever, produce latency. It is important to remember that neonates produce thymidine kinase in their CNS until about 10 days after birth, so even TK-negative viruses may survive and proliferate there [15].

## Complications

### Transplacental Infection

One of the most feared complications is prenatal and perinatal herpes infection. Among pregnant women who, either because of immunosuppression or innate inability to handle the virus, develop a generalized herpes infection, there is a 50% infant mortality rate. While many pregnant women symptomatically shed virus, only about 0.5% of pregnant women actually develop clinical genital herpes. If the infection occurs before 20 weeks of gestation there is about a 25% spontaneous abortion rate. Transplacental infections are rare, but do occur, and are associated with microcephaly, encephalitis, chorioretinitis, intrauterine growth retardation, psychomotor retardation, recurrent cutaneous herpes, hepatic and intracranial calcifications, abnormal digits, cataracts, osseous lesions, and congenital heart disease.

Infection toward the end of the third trimester is associated with prematurity in 50% of infants, which in and of itself increases the risks for respiratory distress, bacterial infections, and hypoglycemia.

### Neonatal Herpes

HSV infections of the neonate, 70% of which are type 2, are usually acquired in passage through an infected birth canal. Even allowing for better reporting, neonatal herpes is clearly becoming more common; in one study it increased from 2 in 100,000 in 1969 to 10 to 14 in 100,000 in 1982. One major problem is that from 66 to 90% of the mothers of neonates with herpes were totally asymptomatic at time of delivery; 35% of them never had a history of genital herpes! Most studies indicate that from 0.2 to 7.4% of pregnant women symptomatically shed herpesvirus vaginally, though one longitudinal study documented a 43% overall incidence.

Neonatal infections usually begin 5 to 7 days postpartum. Since many infants are already at home by that time, over two thirds of infants have a normal hospital nursery course. Seventy percent of neonates present with skin findings, (though 20% may never have skin involvement) [16] usually with associated fever, malaise, diarrhea, and poor weight gain; rarely may they have consumptive coagulopathy. The skin is usually studded with vesicles and pustules that are teeming with virus. Overall, before adequate treatment was available, 50% of affected neonates died and 50% were severely developmentally affected. Usually neonatal herpes is divided into the three clinical groups of skin, eyes, and mouth (SEM), CNS, or generalized. Even in the most benign category, SEM (one third to one half of all patients), 20% died, 20 to 50% had CNS sequelae, and 20% had eye damage. The chance of an individual neonate developing a herpesvirus infection is a function of the amount of virus in the genital tract, the duration of exposure, the use of scalp electrodes, gestational age, and the infant's antibody status.

A true primary genital infection in the mother carries the worst prognosis, as about 50% of neonates will be affected. Among the reasons for this dismal picture are the approximately 1000-fold increase in viral titers in the birth canal (compared with the titer in recurrent lesions) and the low maternal, and thus low neonatal, antibody status. Depending on the study, neonatal antiherpes antibody levels of 1:20 to 1:80 have been found to be protective, dramatically lessening the chance of neonatal infection [17]. If the mother has a recurrent genital herpetic infection, about 4 to 8% of neonates will be affected. If the membranes have been ruptured for more than 4 hours, viral exposure time and the risk of neonatal herpes are tremendously increased. Scalp monitoring, often done with premature infants, also provokes a ready pathway for neonatal viral infection. Postnatal infections, often type 1, can be contracted from mothers, visitors, and even hospital staff. One study found that about 10% of nursery personnel asymptomatically secreted HSV type 1 in their saliva.

Pregnant patients with a personal or consortial history of genital herpes should have a culture done weekly from the 34th week. If the virus is found at the time of delivery, and if the membrane has not been broken for more than 4 hours, a cesarean section should probably be performed, though the risk of infection is only about 5% and c-sections carry their own risks for both mother and child.

## Encephalitis and Meningitis

Each year there are about 250 to 500 cases of herpes simplex encephalitis in the United States, usually secondary to a TK positive HSV type 1 virus. The condition is characterized by fever, aphasia, confusion, and localizing neurologic signs in the temporal and frontal lobes. It has a 70% fatality rate. AIDS patients may develop a subacute progressive encephalomyelitis or chronic encephalitis.

About 4 to 8% of patients with primary HSV type 2 genital infections get meningitis, with nuchal rigidity, photophobia, vomiting, headaches, CSF pleocytosis (with normal sugar level), and a positive CSF culture. It usually runs a benign course, even without therapy.

## Herpes Proctitis

Herpes proctitis patients may develop urinary dysfunction and/or impotence 2 to 14 days after the rectal pain begins. The symptoms may last 4 to 20 days. The probable etiology is a virally induced lumbosacral radiculomyelopathy.

## Erythema Multiforme

One of the more benign but interesting complications of herpesvirus infections is erythema multiforme (EM). The classic target or iris lesions, usually centrifugal, often involving the palms, occur 1 to 2 weeks after a HSV infection. While the etiology of EM is unknown in about one half of cases, in one study 20% of EM patients had an HSV type 1 antecedent infection. Other causes included drugs, other viral and fungal infection, x-ray, and autoimmune disease. While steroids were the drug of choice in this study, it is probably better to treat the herpes patient who gets EM with oral acyclovir at the time of the herpes outbreak. Skin tests with inactivated HSV antigens have reproduced EM in some patients.

## Herpetic Whitlow

The herpetic whitlow, or distal digital infection, is often misdiagnosed and mistreated as a bacterial cellulitis. The patient's occupation, as doctor, dentist, nurse or respiratory therapist, as well as the viral vesicles and recurrent nature, are good clues that the edematous, erythematous digit is herpetically infected.

## Other

Complications of herpes infections are rarely seen in adults, in the absence of other local or systemic disease. Patients at risk include those with local diseases such as atopy, Darier's disease, pemphigus, and Sezary's disease, or with dermabraded areas and burns.

The following systemic problems also put patients at increased risk: malnourishment, cancer, thymus disease, immunosuppression, transplant, Wiskott-Aldrich syndrome, exposure to ultraviolet light or to tetrahydrocannabinol, and AIDS.

Tetrahydrocannabinol has been documented to decrease interferon responses to HSV infections in mice, and ultraviolet light not only increases prostaglandin E levels but also decreases both skin and systemic immunity. AIDS patients who have decreased natural killer cell activity often get localized deep, painful ulcers that extend from the tongue into the throat and even into the lungs, and from the buttocks into the anal canal. These ulcers heal slowly, even with acyclovir therapy, and continue to shed virus for a long time.

Kaposi's varicelliform eruption can be caused by several viruses (such as Coxsackie A-16 and vaccinia) but is often caused by herpesvirus. Those with abnormal epithelial surfaces are most at risk. Involved areas and occasionally all of the skin becomes covered with sheets of vesicles that become pustules, with new lesions occurring for 5 to 7 days. Fever, malaise, and regional adenopathy develop. Lesions heal slowly over 1 to 2 weeks, usually leaving little permanent scarring.

Generalized herpes, with involvement of all the major organs, can occur. If untreated it has a very high mortality rate.

## HSV and Cancer

Herpesvirus has been implicated as a cause of cancer of the cervix. In laboratory experiments, 123 HSV base pairs have transformed NIH 3T3 cells in vitro, and statistically many studies have shown a relationship between the presence of HSV type 2 antibodies and cancer of the cervix. In actuality, it is probably only guilt by association, as several sophisticated restrictive endonuclease analyses have now isolated human papillomavirus (HPV, the cause of genital warts) types 16, 18, 31, and 33 DNA sequences from cervical cancer specimens [18].

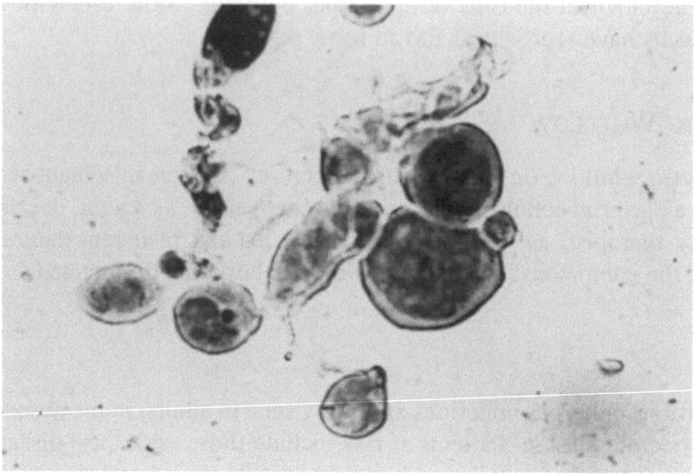

FIGURE 13.4. Multinucleated giant cells seen on Tzanck smear.

## Diagnosis and Differential Diagnosis

### Tzanck Smear

The simplest test to confirm the clinical diagnosis of herpes simplex is the Tzanck smear. If this test is properly performed, multinucleated giant cells and/or intranuclear inclusion bodies are seen in up to 75% of early herpes cases (Fig. 13.4). If Wright's or Giemsa's stain is used, intranuclear inclusions are rarely seen. Pap smears are useful in genital herpes in the female but are only one third as sensitive as cultures.

A newer technique uses monoclonal antibodies tagged with immunofluorescent markers. In symptomatic patients with early lesions it has a combined sensitivity and specificity of 87% [19]. It is not as useful in asymptomatic patients with low viral counts. Barr and Graham [20] devised a neat, practical technique using paragon multiple stain. Scrapings from the vesicular base are spread on a slide and 2 to 3 drops of PMS are added immediately. After 5 seconds the slide is washed, blotted dry, another drop of tap water and a coverslip are added, and the slide is examined under the microscope. This technique requires very little time, space, or equipment and provides very nice staining [20].

### Viral Culture

Actual culture of the herpesvirus represents the gold standard of diagnostic tests. Early researchers used mice, rat, and rabbit corneas and embryonated eggs. They then switched to cell cultures of rabbit kidney, human amnion, chorioallantoic membrane, HeLa cells, or Vero cells. Various transport media may be used, such as the

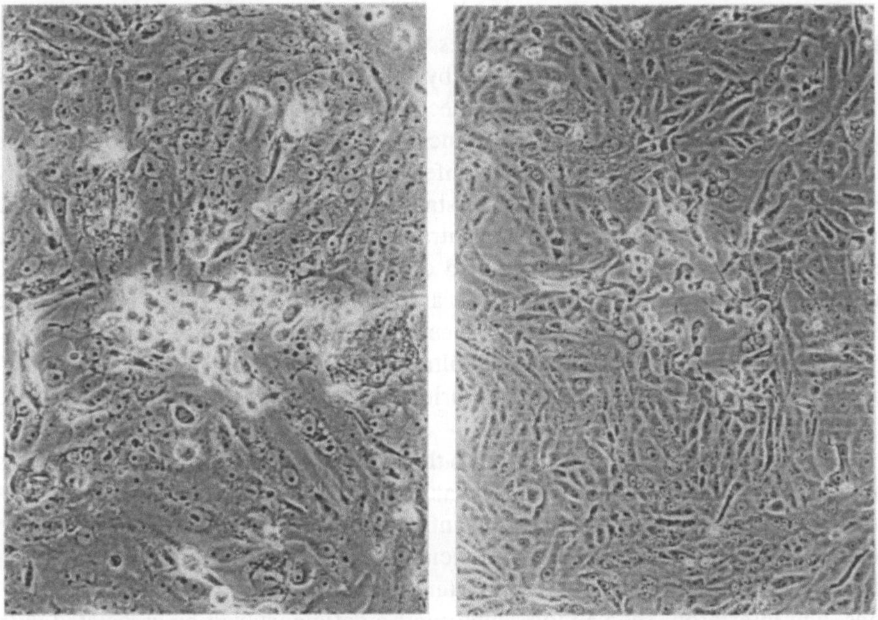

FIGURE 13.5. Cytopathic effects. Left: HSV type 1. Right: HSV type 2.

Leibovitz-Emory, modified Stuart's, or Hanks' balanced salt solution. The medium must be kept at 4°C, as freezing may lower the viral recovery rate significantly. The cell cultures show characteristic cytopathic effects: These begin with granulation; cells enlarge and balloon, become rounded, refractile, and finally lyse. Some strains promote cellular fusion with multinucleated cells; herpes simplex types 1 and 2 are usually readily identifiable from their characteristic cytopathic effects (Fig. 13.5). Cell culture is a relatively rapid technique; 40% of cultures are positive at 24 hours, 82% at 45 hours, and 90% by 3 days.

## HSV Typing

To absolutely differentiate HSV type 1 from 2, neutralization tests, restrictive endonuclease examination, and monoclonal antibody test with either immunofluorescence or immunoperoxidase analyses may be performed. A recent modification has been to perform cell culture (to enhance viral recovery) and then at 24 hours to use a biotin-labeled herpes simplex virus monoclonal antibody with a fluorescent-tagged avidin stain. This is said to have very low false-negative and -positive results. Within the two main HSV types there are many different strains that can be detected via restriction endonuclease analysis. While patients can have both types 1 and 2 and various subtypes either coevally or serially, usually they have only one strain. These data can be used to pinpoint sources of herpes infections, both medically and medicolegally.

### Serologic Tests

Early serologic tests for herpes antibodies were not specific for type 1 or 2. It was noted that acute infections were followed by a relatively rapid rise in IgM antibodies followed by a slower increase in IgG. Recurrent herpes simplex and even herpes zoster infection can be associated with increases in IgM levels, so antibody levels cannot be used to diagnose a primary infection. Maternally derived IgM usually decreases markedly within 6 months postnatally. The antibodies may be detected through a number of tests, including neutralization, complement-fixation, passive hemagglutination, complement-mediated cytolysis, indirect immunofluorescence, and ELISA. To differentiate HSV types 1 and 2 antibodies, the following tests have been used: microneutralization, kinetic neutralization, multiplicity analysis, inhibition passive hemagglutination immunofiltration, ELISA, solid-phase radioimmunoassay, immunoperoxidase, DNA hybridization, and restrictive endonuclease examination.

At the time of the initial infection, both the humoral and cellular immune systems are martialed in the body's defense. The antibodies apparently cannot prevent cell-to-cell spreading, but instead assist with antibody dependent cellular cytotoxicity. In fact, antibody and even complement-deficient patients usually handle herpes infections fairly well. The cellular immune system, including natural killer cells, lymphocytes, and interferon, seems more important; a deficiency can be associated with generalization and prolonged recovery.

## Differential Diagnosis

The differential diagnosis of herpetic pharyngitis includes thrush, aphthous stomatitis, Stevens-Johnson syndrome, other viral and bacterial infections, Behçet's syndrome, and pemphigus. Genital lesions have as their differential diagnosis syphilis, gonorrhea, chancroid, folliculitis, lichen planus, pemphigus, and pemphigoid. The list of vesicular and pustular eruptions in the neonate is much longer: herpes simplex, cytomegalovirus, acne, varicella, miliaria, bullous impetigo, acropustulosis of infancy, erythema toxicum neonatorum, and syphilis [21].

## Management

The types of therapy performed by the medical establishment in an attempt to treat HSV infection have led to a long and often acrimonious debate between partisans and detractors. The list of treatments runs page after page, with each still being used after so-called experts have gone to the next elusive "cure." Some of the more dangerous that should definitely be abandoned are red dye plus light and BCG and vaccinia vaccinations. It should not be necessary to add that levamisole, lysine, zinc, and gamma globulin are equally useless.

## Antiviral Agent

One of the first truly successful therapies was vidarabine (9-B-D-arabinofuranosyl-adenine, adenine arabinoside, Ara-A), a purine nucleoside analogue that is phosphorylated by cellular kinases to a triphosphate, which relatively selectively inhibits viral DNA polymerase. Over 60% of the drug is excreted via the kidneys, and it is widely distributed throughout the body; CNS levels are one third to one half serum levels. Because it is relatively insoluble, it must be administered intravenously with a large amount of fluid over a 12-hour period, daily. Side effects include nausea, vomiting, diarrhea, tremors, parathesias, ataxia, and seizures. Pre-existing neurologic, liver, or kidney problems, or the use of allopurinol, puts the patient at risk for megaloblastic anemia, leukopenia, and thrombocytopenia. While obviously not an ideal drug, it has cut neonatal mortality (from HSV) from 74 to 34% and has been successfully used to treat herpetic encephalitis [22].

Acyclovir, 9-(2-hydroxyethoxymethyl) guanine, is a nucleoside analogue of deoxyguanosine. Reports of its efficacy appeared as early as 1979 [23]. Acyclovir is phosphorylated 30 to 120 times faster (than cellular enzymes) by herpes viral thymidine kinase to acycloguanosine monophosphate. Cellular kinases then phosphorylate it to the active triphosphate form, which inhibits viral DNA polymerase 10 to 30 times more effectively than cellular DNA polymerase. Twenty percent of the oral dose is absorbed; excretion is via glomerular filtration and tubular secretion, so lower doses should be used in patients with renal insufficiency. Intravenous administration may be associated with nausea, vomiting, diarrhea, anorexia, dizziness, and headache, and high doses rarely have been associated with both neurotoxicity and nephrotoxicity. It does not appear to be teratogenic or carcinogenic in animals.

Studies with topical acyclovir in a variety of bases showed that it did decrease viral shedding but only questionably sped healing and decreased pain [24]. Oral acyclovir, five 200-mg capsules per day for 5 days, has been shown to be effective in both primary and recurrent herpes infections:

| | Primary | Recurrent |
|---|---|---|
| Viral shedding | ↓ 70–80% | ↓ 40–50% |
| Duration of symptoms | ↓ 40–50% | ↓ 15–20% |
| Time to heal | ↓ 30–40% | ↓ 20–30% |

Therapy in both primary and recurrent herpes does not prevent further recurrences. As most recurrent lesions, both oral and genital, heal in an average of 4 to 8 days, even a 25% reduction in duration of symptoms and time to heal is at best 2 days, so acyclovir's use in otherwise uncomplicated recurrent herpes simplex infection is not to be encouraged. In patients with frequent recurrences, perhaps monthly or more often, acyclovir may apparently be safely used on a daily basis for 6 months or longer. Some patients may need as little as two 200-mg capsules a day. Use of the drug should periodically be discontinued, as some patients then have fewer recurrences and may not need it. In AIDS patients, 400 to 800 mg five times a day may be necessary for 4 weeks or longer.

In vitro experiments have documented the presence of both TK-negative and polymerase mutants that are resistant to acyclovir. To date, only TK mutants have been seen in humans, and as these TK mutants have a much lessened chance of becoming latent, they have not been a clinical problem.

Foscarnet and phosphonacetic acid (PAP) both act directly on DNA polymerase, and topical foscarnet has been shown to reduce time to crusting if therapy is initiated early enough. Other drugs that are being tested both in the laboratory and in limited field trials include Arildone, BVDU, FIAC, DHBG, EDU, TFT, and 2'-nor-2 deoxyguanosine. Interferon is a species-specific but not viral-specific agent that works against both RNA and DNA viruses. It induces enzymes that block viral reproduction by inhibiting translation of viral mRNA and viral protein. It also enhances NK activity and macrophage activation. It is effective in delaying the onset of perioral herpes after trigeminal ganglion surgery and has been used topically in herpetic keratitis, but the side effects of fever, local pain, anorexia, fatigue, confusion, malaise, alopecia, and hematologic toxicity preclude its systemic use in most cases. In addition, infected cells spontaneously develop high levels of interferon, and it is doubtful if additional exogenous interferon would be of further help.

### Vaccine

Obviously much research is now being dedicated to finding a vaccine to prevent herpes, and the following types are under active investigation: inactivated whole HSV type 2 virus, protein subunits, glycoprotein, HSV type 2 genes inserted into vaccinia virus, and live nonvirulent strains. One of the most promising avenues of research is use of cloned, truncated gB and gD glycoproteins; these have been shown to protect mice and guinea pigs from HSV infections. Human experiments are now under way. Obviously, once a patient has latent herpes, vaccines will not eradicate or prevent recurrences. The problem of the multiplicity of antigenic types and subtypes must also be dealt with.

## Prognosis

The prognosis in the otherwise healthy patient is excellent. With time, recurrence becomes less frequent. Thus, the usual natural course of the disease is encouraging, even though it may take several years for recurrences to diminish to a relatively insignificant frequency.

### References

1. Beswick TSL: The origin and the use of the word herpes. *Med Hist* **6**:214–232, 1962.
2. McNair Scott TF: Historical aspects of herpes simplex infection. *Int J Dermatol* **25**:63–69, 1986.
3. Chang TW: Herpes simplex virus infection. *Int J Dermatol* **22**:1–7, 1983.
4. Reichman R: Herpes simplex virus. In R Belshe (Ed): *Textbook of Human Urology.* Littleton, Mass.: PSG Publishing, 1984, pp. 811–829.

5. Corey L, Spear P: Infections with herpes simplex virus. *N Engl J Med* **313**:686–691; **314**:749–757, 1986.
6. Nerurkar L, et al: Survival of herpes simplex virus. *JAMA* **250**:3081–8083, 1983.
7. Oxford JS, Oberg B: Herpes simplex virus infections. In *Conquest of Viral Diseases*. New York: Elsevier, 1985, pp. 463–536.
8. Nahmias A, Josey W: Herpes simplex viruses 1 and 2. In AS Evans (Ed): *Viral Infections of Humans*. New York: Plenum Medical Books, 1982, pp. 351–372.
9. Stagnno S, Whitley R: Herpes virus infection of Pregnancy. *N Engl J Med* **314**:749–757, 1985.
10. Adam E: Herpes simplex virus infections. In R Glaser, T Gotlieb-Stematsky (Eds): *Human Herpes Virus Infections*. New York: Marcel Dekker, 1982, pp. 1–57.
11. Reeves W, et al: Risk of recurrence after 1st episodes of genital herpes. *N Engl J Med* **305**:**306**:315–319, 1981.
12. Rawls W: Herpes simplex virus infections. In E Lonnette (Ed): *Laboratory Diagnosis of Viral Infections*. New York: Marcel Dekker, 1985, pp. 313–329.
13. Lever W, Schaumburg-Lever G: *Histopathology of the Skin*. 6th ed. New York: Lippincott, 1983, pp. 361–365.
14. Mclean D, Wong K: *Same Day Diagnosis of Human Virus Infections*. Florida: CRC Press, 1984, pp. 46–56.
15. Becker Y: Herpes simplex virus type 1. Thymidine kinase controls virus pathogenesis and latency in the nervous system. In A Kohn, P Fuchs (Eds): *Mechanisms of Viral Pathogenesis*. Boston: Nijhoff, 1984, pp. 293–308.
16. Stagnno S, Whitley R: Herpes virus infection of pregnancy. *N Engl J Med* **313**:1327–1330, 1985.
17. Prober CG, Hensleigh PA, Boucher FD, et al: Low risk of herpes simplex Infections in Neonates. *N Engl J Med* **316**: 240–244, 1987.
18. Tomita Y: Detection of Human papilloma virus DNA in genital warts, cervical dysplasia and neoplasms. *Intervirology* **25**:151–157, 1986.
19. Lopez C, Roizman B: *Human Herpes Virus Infections*. New York: Raven Press, 1986.
20. Barr R, Herten J, Graham J: Rapid method for Tzanck preparations. *JAMA* **237**: 1119–1120, 1977.
21. Behlmer S, Anderson P: Herpes simplex infections complicating parturition. *Int J Dermatol* **20**:242–248, 1981.
22. Hirsh M, Schooley R: Treatment of herpes simplex infections. *N Engl J Med* **309**:963–970, 1983.
23. Collins P, Baker DJ: Activity in vitro against herpes virus of acycloguanosine. *J Antimicrob Chemother* **5**:431–436, 1979.
24. Hirsh M, Schooley R: Treatment of herpes virus infections. *N Engl J Med* **309**:1034–1039, 1983.

CHAPTER 14

# Condyloma Acuminatum

Barbara M. Rock

## Overview

Condyloma acuminatum has been of increasing interest and concern in recent years. The incidence of infection increased fivefold in the 15-year period between 1966 and 1981 [1]. Estimates of the prevalence of genital tract human papillomavirus (HPV) infection in women vary from 3 to 28%, depending upon the population studied [2].

Although condylomata acuminata are benign growths, there is a well-established association of wart virus infection with genital tract malignancies. HPV DNA sequences can be found in approximately 90% of cervical carcinomas and probably an equal number of vulvar carcinomas. A significant number of penile carcinomas have also been shown to contain HPV DNA sequences [3].

Hampering study of HPV infection has been the difficulty in producing in vitro multiplication of the complete, infective virus. The papillomavirus requires a stratified epithelium for normal growth and differentiation. Keratinocytes in tissue culture do not mimic the in vivo pattern of growth. New laboratory methods for DNA hybridization that use in situ and extraction techniques have widely expanded the current understanding of papillomavirus infection.

## Synonyms

Synonyms for condyloma acuminatum are venereal warts, genital warts, penile warts, anogenital warts, and acuminate warts.

## Definition

Condylomata acuminata are papillomatous growths found in the urogenital, perineal, and perianal regions caused by infection with the human papillomavirus. Papillomavirus is one of two genera in the papovavirus family (the other being polyomavirus). HPV is characterized by a 55-nm virion size, an icosahedral capsid, and double-stranded circular DNA of 8,000 base pairs. HPV infects epithelial tissue and

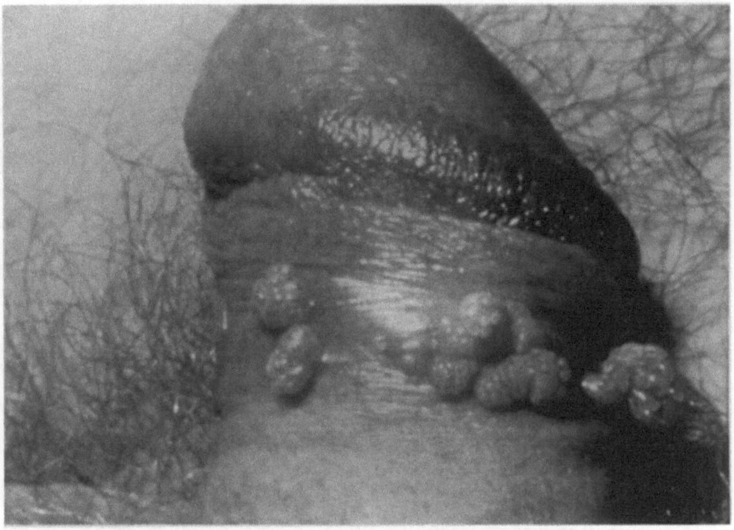

FIGURE 14.1. Typical penile condylomata acuminatum.

multiplies in the nucleus of infected cells. There is no good evidence for a viremia in patients with HPV infection. The abnormal cellular proliferation caused by this virus occurs at the site of inoculation. The virus requires a differentiating squamous epithelium for growth and production of mature viral particles capable of infecting other epithelial tissue. The HPV types causing condylomata acuminata infect both skin and mucous membranes, particularly of the intertriginous areas.

Currently more than 40 HPV types have been described. Only a few of these are generally associated with condylomata acuminata–HPV types 6, 11, 16, 18, and 31. Other HPV types are more rarely seen. Types 6 and 11 are the most commonly seen in condylomata acuminata. Types 16 and 18 are seen more rarely, but these lesions have more potential for malignant transformation [3]. There is no well-established way to distinguish clinically which condylomatous lesions are caused by those HPV types more often associated with malignant transformation [4].

## Clinical Findings

Condylomata acuminata are seen most often in young, sexually active adults. The age distribution parallels that of other sexually transmitted diseases. The incubation period varies from several weeks to several months. In some cases an inconspicuous infection may last for years in the form of cervical flat warts, penile flat condylomata [5], or other subclinical eruptions.

In men, condylomata acuminata are typically skin colored to slightly pink or white verrucous papules. The lesions may be solitary or confluent, taking on the typical "cauliflower" appearance (Fig. 14.1). They are often seen at the frenulum

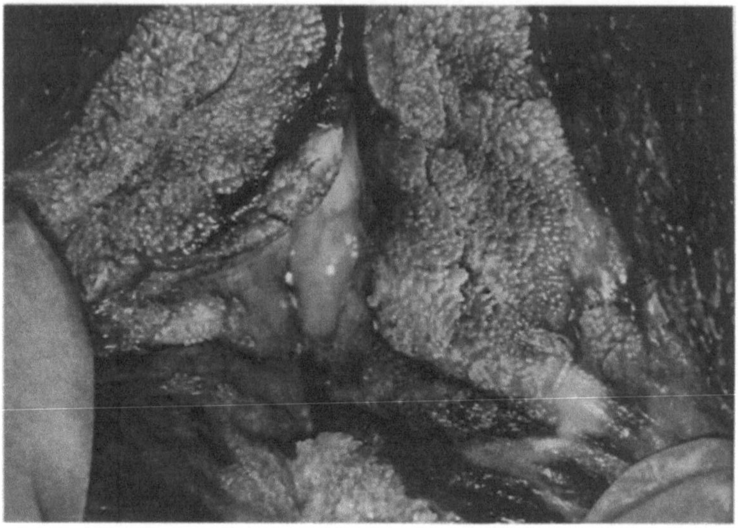

FIGURE 14.2. Extensive vulvar condylomata acuminata.

and coronal sulcus but may be seen anywhere along the penile shaft as well as on the glans, particularly the meatal region. When meatal involvement is seen, urethral involvement should be suspected. Anal and perianal lesions are common, particularly in homosexuals but also in heterosexuals. Direct extension from genital lesions as well as inoculation during anal intercourse can occur.

In women, the condylomata are morphologically similar to those in men. They are found in the introital region, labia minora, and labia majora (Fig. 14.2). Involvement of the perianal and perineal regions may be seen. Extension onto the thigh is unusual. Vaginal and cervical condylomata (Fig. 14.3) should be suspected whenever vulvar lesions are seen.

In both men and women, papillomavirus infection can range from a mild eruption that is asymptomatic to large papillomatous growths with a tendency to irritation, traumatic ulceration, and secondary infection. The lesions may be associated with pruritus and burning. With large exophytic lesions, pain and fissuring can occur.

## Histology

Characteristic histologic features of condyloma acuminatum include acanthosis, papillomatosis, and parakeratosis overlying the epithelial projections (Fig. 14.4). Perinuclear vacuolization forming the classic koilocytic cells are predominantly seen in the upper stratum malpighii. The koilocytic cells should be distinguished from the normal vacuolization seen in the superficial portion of all mucosal surfaces. Immunoperoxidase staining for HPV antigens demonstrates positivity pre-

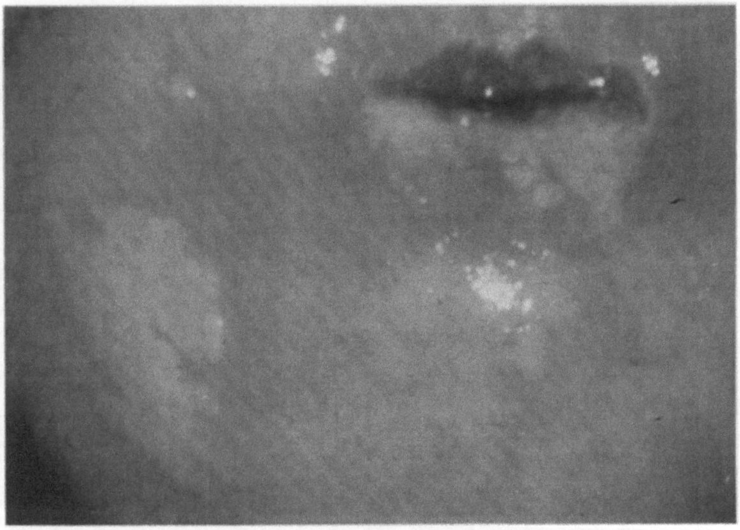

FIGURE 14.3. Cervical flat warts.

dominantly in the koilocytic cells. Vascular dilatation and a lymphohistiocytic infiltrate are generally present in the dermis.

Mitotic figures may be seen in condylomata acuminata, but other features of carcinoma generally are not found. Features indicative of Bowen's disease, erythroplasia of Queyrat, or vulvar intraepithelial neoplasia include atypical mitotic figures, pleomorphic nuclei, and a disorganized growth pattern. Koilocytic cells may be seen in benign, premalignant, and malignant lesions with diminishing frequency from benign to malignant. Occasionally condylomata are biopsied shortly after podophyllin treatment. The specimen may then have arrested mitotic figures and other atypical features including unusually large and atypical keratinocytes in the upper layers of the epidermis (so-called podophyllin cells). Because these changes simulate malignancy it is important for the pathologist to have a good clinical history to prevent the misdiagnosis of neoplasia.

There are two other clinical entities in the histologic differential of condyloma acuminatum: bowenoid papulosis and verrucous carcinoma. Bowenoid papulosis is the current designation given to an HPV infection of the genitalia that clinically resembles condyloma but histologically is more consistent with squamous cell carcinoma in situ [6]. These lesions have the features of vulvar intraepithelial neoplasia along with prominent koilocytic cells and evidence of viral change. They have been shown to spontaneously resolve in some cases, but generally should be treated as premalignant lesions.

Verrucous carcinoma, previously known as giant condyloma of Buschke and Lowenstein, shares some of the histologic features of condyloma acuminatum. Distinguishing features include much more extensive papillomatosis, deep penetration

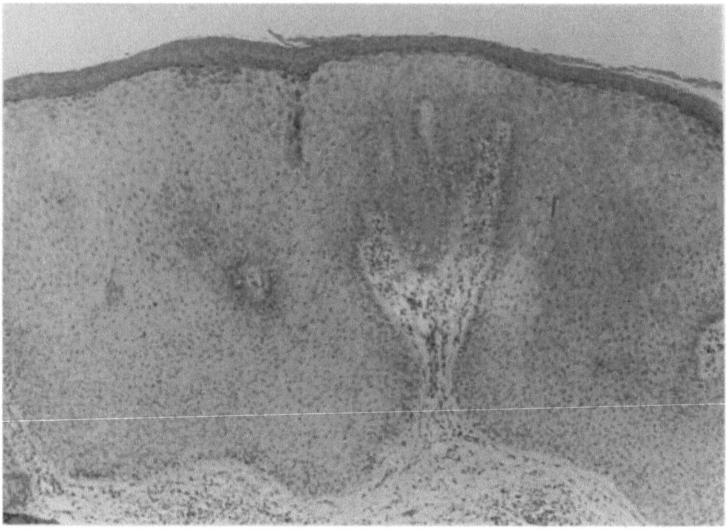

a

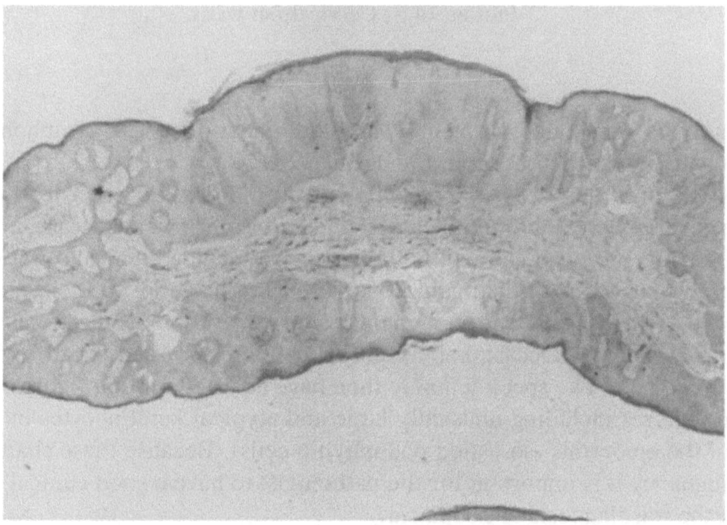

b

FIGURE 14.4. (a) Histology of condyloma acuminatum including acanthosis, papillomatosis, parakeratosis, and koilocytosis, (b) higher magnification of (a).

of the underlying tissue with broad epithelial strands, and tendency to recur after excision. Verrucous carcinoma is a low-grade squamous cell carcinoma associated with HPV infection [7].

## Natural History

Papillomavirus infection causing condyloma acuminatum is spread by direct contact in the genital area with an infected individual. The trauma of sexual intercourse may play a role in inoculation. The reservoir of papillomavirus infection is generally, but not always, in clinically apparent condylomata. Lesions inapparent on external exam in the female include cervical flat warts or papillomas and vaginal papillomas. In the male they include urethral papillomas and penile flat condylomata. There is no convincing evidence that condylomata acuminata are spread from common hand warts. Studies of G-6PD heterozygous women support a monoclonal etiology of genital warts [8]. The finding of multiple HPV types in individual lesions relates to infection with more than one viral type and the confluence of discrete monoclonal papillomas.

Several studies have assessed the infectivity rate of papillomavirus. Most of these studies have evaluated male partners of women with condylomata acuminata or with viral changes in Papanicolaou smears. Sand et al [9] evaluated 91 male partners of women with biopsy-proven condyloma and found that 69% of the men were affected. Schneider et al [4] evaluated male consorts of 40 women with cervical HPV infection and found 65% to be infected. Interestingly, only 48% shared the same viral type that was found in the woman. Sedlacek et al [10] demonstrated the value of magnification during examination after acetic acid swabbing of the penis. In 51 men who were partners of women with condyloma, only 8 had grossly visible lesions. Thirty-five additional cases were diagnosed when magnification was used. This brought the total percent of partners affected to 88%. These data of course do not take into consideration the number of sexual encounters before infection, history of antecedent infection, number of sexual partners, and other possible risk factors. Host immunity probably plays a role in those partners who are found to be free of infection after thorough evaluation.

Children may develop condyloma acuminatum (Fig. 14.5). Most often this is the result of sexual abuse by an infected adult. If the child is less than 1 year old at the time of infection, exposure to the virus during passage through an infected birth canal is possible. "Innocent" inoculation through close contact such as bathing together has been speculated but not proven. The viral types causing condyloma acuminatum in children are the same as those causing disease in adults [11].

Immunity to papillomavirus infection involves both humoral and cell-mediated factors [12,13]. Cell-mediated immunity is felt to be the most significant. Warts may resolve after dinitrochlorobenzene sensitization and treatment, and also with other immune adjuvants. Patients with depressed cell-mediated immunity, such as renal transplant recipients, patients with lymphoproliferative disease, and AIDS patients, tend to have more extensive disease. Spontaneous resolution of other HPV infections such as verruca vulgaris is a well-known phenomemon, even without

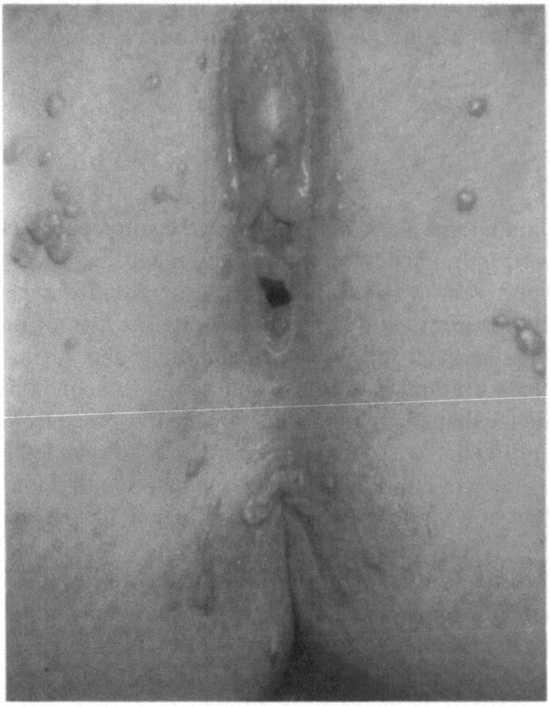

FIGURE 14.5. Condylomata acuminata in a 2-year-old child.

obvious trauma or inflammation. Improvement of condyloma acuminatum post partum has been seen. The exact incidence of spontaneous remission in condyloma acuminatum is not known. Because of the known risk of malignancy associated with HPV infection, a long-term prospective study of untreated condyloma acuminatum would be difficult.

## Complications

Condyloma acuminatum may be asymptomatic in many patients. As the lesions enlarge, or become more numerous, the patient may complain of pruritus or irritation. Still larger lesions may fissure, ulcerate, and become superficially infected. Urethral or meatal lesions may cause urinary burning and rarely, urinary retention. Large anal and perianal lesions may cause painful or difficult defecation with blood streaking of stools.

Extensive involvement of the cervix, vagina, or vulva in a pregnant woman may necessitate cesarean section because of the difficulty of delivery [14]. One serious complication of spontaneous delivery through an infected birth canal is the rare possibility of the development of respiratory papillomatosis in the child [15]. For this reason most obstetricians do not delay appropriate treatment of condylomata acuminata during pregnancy. Cesarean section is considered if treatment of extensive disease has not been possible prior to delivery.

The HPV types causing condylomata acuminata also cause mucosal papillomas at nongenital body sites. These include conjunctival papillomas [16] and some types of oral papillomas [17]. Presumably these are spread by direct contact with infected body sites.

Malignancy is certainly the most significant complication of HPV infection. As noted in the overview, the vast majority of cervical and vulvar carcinomas tested by nucleic acid hybridization techniques have been associated with HPV genetic material. The viral genetic material tends to be integrated into host DNA in malignant cells. The number of patients with clinically uncomplicated condyloma acuminatum who will go on to develop carcinoma of the genital tract is not known. The ability to do viral typing in a routine fashion would be somewhat predictive because of the greater association of types 16 and 18 with malignancy. These types, of course, are not often found in benign lesions [3,4].

The precise mechanisms for virally induced transformation in HPV infection is not known. Certain cofactors or cocarcinogens may play a significant role as well as host immune surveillance.

## Differential Diagnosis

The differential diagnosis of condyloma acuminatum includes both benign and malignant lesions. A frequently misdiagnosed anatomic variant in men is the group of lesions known as pearly penile papules [18]. These are firm, 1- to 2-mm papules found in rows at the edge of the corona. They are most often seen in uncircumcised men. Pearly penile papules are histologically differentiated from warts by lack of significant acanthosis and lack of koilocytic cells. Sebaceous hyperplasia, epidermal inclusion cysts, syringomas, nevi, fibroepithelial polyps, and various adnexal tumors should all be differentiated from condylomata. Some inflammatory dermatoses such as lichen nitidus, lichen planus, and psoriasis may initially be confused with condyloma. Condyloma lata, or secondary syphilis in the genital region, may mimic condyloma acuminatum as well.

In women, similar sorts of benign tumors occur and should be differentiated from condyloma acuminatum. Another benign condition is Fordyce spots, or ectopic sebaceous glands, which occur on oral and genital mucosa. They are 1- to 2-mm slightly yellow papules that are generally symmetric and evenly distributed on the mucosal surface. Vulvar porokeratosis may rarely resemble and be confused with condylomata. In both men and women, if there is any doubt at all about the diagnosis of condyloma acuminatum, a simple biopsy with the patient under local anesthesia should be done. This will help avoid unnecessary and inappropriate treatment.

Malignant conditions must also be differentiated from benign HPV infection. Any ulcerated lesion, abnormally large lesion, or clinically suspicious lesion should be evaluated for in situ or invasive carcinoma. Lesions that do not respond to treatment should similarly be evaluated. Verrucous carcinoma, which may also be virally induced, should be suspected in large, destructive lesions [7]. Bowenoid papulosis clinically resembles condyloma but histologically has features of vulvar intraepithelial neoplasia. It has been associated with HPV-16 [6].

## Management

Several factors have to be considered in managing patients with condyloma acuminatum. Because it is a sexually transmitted disease, evidence for other sexually transmitted diseases must be sought. The patient should be educated to the mode of transmission and his or her likelihood of spreading the infection. A condom is generally recommended as a form of barrier protection. Though the precise number of patients who might go on to develop malignancy related to the HPV infection is not known, the patient should be informed of this association. Recurrence rates are high in HPV infection partly because of "subclinical" infection and also because of the persistence of viral genome in clinically normal-appearing skin adjacent to areas of condylomatous involvement [19,20].

Careful physical examination with a high index of suspicion for internal involvement is important. All women with external lesions of condyloma acuminatum need to be evaluated for cervical and vaginal involvement. This of course includes a Pap smear looking for early signs of dysplasia. Anoscopy is indicated for patients with perianal disease. Urethroscopy may be indicated when meatal condylomata are present, particularly if abnormalities are seen on voiding cystourethrography [21]. Soaking the genital region with 3 to 5% acetic acid for 5 minutes before evaluation may highlight some of the more subtle lesions, particularly when magnification with a hand lens or a colposcope is used. If there is any doubt in the diagnosis, a simple biopsy with the patient under local anesthesia should be done.

There are several modes of treatment in men and women depending on the clinical setting and patient preference. External exophytic warts may be treated with podophyllin resin 25% in tincture of benzoin. Podophyllin is a resin obtained from the rhizome of the plant *Podophyllin peltatum* in North America. Its primary action is to arrest mitosis in metaphase, thus causing epithelial cell death. Additionally, it has an irritant effect. Podophyllin is most effective on individual, new, moist lesions. It is somewhat less effective on keratinized lesions of the penile shaft and vulvar skin. Podophyllin is applied to individual lesions by the physician and allowed to dry. The treated area is washed off 4 to 6 hours later. The expected response is sloughing of the treated epithelium. Local side effects include pain, edema, and ulceration. Systemic toxicity includes gastrointestinal distress, peripheral neuropathy, tachycardia, acute renal disease, cytopenias, coma, and death. Podophyllin is a teratogen and should not be used in pregnancy. To reduce side effects the area treated should be limited to 2 $cm^2$ and application repeated no more frequently than once per week. Treatment of internal mucous membranes and treatment during pregnancy should be avoided [22].

Solitary lesions on the penis and vulva can be treated with cryotherapy, electrodessication, or, least often, surgical excision. Flat condylomata of the vagina, vulva, and penis can be treated with trichloracetic acid 50 to 90% that is applied by the physician directly to the lesions. Cervical lesions can be treated with cryosurgery or laser photocoagulation after appropriate biopsy.

Extensive condylomatous lesions require more definitive treatment. Fulguration with the $CO_2$ laser is very effective for lesions at most body sites. This can be done with regional or general anesthesia, depending on the site treated. Alternatively, for vaginal warts topical 5% 5-fluorouracil cream may be instilled into the vagina on a daily or alternate-day regimen as tolerated for five treatments. Even with barrier cream protection to the urinary meatus and vulva, severe irritation often develops. 5-Fluorouracil is an antimetabolite and should not be used in pregnancy [23]. In general, urethral, vaginal, cervical, and intraanal lesions should be treated by the appropriate specialist. Often a combination of treatment modalities is needed.

There have been several reports of the use of interferon in the treatment of warts. A large, double-blind, randomized trial of interferon alpha-2b with placebo showed a statistically significant decrease in wart size was found in the interferon group [24]. Side effects in the treated group included fever and malaise, as well as a mild to moderate transient leukopenia in 26 of 89 patients. Similar results were seen in a recent study of natural interferon alpha [25]. The role of interferon as an adjuvant to treatment in resistant condylomata versus as a primary mode of therapy has yet to be determined. Interferon ALFA-26 (Intron A) is now commercially available from Schering-Plough (Kenilworth, NJ).

Whatever the mode of therapy chosen, close follow-up is essential. Patients not responding to treatment should be reevaluated for possible misdiagnosis either for other benign genital eruptions or for malignancy.

## Prognosis

Condylomata acuminata are benign growths induced by HPV infection that have premalignant potential in a small percentage of patients over a long period of time. Recurrence rates may be as high as 33% after appropriate therapy, probably because of persistence of latent papillomavirus infection in clinically normal-appearing skin [19]. Because the lesions may be clinically subtle and asymptomatic and do not threaten the overall health of the individual, treatment may be unfortunately delayed. Eradication of the infection should be sought. This may require multiple patient visits and treatment modalities. Follow-up visits are essential to treat recurrences early on and to monitor for changes suggestive of malignancy.

### References

1. Condyloma acuminatum—United States, 1966–1981: Current trends. *MMWR* **32**:306–308, 1983.
2. Shah KV, Gissman L: Papovaviruses. In NJ Schmidt, RW Emmons, et al (Eds): *Diagnostic Procedures for Viral, Rickettsial and Chlamydial Infections*. 6th ed. American Public Health Association, Washington, DC. (in preparation.)
3. Gissman L, Schneider A: Human papillomavirus DNA in preneoplastic and neoplastic genital lesions. In R Peto, H zur Hansen (Eds): *Banbury Report 21*. New York: Cold Spring Harbor, 1986, pp. 217–224.
4. Schneider A, Sawada E, Gissman L, et al: Human papillomavirus in women with a history of abnormal papanicolaou smears and in their male partners. *Obstet Gynecol* **69**:554–562, 1987.

5. Rosemberg SK: Subclinical papilloma viral infection of male genitalia. *Urology* **26**:554–557, 1985.
6. Obalek S, Jablonska S, Beaudenon S, et al: Bowenoid papulosis of the male and female genitalia: Risk of cervical neoplasia. *J Am Acad Dermatol* **14**:433–444, 1986.
7. Kao GF, Graham JH, Helwig EB: Carcinoma cuniculatum (verrucous carcinoma of the skin). *Cancer* **49**:2395–2403, 1982.
8. Buscema J, Shah K, Hsu S, et al: Genetic investigation of the cellular origin of vulvovaginal condylomata acuminata. In B Steinberg, Brandsma J, Taichman L (Eds): *Cancer Cells*. Vol. 5, *Papillomavirus*. New York: Cold Spring Harbor, 1987, pp. 245–247.
9. Sand PK, Bowen LW, Blischke SO, et al: Evaluation of male consorts of women with genital human papilloma virus infection. *Obstet Gynecol* **68**:679–681, 1980.
10. Sedlacek TV, Cunnane M, Carpiniello V: Colposcopy in the diagnosis of penile condyloma. *Am J Obstet Gynecol* **154**:494–496, 1986.
11. Rock B, Naghashfar Z, Barnett N, et al: Genital tract papillomavirus infection in children. *Arch Dermatol* 122:1129–1132, 1986.
12. Kienzler J: Humoral immunity to human papillomavirus. *Clin Dermatol* **3**(4):144–155, 1985.
13. Chardonnet Y, Viac J, Thivolet J: Cell-mediated immunity to human papillomavirus. In S Jablonska, G Orth (Eds): *Warts/Human Papillomavirus. Clin Dermatol* **3**(4):156–164, 1985.
14. Young RL, Acosta AA, Kaufman RH, et al: The treatment of large condylomata acuminata complicating pregnancy. *Obstet Gynecol* **41**:65–73, 1973.
15. Mounts P, Shah KV, Kashima H: Viral etiology of juvenile- and adult-onset squamous papilloma of the larynx. *Proc Natl Acad Sci* **79**:5425–5429, 1982.
16. Lass JH, Grove AS, Papale JJ, et al. Detection of human papillomavirus DNA sequences in conjunctival papilloma. *Am J Ophthalmol* **96**:670–674, 1983.
17. Naghashfar Z, Sawada E, Kutcher MJ, et al. Identification of genital tract papillomaviruses HPV-6 and HPV-16 in warts of the oral cavity. *J Virol* **17**:313–324, 1985.
18. Johnson BL, Baxter DL: Pearly penile papules. *Arch Dermatol* **90**:166–169, 1964.
19. Ferenczy A, Mitao M, Nagai N, et al: Latent papillomavirus and recurring genital warts. *N Engl J Med* **313**:784–788, 1985.
20. Macnab JCM, Walkinshaw SA, Cordiner JW, et al: Human papillomavirus in clinically and histologically normal tissue of patients with genital cancer. *N Engl J Med* **315**: 1052–1058, 1986.
21. Pollack HM, DeBenedictis TJ, Marmar JL, et al: Urethrographic manifestations of venereal warts (condyloma acuminatum). *Radiology* **126**:643–646, 1978.
22. Miller RA: Podophyllin. *Int J Dermatol* **24**:491–498, 1985.
23. Ferenczy A: Comparison of 5-fluorouracil and $CO_2$ laser for treatment of vaginal condylomata. *Obstet Gynecol* **64**:773–778, 1984.
24. Eron LJ, Judson F, Tucker S: Interferon therapy for condylomata acuminata. *N Engl J Med* **315**: 1059–1064, 1986.
25. Friedman-Kien AE, Eron LJ, Conant M: Natural interferon alpha for treatment of Condylomata acuminata. *JAMA* **259**: 533–538, 1988.

CHAPTER 15

# Molluscum Contagiosum

R.F.E. de Wit

## Overview

Molluscum contagiosum (Latin *molluscus* [soft], *contagiosum* [infectious]) is, as the name suggests, a contagious soft tumor. Proof for the contagiousness of the affliction is available from different sources. Koebner's phenomenon, an autoinoculation resulting in a linear distribution of the lesions, is seen in children (Fig. 15.1). Small epidemics of molluscum contagiosum in families, school classes, and a small group of wrestlers [1] show further evidence for an infectious nature. The presence of similar lesions on the genitals of both partners suggests the possibility of transmission by sexual contact. In most STD clinics, however, molluscum contagiosum is a minor problem, affecting fewer than 1 in 1,000 new patients, mostly young adults. Conclusive inoculation experiments on volunteers, unfortunately, are not mentioned in the literature. Spontaneous healing without scar formation occurs after 6 to 12 months. Often secondary impetiginization due to scratching is seen. Sometimes the lesion is solitary and more persistent.

## Synonyms

Synonyms for molluscum contagiosum are epithelioma contagiosum, condyloma porcelaneum, and molluscum epitheliale.

## Definition

Molluscum contagiosum is a benign hemispherical tumor of the skin caused by the 200-μm poxvirus mollusci. This virus has no cross-antigenicity [2] with other members of the poxvirus group. Culture is possible on human chorion-allantoin membrane. Inoculation on HeLa cells results in cytopathic changes without viral duplication.

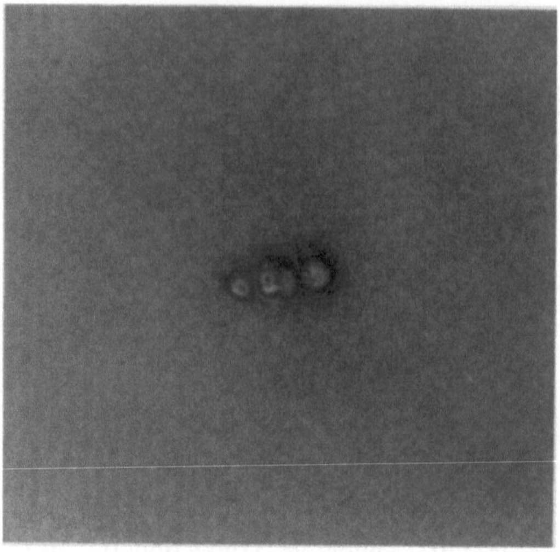

FIGURE 15.1. Linear distribution (Koebner's phenomenon) of molluscum contagiosum lesions in a child.

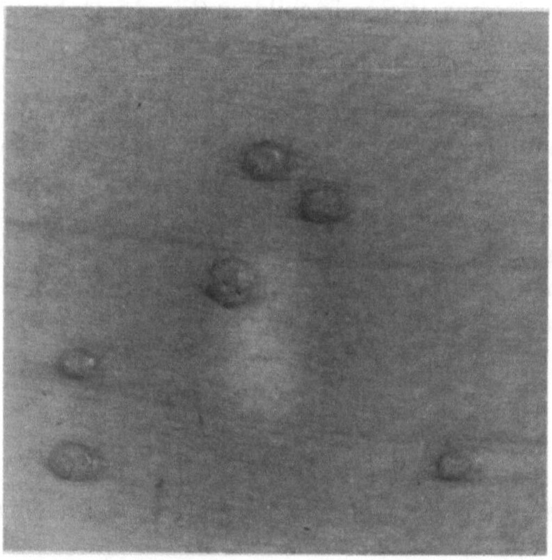

FIGURE 15.2. Molluscum contagiosum. Umbilicated pearly white or pink papulonodules.

FIGURE 15.3. Numerous umbilicated lesions of molluscum contagiosum in a patient with AIDS.

## Clinical Findings

Principle sites of involvement are the genitals, face, and hands; however, all parts of the skin may be affected, even the soles of the feet [3]. In some widely spread infections, lesions are seen on the buccal mucosa, lips, and tongue. The papulonodular lesions are often grouped and consist of hemispherical, pearly pinkish white, shining, 3- to 10-mm large tumors with a central "delle" (Fig. 15.2). A whitish paste is easily squeezed out of this delle. The paste is composed of degenerated epithelial cells and keratin. When the papules are small, they are easily overlooked or misinterpreted as vesicles. A pathologist's diagnosis may then surprise the clinician. To prevent this, the dermatologist can accentuate the central delle of the mollusk by ethyl chloride freezing, an easy diagnostic procedure. The number of lesions per patient varies. In a widely spread infection, as is often seen in atopic patients [4] and in immunocompromised hosts (Fig. 15.3) up to 1,000 papules may be found. On the other hand, solitary papulonodules exist (Fig. 15.4) with diameters as large as a giant 20 mm.

## Histopathology

The target cells for the virus are those in the basal layer of the epidermis [5]. These cells become swollen, while inclusion bodies—virus particles—are visible in the cytoplasm. The nucleus of affected cells is pressed aside. The resulting gigantic cells with inclusion bodies are known as molluscum cells.

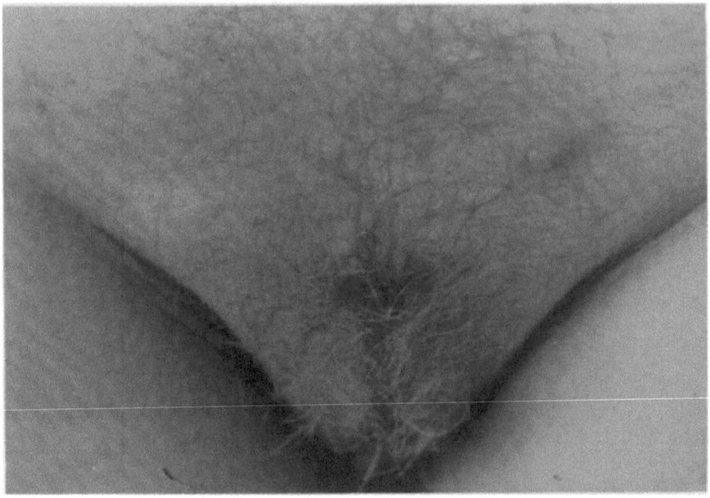

FIGURE 15.4. Solitary molluscum contagiosum lesion in pubic region.

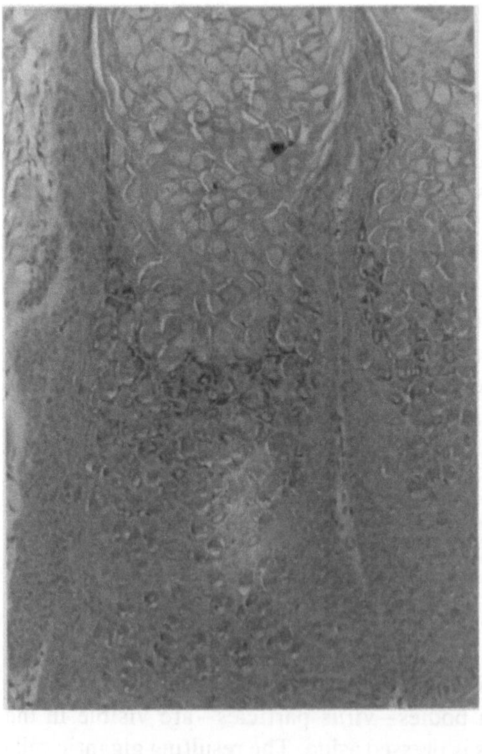

FIGURE 15.5. Typical pear-shaped lobules of molluscum contagiosum in the basal keratinocytes. Development of molluscum bodies can be observed.

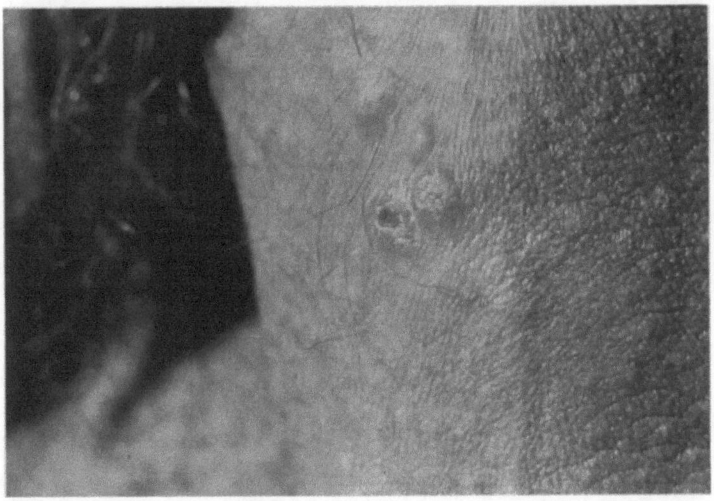

FIGURE 15.6. Herpetiform distribution of molluscum contagiosum lesions on penis.

Proliferation of basal cells occurs also, leading to hyperplasia of the epidermis that invaginates the dermis as lobules (Fig. 15.5). These lobules are separated from each other by thin septa of fibrous tissue. In the center of a lobule the molluscum cells are surrounded by granular keratinocytes. Together, they form the paste that may be squeezed out of the delle.

Newer studies have revealed changes in the basal cells such as abortive differentiation toward hairs or new pilosebaceous units [5]. The way by which the virus particles reach the target basal cells is unknown.

## Natural History

Molluscum contagiosum is found throughout the world, but reliable data on its incidence are not available. Age peaks are influenced by communal living conditions, and vary from 1 to 4 years of age in Zaire to 10 to 15 years in Western Europe.

In sexually transmitted infections, the anogenital region is usually involved [6] (Figs. 15.6, 15.7). In other cases, the distribution of the lesions over the body seems to be influenced by climate and the resulting clothing patterns. Most mollusks are found on exposed skin areas.

In typical cases, 10 to 50 nodules appear after an estimated incubation period of 2 to 7 weeks. These tend to enlarge for the next 1 to 3 months. The attained maximal diameter measures 3 to 10 mm, rarely 20 to 25 mm (usually in solitary cases). Some 6 to 12 months (rarely several years) later, spontaneous involution results in a cure without scar formation. In the last months of the disease, inflammatory changes may occur (Fig. 15.8), resulting in suppuration or eczematous reactions. In most

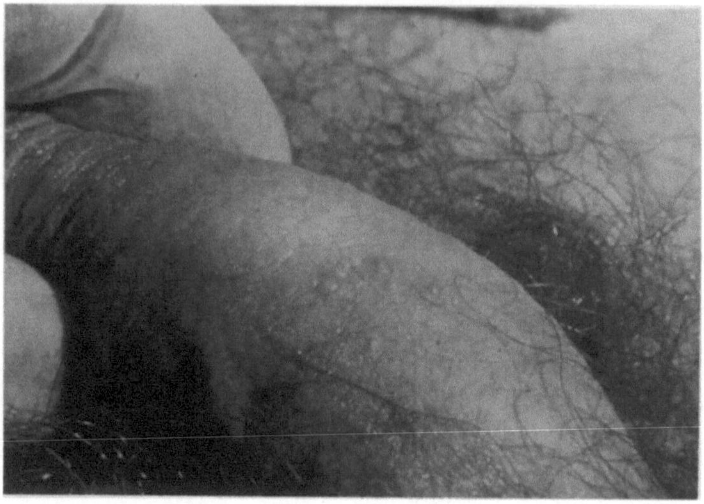

FIGURE 15.7. Typical cluster of molluscum contagiosum lesions as seen in transmission by sexual contact.

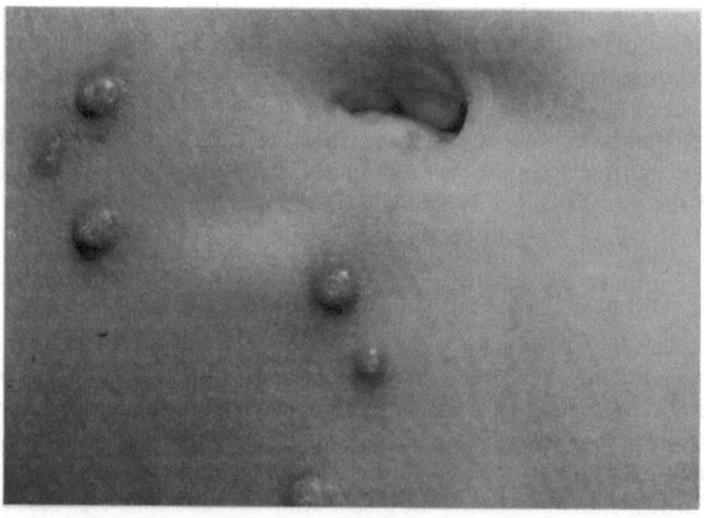

FIGURE 15.8. Lesions of molluscum contagiosum with surrounding local inflammation.

FIGURE 15.9. Dense inflammatory reaction around a lesion of molluscum contagiosum, indicating cellular immune response.

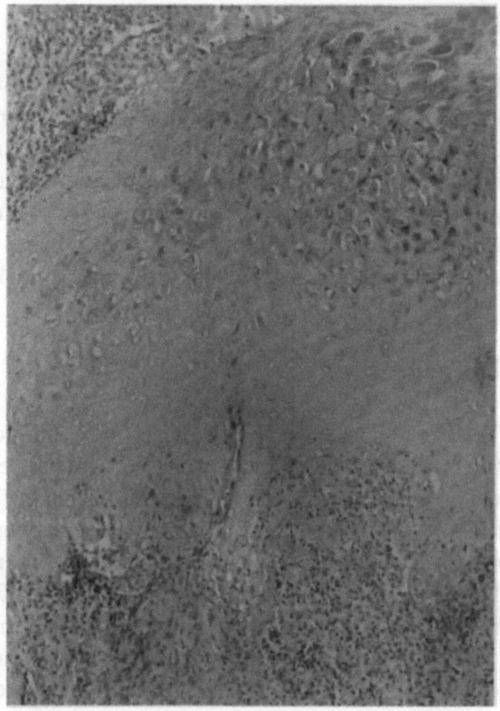

cases the attack of molluscum contagiosum is self-limiting within the first year, and only after a secondary infection has occurred should scar formation be feared.

## Complications

In some 10% of cases, an irritating nummular dermatitis is found around the nodules. This will lead to secondary infection after scratching, and may induce spreading of the mollusks to various parts of the skin. This dermatitis will fade quickly after the mollusks are removed. Infection of the eyelids sometimes results in conjunctivitis and keratitis punctata. Patients receiving immunosuppressive drugs or corticosteroids, as well as patients with AIDS [7] may show an extensive eruption (Fig. 15.3).

A few cases of perinodular depigmentation around a lesion, or the development of a halo nevus, have been reported. In the last event, the mollusk formed on top of a nevus pigmentosus. The immune mechanisms are uncertain. In 85% of patients with molluscum contagiosum, humoral antibodies are demonstrated. In patients with an expected sexual transmission, examination for other sexually transmitted diseases is advisable.

## Differential Diagnosis

Diagnosis of molluscum contagiosum is obvious when multiple lesions are present. In case of solitary giant lesions, secondary infected lesions, or small lesions, the differential diagnosis with the following ailments may pose a problem: herpes infection (in case of inflammation), ulcus durum, verruca vulgaris, verruca plana juvenilis, condyloma acuminatum, condyloma latum, syringoma, hydrocystoma, fibroma, milium, pyogenic granuloma, basal cell carcinoma, and furunculus. The effect of superficial freezing with ethyl chloride may help to discriminate.

## Management

Treatment is necessary because of the contagiousness of the disease and sometimes the long-standing itch or cosmetic disturbances. The treatment of choice in individual cases will depend on the localization of the lesions. It may also vary individually.

Removal with a curet under local hypesthesia by freezing with ethyl chloride is very effective, as is electrocoagulation or cryocoagulation with liquid nitrogen. Painting with liquor iodii fortior or with 20% podophyllin in acetone gives good results but may have to be repeated for a rather long period.

Another effective possibility is the application of retinoic acid, 0.1% solution (contraindicated for the skin area around the eyes). In widely spread infections, etretinate 0.25 to 1 mg/kg body weight, has been successfully used but with much caution. In some cases removal under total anesthesia may be advisable.

## Prognosis

Prognosis is good. Complete spontaneous involution of the papules can be expected in 6 months to 1 year.

## References

1. Overfield ThM, Brody JA: An epidemiologic study of molluscum contagiosum in Anchorage, Alaska. *J Pediat* **69**:640–642, 1966.
2. Naseman TH: Molluscum contagiosum. In *Viral Diseases of the Skin, Mucous Membranes and Genitals*, Stuttgart: Georg Thieme, 1977, p. 67.
3. Dickinson A, Tschen JA, Wolf JE: Giant molluscum contagiosum of the sole. *Cutis* **32**:239–1243, 1983.
4. Solomon LM, Telner P: Eruptive molluscum contagiosum in atopic dermatitis. *Canad Med Assoc J* **95**:978–979, 1966.
5. Reed RJ, Parkinson RP: The histogenesis of molluscum contagiosum. *Am J Surg Pathol* **1**:161–166, 1977.
6. Menke HE: Molluscum contagiosum. In JRW Harris (ed): *Recent Advances in Sexually Transmitted Diseases*. Vol 2. Edinburgh: Churchill-Livingstone, 1981, p. 247.

7. Redfield RR, James WD, Wright DC et al: Severe molluscum contagiosum infection in a patient with human T cell lymphotrophic (HTLV-III) disease. *J Am Acad Dermatol* **13**:821–824, 1985.

CHAPTER 16

# Behçet's Disease

Reynold C. Wong

## Overview

Although recognized as a clinical entity in 1937, Behçet's disease (also called Behçet's syndrome) was described by Hippocrates as well as by others early in this century [1]. In 1937, Hulusi Behçet, a Turkish dermatologist, described a triad of recurrent oral and genital ulcerations and relapsing uveitis [2]. Over the ensuing 45 years, the multisystem nature of this disease has been appreciated and much research has been done, but the etiology is still unknown, the diagnosis is often difficult to make, and really safe and effective therapy still needs to be found [1]. Behçet's disease can present to physicians in many different disciplines, including the gynecologist and venereologist.

The disease has an unusual distribution in that it is most common in Japan, Korea, China, the eastern Mediterranean basin, and the Middle East. The prevalence in Japan is 1 in 1,000 and in Olmsted County, Minnesota, 1 in 25,000 [3]. The disease usually begins in early adulthood, but the age range of time of onset is large [3,4]. The disease occurs more often in men than in women in most series, with the exception of North America and Australia [1,3].

## Definition

Behçet's disease is a chronic and recurring systemic small-vessel vasculitis, characterized by oral and genital ulcers, relapsing uveitis, and cutaneous, articular, intestinal, urogenital, cardiovascular, and neurologic abnormalities [1,4,5]. The diagnosis is based on a constellation of clinical signs and laboratory findings, and no one single feature is pathognomonic [1,4]. In fact, there are three main sets of criteria for the diagnosis of Behçet's disease: the Barnes criteria, the Shimizu criteria, and the O'Duffy criteria [1,6–8]. All three sets use various major and minor criteria to establish the diagnosis (Table 16.1) [9]. The diagnosis may be made with confidence if all four major symptoms (Table 16.1) are present sometime during the disease process and inflammatory bowel diseases and collagen vascular diseases are ruled out. Combinations of major and minor criteria are less reliable, but may be reasonably specific.

TABLE 16.1. Diagnosis of Behçet's Disease: Diagnostic Criteria.

| Major criteria | Minor criteria |
|---|---|
| Recurrent oral ulcerations | Arthralgia/arthritis (large joints)/synovitis/ femoral head aseptic necrosis |
| Recurrent genital ulcerations | Intestinal ulcers |
| Eye lesions | Central nervous system involvement |
| Recurrent uveitis | Meningoencephalitis |
| Chorioretinitis | Brainstem involvement |
| Optic nerve atrophy | Psychiatric symptoms |
| Skin lesions | Vascular lesions |
| Cutaneous vasculitis (leukocytoclastic or Sweet's-like) | Arterial occlusions |
| Erythema nodosum | Venous occlusions |
| Thrombophlebitis | Aneurysms |
| Pathergy lesion (sterile pustules induced by needle prick, injection of intradermal saline or histamine) | Epididymitis |

Data from Wong et al [1], Schiffman et al [5], and Plotkin et al [14].

# Clinical Findings

## RECURRENT ORAL ULCERATIONS [1,4,5]

Recurrent aphthous stomatitis is the most common clinical manifestation of Behçet's disease, occurring with a frequency of 99%. It constitutes the initial symptom in 75% of patients. Ulcerations involve the lips, gingiva, cheeks, tongue, and palate. The oral ulcers tend to occur in crops at irregular intervals, tend to be painful, but generally do not scar. They begin as erythematous macules that develop into shallow and sharply delineated 2- to 10-mm ulcers with erythematous borders within 1 to 2 days (Figs. 16.1, 16.2). A white or yellowish necrotic pseudomembrane is usually present. The ulcers heal within 4 weeks. The ulcers are identical in appearance to ordinary canker sores.

## RECURRENT GENITAL ULCERATIONS [1,4,5]

Genital ulcers occur with a frequency of 67%, usually on the scrotal or vulvar surfaces, but also on the glans penis, in the vagina, and in the perianal region (Fig. 16.3). They resemble the oral ulcers except for being much deeper. The genital ulcers generally recur less than the oral ones.

## EYE LESIONS [1,3–5]

Uveitis occurs in about 70% of Behçet's patients, with some form of ocular lesion occurring in up to 90% of patients. Typically, 6 years elapse between the first manifestation of Behçet's disease and the onset of uveitis. The uveitis is usually bilateral. Lesions in the anterior chamber of the eye are generally transient and benign. These

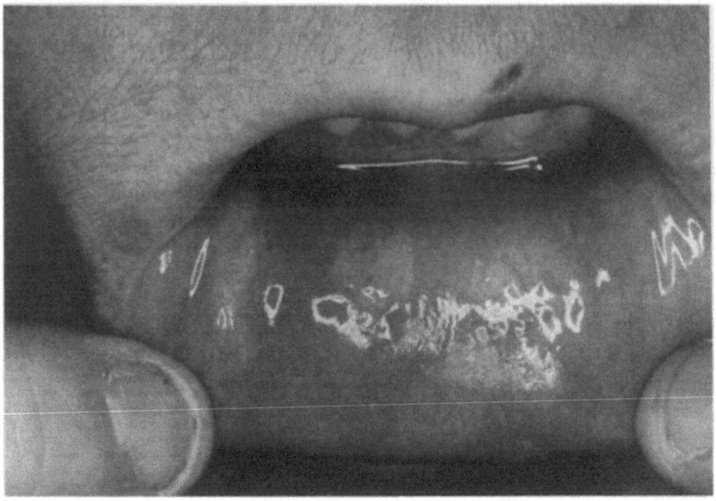

FIGURE 16.1. Aphthous ulcer in Behçet's disease.

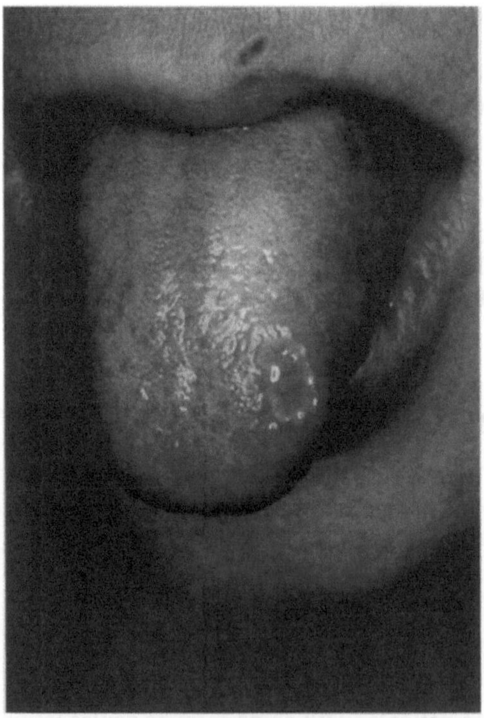

FIGURE 16.2. Aphthous ulcer in Behçet's disease.

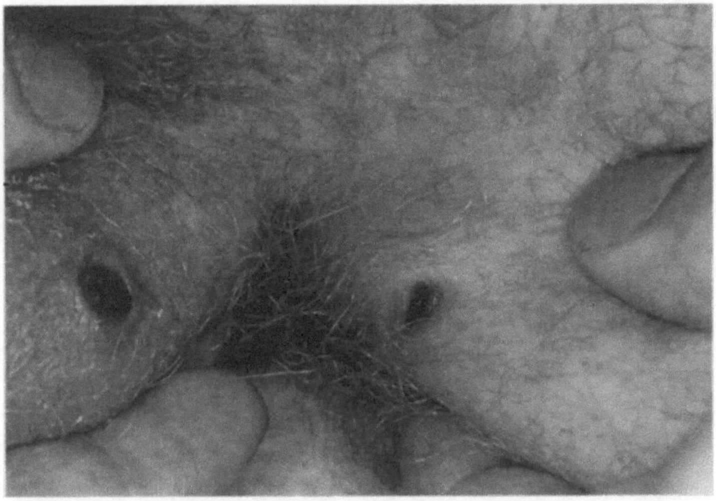

FIGURE 16.3. Genital ulcer in Behçet's disease.

include iridocyclitis, neovascularization of the iris, and hypopyon (Fig. 16.4). In contrast, posterior-chamber involvement is more serious and can lead to blindness. Manifestations include chorioretinitis, retinal vasculitis, optic papillitis, neovascularization of the retina, and vitreous hemorrhage.

## Skin Lesions [1–3,4,9,10]

In adults, skin lesions are found in about 85% of patients at some time during the course of the disease. Tender, nodular, bluish lesions on the lower extremities resembling erythema nodosum are often found (Fig. 16.5). They may also be present on the neck, face, and buttocks. Lesions may be grouped or may become ulcerated. They tend to resolve within 2 weeks, but recurrences do occur. Superficial and deep thrombophlebitis is not uncommon. A host of other cutaneous lesions include papules, pustules, pyoderma, vesicles, folliculitis, acne, and erythema multiforme. Dermographism is common. Incontinentia pigmenti has also been described in association with Behçet's disease in pediatric patients.

A distinctive feature of Behçet's disease is the development of an erythematous papule or pustule 24 to 48 hours after cutaneous trauma. The prevalence of pathergy in Mediterranean countries ranges from 40 to 88%. False-positives do occur.

## Joint Manifestations [1,4,5]

About half of patients will develop articular manifestations such as arthralgias, arthritis, and synovitis. These are often asymmetric and migratory. The large joints such as the knees, wrists, elbows, and ankles are the most frequently involved.

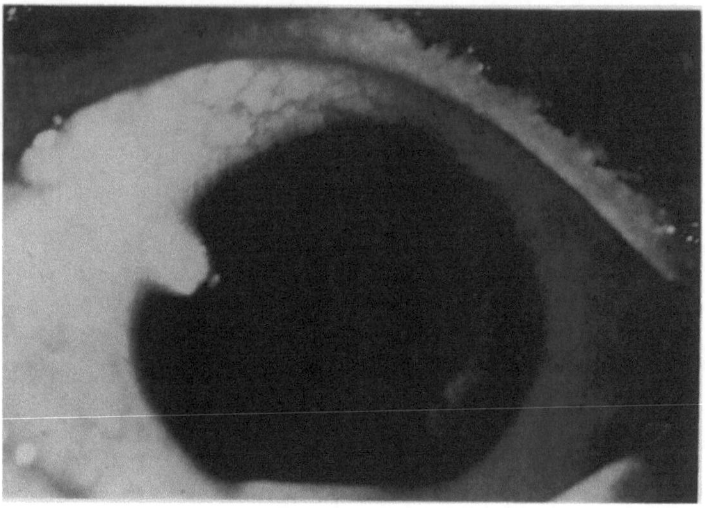

FIGURE 16.4. Hypopyon in Behçet's disease.

### Gastrointestinal Symptoms [1,4,5]

Gastrointestinal symptoms occur in about 50% of patients, are usually nonspecific, and include nausea, vomiting, loss of appetite, abdominal pain, distention, flatulence, diarrhea, and constipation. Shallow ulcers may occur in any part of the gastrointestinal tract, but are most common in the ileocecal area.

### Central Nervous System Involvement [1,3–5,9]

Neurologic involvement occurs in up to 50% of patients. In the presence of headaches, fever, a stiff neck, and focal neurologic deficits, meningoencephalitis is likely. Other clinical findings include corticospinal tract disease, cerebellar ataxia, pseudobulbar palsy, and transient cranial nerve palsies.

### Involvement of Other Systems [1,5,9,11]

Other abnormalities include vertigo, thrombosis of large veins and arteries, arterial aneurysms, arteritis, phlebitis, pulmonary opacities, and hepatomegaly. A syndrome with features of relapsing polychondritis and Behçet's syndrome has also been described. The name "MAGIC syndrome" has been proposed.

## Histopathology

A neutrophilic vascular reaction, either leukocytoclastic vasculitis (Fig. 16.6), or Sweet's-like vasculitis, is usually found in early cutaneous lesions (e.g., aphthous ulcers) and pathergy lesions from patients with Behçet's syndrome. Areas of ulcera-

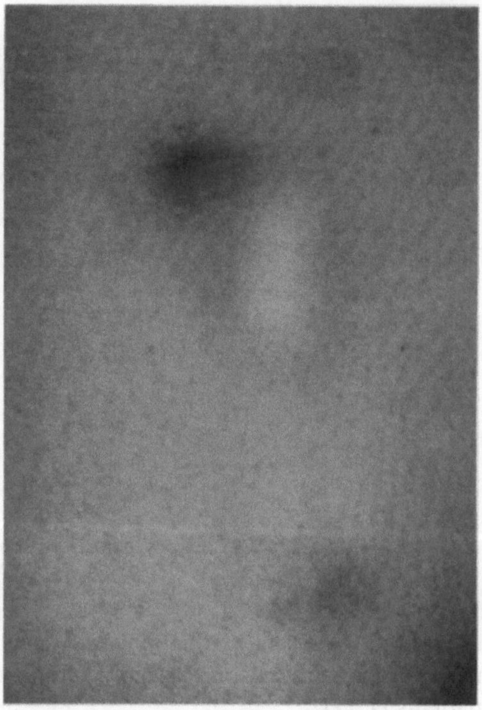

FIGURE 16.5. Erythema nodosum-like lesions on the tibial surface in patient with Behçet's disease.

tion in Behçet's disease may also initially show a perivascular mononuclear cell infiltrate, which evolves into a neutrophilic vascular reaction. A lymphocytic infiltrate is usually found in older lesions. Plasma cells and mast cells may also be present in Behçet's lesions. Erythema nodosum-like lesions in Behçet's disease show a perivascular lymphoid infiltrate in the deep dermis and a septal panniculitis similar to erythema nodosum. There is a preponderance of T helper-inducer cells over T suppressor-cytotoxic cells in lesions of oral aphthae and erythema nodosum [9,10,12–14].

Histologic studies of cardiovascular lesions have revealed splitting and degeneration of the elastic fibers of the media, perivascular lymphocytic cuffing of the vasa vasorum, aneurysmal dilatation, and granulomas involving the endocardium. Secondary amyloidosis involving the kidney has been described. In meningoencephalitis, histologic studies show a perivascular lymphocytic infiltrate, demyelinization, and a meningeal lymphocytic infiltrate, especially in the brainstem [3,7,15].

## Natural History

The natural history of the disease is variable. In some patients it follows a fairly benign course with recurrent aphthous ulcers and genital ulcers despite therapy, while in others severe central nervous system involvement, bowel perforation, or

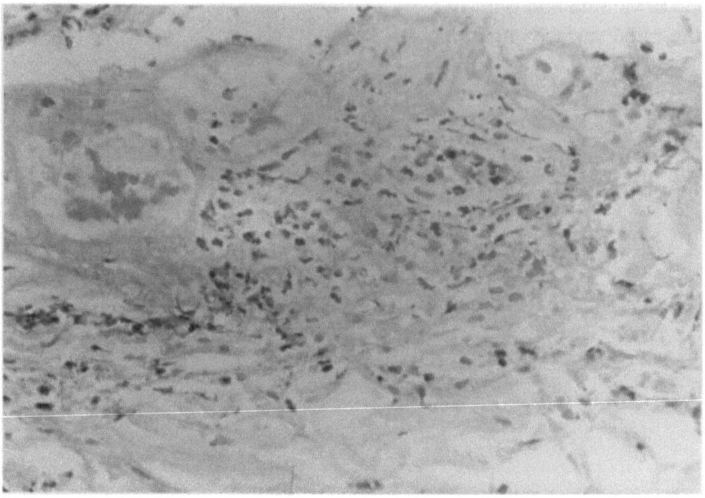

FIGURE 16.6. Leukocytoclastic vasculitis (mild) in Behçet's disease.

arteritis develops and the patient dies. Ocular involvement may progress to blindness. A slower rate of recurrent symptoms after several years is common in many patients [1,12].

## Complications

The complications of Behçet's disease are many and diverse, depending on the organ system involved. Recurrent genital ulcerations can scar, especially in women. Blindness is the most dreaded ocular complication of Behçet's disease, but glaucoma and cataracts can also occur. Some of the other more serious sequelae of Behçet's disease include cochlear or retrocochlear disease (resulting in hearing loss), epididymitis, acute proliferative glomerulonephritis, necrotizing myositis, destruction and atrophy of bone and cartilage, intestinal perforation, phlebitis (resulting in such entities as Budd-Chiari syndrome, venocaval occlusion, and benign intracranial hypertension), arterial occlusion or ruptured aneurysms (resulting in limb ischemia, stroke, renovascular hypertension, avascular necrosis of the femoral head, intermittent claudication, and massive hemoptysis), pericarditis, myocarditis, endocarditis, myocardial infarction, and endocardial fibrosis. Successive attacks of meningoencephalitis can cause extensive neurologic defects [1,3–5,9,11,15].

## Differential Diagnosis

It is important to note that the symptoms and signs of Behçet's disease can occur individually and may be separated by months or even years. Spontaneous remissions are common. This has resulted in the diagnosis often being considered only late in the course of the disease [1,3].

Oral ulcerations are common, but if genital ulcers occur with them, the diagnosis of Behçet's disease should be considered. However, there is the rare patient with recurrent oral and genital ulcers or with very frequent oral aphthae who will not develop Behçet's disease. Such a patient has an entity labeled complex aphthosis. This occasionally presents in female adolescents with temporary aphthous ulcers and vulvitis [1,5,16]. Herpes simplex virus infection should be considered in any patient with recurrent oral ulcerations and especially in patients with recurrent genital ulcerations. A viral culture should be performed to exclude herpes infection.

Inflammatory bowel diseases can present with some of the major and minor criteria for Behçet's disease such as oral aphthous ulcers, iritis, erythema nodosum, arthritis, and gastrointestinal symptoms. A proctoscopic examination and barium enema may be required to exclude ulcerative colitis and regional enteritis. A few patients may have both Behçet's disease and Crohn's disease [1,3,5,10].

Reiter's syndrome can sometimes be confused with Behçet's disease in that both can present with oral ulcerations, genital lesions, iritis, and arthritis, but the oral ulcerations in Reiter's syndrome are typically superficial and painless; the genital lesion is a circinate balanitis rather than an ulcer; and urethritis, hyperkeratotic lesions of the palms and soles (keratodermia blennorrhagica), heel pain, and sacroileitis do not occur in Behçet's disease [5].

Systemic lupus erythematosus, erythema multiforme, sarcoidosis, and multiple sclerosis encephalitis may occasionally be confused with Behçet's disease [1,17].

## Genetics, Immunology, and Etiologic Agents

The cause and pathogenesis of Behçet's disease are unknown; various theories are discussed below.

### Genetic Studies

A genetic predisposition has been proposed because of an increased frequency of HLA-B51 and HLA-DRW52 as well as familial clustering in a few cases. Previous reports of an increase in HLA-B27 have been in error [1,9,18].

### Virologic Studies

Many studies throughout the years have demonstrated nonspecific evidence for a viral etiology in Behçet's disease. Behçet himself reported the finding of inclusion bodies in oral exudate and hypopyon fluid. Several investigators have isolated an agent(s) from lesions or internal organs in Behçet's disease that produced pock lesions on egg membrane and resulted in a disease similar to Behçet's disease in laboratory animals. Decreased levels of both the free and the bound secretory component of IgA in the saliva of patients with Behçet's disease support the theory that a virus enters the body via the mucosal route because of impaired defenses. Secretory IgA as well as the secretory component is important for host defenses at the mucous membrane level. Recently, nonspecific evidence has been presented implicating herpes simplex virus type 1 (HSV-1) in the pathogenesis of Behçet's disease. There appears to be an increased incidence of HSV-1 homologous DNA in the peripheral blood lymphocytes and HSV-1 specific, IgG1-subclass circulating immune complexes in patients with Behçet's disease [1,9].

However, numerous other studies have failed to isolate a virus. Arguments against a viral etiology include lack of infectivity and epidemics, absent immunity, and only rare familial cases [1].

## Immunologic Findings

The literature is replete with immunologic studies of active Behçet's disease, and it is often difficult to ascertain the significance of various abnormalities. Evidence of autoimmunity includes circulating antibodies to human mucous membranes; lymphocytotoxicity to oral mucosa; lymphocyte transformation by fetal oral mucosa; elevated levels of serum IgA, IgM, and C9; T suppressor cell dysfunction; imbalance of T cell subsets; deficient interleukin-2 activity; and markedly increased numbers of natural killer cells, but decreased activity [1,3,19,20]. Recently, an assay for detecting serum antibodies to oral mucosal cytoplasmic antigens in patients with Behçet's disease and uveitis has been described [21]. Abnormalities in B cell activation and regulation at the level of the B cell, and T cell control of B cell function, may also be involved in the pathogenesis of Behçet's disease [20].

While some investigators feel that mononuclear cells are of primary immunopathogenic importance, others feel that neutrophils and circulating immune complexes (CIC) are important [9,10,12,14,16,22]. CIC are found in 44 to 60% of patients with Behçet's disease. One theory on the pathogenesis of Behçet's disease proposes that the lesions result from an interaction between CIC-mediated vessel damage and enhanced neutrophil migration. Jorizzo and others have been able to tentatively validate this theory clinically by using it to predict which patient out of six with complex aphthosis would eventually develop Behçet's disease. These investigators also feel that examination of pathergy lesions by light and immunofluorescence microscopy is helpful in assessing clinical disease activity and response to experimental thalidomide therapy, as well as being useful in the diagnosis of Behçet's disease [9,10,12,16,22].

## Miscellaneous Findings

C-reactive protein is elevated in active Behçet's disease and may alter the immune response by inhibiting T lymphocytes, promoting phagocytosis, and activating complement [1]. Serum lysozyme and alpha-1 acid glycoprotein are increased, but only with ocular disease [23]. Plasminogen activator activity levels are decreased by Behçet's disease, as are prostacyclin levels. This may contribute to the persistence and organization of blood clots in ocular vessels and elsewhere via low plasma fibrinolytic activity [24,25]. Interferon gamma is higher in the sera of Behçet's disease patients than in those of controls [3]. An elevated erythrocyte sedimentation rate, mild anemia, and hypergammaglobulinemia are common [3].

Ingestion of English walnuts can exacerbate the oral ulcerations and initiate arthritis in Behçet's disease; other foods associated with exacerbation of the disease include chocolate, tomatoes, rice cakes, and oranges. Zinc and organophosphate pesticides have been implicated in the etiology of Behçet's disease [1,26].

## Management

Different treatment regimens and numerous medications have been used, alone and in combination, to treat the various manifestations of Behçet's disease. The effectiveness of any therapy is difficult to evaluate because of the many exacerbations and remissions that characterize the disease. Most studies are not controlled. The treatment and management of patients with Behçet's disease are usually matters of trial and error. Toxic and potentially lethal side effects of the drugs used need to be guarded against, and it follows that the physician should be familiar with the use and toxicities of these agents. Specialists should be freely consulted.

### Topical Therapy [1,3,23,27]

Topical therapeutic agents used in aphthous stomatitis can be used in the aphthous ulcerations of Behçet's disease.

1. *Topical Steroids*. Topical corticosteroids in pastes or gels are useful for aphthous ulcers if applied during the prodromal phase before the ulcer actually occurs. The regimen used is two to four times daily. Topical steroid eye drops have also been used to suppress ocular inflammation.
2. *Tetracycline*. A slurry of 5 ml of water or flavored syrup and one 250-mg capsule of tetracycline can be used to reduce ulcer size, duration, and pain. One regimen advocates packing the ulcer with a soft cotton cloth soaked in a tetracycline suspension three times a day. Topical tetracycline with nystatin may be helpful in preventing candidiasis.
3. *Miscellaneous Agents*. Mouth washes such as chlorhexidine have been shown to be helpful in healing aphthous ulcers. Viscous xylocaine is useful in relieving oral pain. Mydriatics have been reported to be effective in uveitis.

### Systemic Therapy

#### Immunosuppressives and Antiinflammatory Agents

##### *Systemic Corticosteroids [1,3,5,23,28]*

Although it is at best palliative, systemic corticosteroid therapy is the mainstay of therapy for many of the manifestations of Behçet's disease, especially mucocutaneous, ophthalmic, and articular involvement. It can be used to augment the effects of topical steroid eye drops and subconjunctival, retrobulbar, and intraarticular steroid injections. Although prednisone in a dose as low as 4 mg a day can be helpful for mild symptoms, 60 mg daily is usually needed to suppress active mucocutaneous, ocular, joint, and meningeal inflammation. Not uncommonly, however, prednisone is ineffective for oral or central nervous system involvement.

A state of resistance to the beneficial effects of corticosteroids on ocular inflammation can develop, with increasingly more numerous and severe exacerbations. Combination therapy with corticosteroids and other immunosuppressive medications is sometimes helpful in resistant cases of Behçet's disease and is also steroid sparing.

#### *Chlorambucil [1,3,9,27–29]*

Chlorambucil is the least toxic, the best tolerated, and the most effective of the immunosuppressive agents in comparison with azathioprine and cyclophosphamide. In fact, some authors consider chlorambucil the first drug of choice for retinal vasculitis. Several studies have shown that 80% of patients with iridocyclitis and conjunctivitis with decreased visual acuity had an improvement in visual acuity when given chlorambucil. Some patients were recurrence-free over 1 to 5 years. Improvement was also seen in orogenital and cutaneous lesions as well as in arthritis, thrombophlebitis, and neurologic symptoms. Relapses were seen once therapy was stopped. Chlorambucil has also been shown to be useful in preventing meningoencephalitis. Unfortunately, other studies have found chlorambucil not to be effective in Behçet's disease.

#### *Other Drugs [1,23]*

Azathioprine has been effective in lessening ocular symptoms in some patients, but side effects are significant. Prednisone with cyclophosphamide has been reported to help clear aphthous stomatitis and improve vision. Antiinflammatory agents such as indomethacin, oxyphenbutazone, and aspirin have been used with limited success.

### Other Systemic Therapies

#### *Colchicine [1,14,22,23,27,30]*

The chemotactic activity of polymorphonuclear (PMN) leukocytes is increased in Behçet's disease, and this provides the rationale for using colchicine, an antichemotactic agent that interferes with cytoskeletal function by binding microtubular protein. There are conflicting reports regarding the efficacy of colchicine in Behçet's disease. Some reports show that colchicine has beneficial effects on oral aphthous ulcerations, genital ulcers, ocular inflammation, erythema nodosum, and other skin lesions; arthritis; and gastrointestinal manifestations. Other investigators have found no beneficial effect of colchicine in Behçet's disease.

#### *Thalidomide [9,27,31]*

Oral thalidomide has been reported to be dramatically beneficial for the mucocutaneous ulcers and arthritis of Behçet's disease. It is not effective alone in the treatment of iridocyclitis, but may permit a reduction in steroid dosage if patients are already receiving systemic corticosteroids.

*Miscellaneous [1,23,27,32,33]*

Other medications such as levamisole, cyclosporine, fibrinolytic drugs, transfer factor, poliomyelitis vaccine, prostacyclin, acyclovir, dapsone, chloroquine, hydroxychloroquine, tripterygium, alpha-interferon, ketoconazole, and 13-cis retinoic acid have been reported to be helpful in Behçet's disease.

## Prognosis

The prognosis for patients with Behçet's disease depends upon the organ systems involved. Involvement of the eyes, especially with posterior uveitis, is particularly worrisome, often resulting in loss of visual acuity and ultimately blindness within 5 to 6 years [1,15]. Central nervous system, bowel, or large artery involvement may result in death from meningoencephalitis, intestinal perforation, arteritis, or rupture of an aneurysm [1,15]. The progression of the disease may be altered with immunosuppressive agents.

### References


1. Wong RC, Ellis CN, Diaz LA: Behçet's disease. *Int J Dermatol* **23**:25–32, 1984.
2. Behçet H: Uber rezidivierende, aphthose, durch ein Virus verursachte Geschwure am Mund, am Auge, und an den Genitalien. *Dermatol Wochenschr* **105**:1152–1157, 1937.
3. O'Duffy JD: Behçet's Disease. In WB Kelly, et al (Eds): *Textbook of Rheumatology.* Philadelphia: WB Saunders, 1985, pp 1174–1178.
4. Ammann AJ, Johnson A, Fyfe GA, et al: Behçet's syndrome. *J Pediatr* **107**:41–43, 1985.
5. Schiffman L, Giansiracusa D, Calabro JJ, et al: Behçet's syndrome. *Comp Therapy* **12**:62–66, 1986.
6. Mason RM, Barnes CG: Behçet's syndrome with arthritis. *Ann Rheum Dis* **28**:95–103, 1969.
7. Shimizu T, Ehrlich GE, Inaba G, et al: Behçet's disease (Behçet's syndrome). *Semin Arthritis Rheum* **8**:223–260, 1979.
8. O'Duffy JD, Goldstein NP: Neurologic involvement in seven patients with Behçet's disease. *Am J Med* **61**:170–178, 1976.
9. Jorizzo JL: Behçet's disease: An update based on the 1985 international conference in London. *Arch Dermatol* **122**:556–558, 1986.
10. Jorizzo JL, Solomon AR, Cavallo T: Behçet's syndrome: Immunopathologic and histopathologic assessment of pathergy lesions is useful in diagnosis and follow-up. *Arch Pathol Lab Med* **109**:747–751, 1985.
11. Firestein GS, Gruber HE, Weisman MH, et al: Mouth and genital ulcers with inflamed cartilage: MAGIC syndrome. Five patients with features of relapsing polychondritis and Behçet's disease. *Am J Med* **79**:65–72, 1985.
12. Jorizzo JL: Behçet's syndrome: Pathogenesis, diagnosis, and treatment. *Cutis* **32**:441–448, 1983.
13. Kaneko F, Takahashi Y, Muramatsu Y, et al: Immunological studies on aphthous ulcer and erythema nodosum-like eruptions in Behçet's disease. *Br J Dermatol* **113**:303–312, 1985.

14. Plotkin GR, Patel BR, Shah VN: Behçet's syndrome complicated by cutaneous leukocytoclastic vasculitis. *Arch Intern Med* **145**:1913–1915, 1985.
15. Huycke EC, Robinowitz M, Cohen IS, et al: Granulomatous endocarditis with systemic embolism in Behçet's disease. *Ann Intern Med* **102**:791–793, 1985.
16. Jorizzo JL, Taylor RS, Schmalstieg FC, et al: Complex aphthosis: A forme fruste of Behçet's syndrome? *J Am Acad Dermatol* **13**:80–84, 1985.
17. Huff JC, Weston WL, Tonnesen MG: Erythema multiforme: A critical review of characteristics, diagnostic criteria, and causes. *J Am Acad Dermatol* **8**:763–775, 1983.
18. Lewis MA, Priestley BL: Transient neonatal Behçet's disease. *Arch Dis Child* **61**:805–806, 1986.
19. Kaneko F, Takahashi Y, Muramatsu R, et al: Natural killer cell numbers and function in peripheral lymphoid cells in Behçet's disease. *Br J Dermatol* **113**:313–318, 1985.
20. Suzuki N, Sakane T, Ueda Y, et al: Abnormal B cell function in patients with Behçet's disease. *Arth Rheum* **29**:212–219, 1986.
21. Michelson JB, Chisari FV, Kansu T: Antibodies to oral mucosa in patients with ocular Behçet's disease. *Ophthalmology* **92**:1277–1281, 1985.
22. Jorizzo JL, Hudson RD, Schmalstieg FC, et al: Behçet's syndrome: Immune regulation, circulating immune complexes, neutrophil migration, and colchicine therapy. *J Am Acad Dermatol.* **10**:205–214, 1984.
23. James DG: Behçet's disease. In TB Fitzpatrick, Eisen AZ, Wolff K, et al (Eds): *Dermatology in General Medicine*. New York: McGraw-Hill, 1987, pp. 1239–1244.
24. Mishima H, Masuda K, Shimada S, et al: Plasminogen activator activity levels in patients with Behçet's syndrome. *Arch Ophthalmol* **103**:935–936, 1985.
25. Hizli N, Sahin G, Sahin F, et al: Plasma prostacyclin levels in Behçet's disease. *Lancet* **1**:1454, 1985.
26. Kikuchi I: The effects of walnuts on Behçet's syndrome in two sisters. *J Dermatol* **12**: 290–291, 1985.
27. Shelley WB, Shelley ED: *Advanced Dermatologic Therapy.* Philadelphia: WB Saunders, 1987.
28. Benezra D, Cohen E: Treatment and visual prognosis in Behçet's disease. *Br J Ophthalmol* **70**:589–592, 1986.
29. Pezzi PP, Gasparri V, deLiso P, et al: Prognosis in Behçet's disease. *Ann Ophthalmol* **17**:20–25, 1985.
30. Sander HM, Randle HW: Use of colchicine in Behçet's syndrome. *Cutis* **37**:344–348, 1986.
31. Hamza M'H: Treatment of Behçet's disease with thalidomide. *Clin Rheumatol* **5**:365–371, 1986.
32. Wenyan X, Jiarun Z, Xeuyu L: Tripterygium in dermatologic therapy. *Int J Dermatol* **24**:152–157, 1985.
33. Tsambaos D, Eichelberg D, Goos M: Behçet's syndrome: Treatment with recombinant leukocyte alpha-interferon. *Arch Dermatol Res* **278**:335–336, 1986.

CHAPTER 17

# Connubial Contact Dermatitis

Jere D. Guin, Dowling B. Stough IV, and Robert L. Rietschel

When the term *sexually transmitted disease* is used, one may think of syphilis, AIDS, gonorrhea, or even herpes. But how often does this term suggest contact dermatitis or urticaria? Case reports of such can be so fascinating that they are not easily forgotten. Some rare types of reactions, for example, anaphylaxis to seminal fluid, have received considerable notoriety, but connubial contact dermatitis and urticaria may not be as rare as one might assume. Reactions related to close contact or sexual activity might include poison ivy dermatitis and other types of contact dermatitis, contact irritant reactions (Fig. 17.1), various results of trauma, and allergic and nonimmunologic contact urticaria.

## Reactions to Seminal Fluid

Of all connubial contact reactions, none is more dramatic than the anaphylactic reaction to seminal fluid. While rare, this has been described several times since the original report by Halpern et al in 1967 [1]. Such reactions may be systemic (anaphylactic) or local [2–4].

Life-threatening anaphylactic reactions are accompanied by symptoms of an immediate hypersensitivity reaction with severe asthmatic dyspnea; generalized urticaria; angioedema of the lips, eyelids, and tongue; violent pelvic or abdominal pain; and hypotension, sometimes with loss of consciousness. Onset typically occurs shortly after ejaculation in sexual intercourse [2].

There is also a more localized reaction comprising erythema, stinging, burning, and pain in the vagina; redness and swelling of the vulva; and labial urticaria, often with generalized pruritus. This begins immediately after ejaculation and persists 2 to 72 hours [2–4]. The cause is almost always recognized, except in milder cases where the association may not be as obvious [3]. This type of reaction was reported in four women in the same family with the same general clinical picture [4], so there may be both familial and nonfamilial types of the local or milder form of the condition.

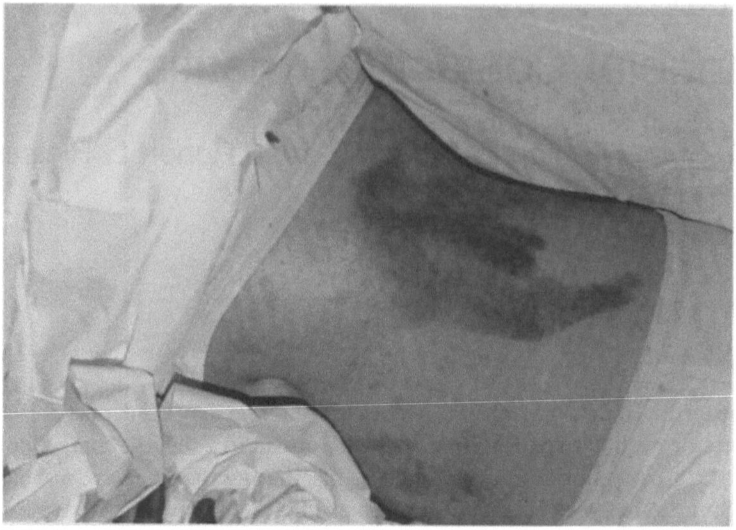

FIGURE 17.1. Hand print on abdomen caused by battery acid on boyfriend's hand during an intimate session that followed automotive battery installation. Courtesy of John Jucas, M.D.

Although antibodies to sperm are known (and are thought to perhaps be one cause of infertility) [5], and specific spermatazoal IgE antibodies have been identified in some patients [2], the causative factor is rather a component of seminal fluid, derived from the prostate or seminal vesicles rather than from the testis or epididymis. It has been characterized as a 14,000- to 30,000-dalton component of seminal fluid protein [1,4,6–9]. The antigen is species specific, because semen from nonhuman sources fails to elicit a reaction [1]. It is present in vasectomized men [6].

Faced with such a patient, however, one should also consider the possibility that the seminal fluid contains a foreign antigen from systemic medications or food. Postcoital urticaria has occurred from ingested dicloxacillin [10] and walnuts [7,11] transferred in semen.

Systemic reactions are IgE mediated, since the antigen is thermolabile with positive passive transfer to humans and monkeys but not nonprimates [1]. This has been confirmed by histamine release from basophilic leukocytes, radioallergosorbent test (with inhibition), and neutralization of passive transfer antibodies [2]. Scratch tests may be positive at up to $10^6$ or $10^7$ dilutions [1,6]. The local reaction, while associated with a cell-mediated immune response [2], is probably caused by a different mechanism, because symptoms and signs appear immediately. Perhaps the cell-mediated response is an associated or concomitant reaction. The reason for an immunologic reaction on first coitus is not clear, but there may be some cross-reacting antigens [2].

Histamine release has been observed when the affected patient's leukocytes are challenged with the implicated seminal plasma [7]. The pathogenesis is unclear, but

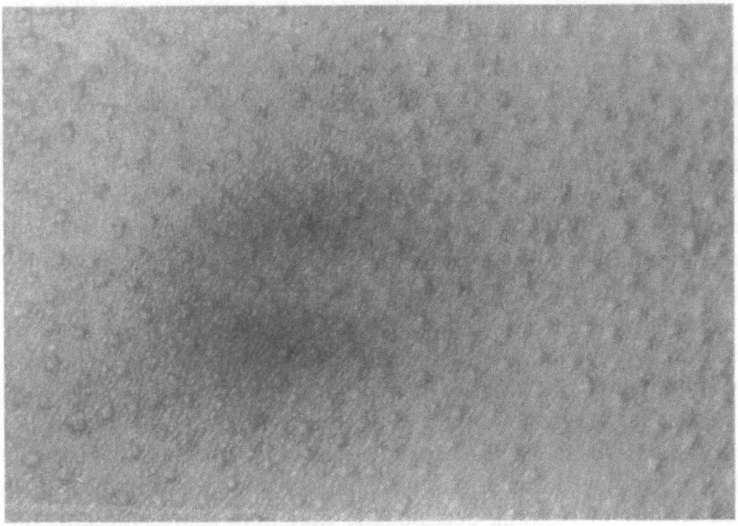

FIGURE 17.2. Follicular papules on trunk of a 24-year-old woman caused by transfer of homosalate in Coppertone lotion used as a sun protectant by her physician boyfriend.

genetic susceptibility appears to be a factor [4]. There may be a history of atopic problems [1,2,6–8] including atopic dermatitis [7].

Hyposensitization may [7] or may not [1] be of benefit. Condom use prevents the reaction [9], but rupture of a condom in one case led to a severe anaphylactic reaction [2]. Antihistamines may reduce symptoms of a mild [8] and localized reaction [4], but not of a more severe systemic reactions [1].

## Connubial Contact Dermatitis

Many allergens can cause connubial contact dermatitis, including perfumes and colognes [12], benzoyl peroxide [13], perfume [14], feminine hygiene sprays [15], hair lotion [16], topical medications [17], nickel [18], hair dye [19], condoms [20–24], lubricating jelly [4,13], sunscreen products [25] (Fig. 17.2), fiberglass in work clothes [4], and other sources of irritation. Uncovering the causative agent often requires careful questioning and patch testing, as the causative allergen is not always obvious.

### *Toxicodendron* DERMATITIS

Poison ivy dermatitis is probably the most common cause of allergic connubial contact dermatitis because of the frequency of exposure, the high percentage of the population that is allergic, and the tendency for the antigen to persist on the skin for up to 3 days after exposure, allowing transfer to sensitized persons.

Poison ivy dermatitis is known to be caused at times by transfer of the antigen between persons. The oil-soluble oleoresin under experimental conditions remains on protected areas for 2 or 3 days at most [26], but it probably disappears much more rapidly under normal activity where moisture is present [26–28], and contact with clothing and other objects tends to remove the oleoresin. Highly sensitive subjects are probably at risk for a much longer time. Classic studies by Shelmire [28] and later by Kligman [26] showed that transfer from the hands is possible after washing. To effectively reduce symptomatology, removal with soap and organic solvents has to be done before the oleoresin has a chance to penetrate the stratum corneum. One can see clear evidence of hand transfer by following patterns and courses of family members with poison ivy dermatitis, sometimes demonstrating hand print and fingerprint patterns on the person originally exposed and the same hand- and finger-shaped lesions in a spouse (connubial contact dermatitis) or a son, daughter, or parent (filial contact dermatitis [29]). While contaminated articles of clothing occasionally may be a source [26,28], the antigen is most often transferred by the hands. Resnick illustrated this in his review of the subject [30].

The penis is a common site for poison ivy dermatitis in the male (again because of hand transfer), but blister fluid does not cause contact dermatitis [26]. Even in those already allergic, the reaction usually does not appear for 1 or 2 days (except perhaps on the face) [31], so by the time the rash appears, it is unlikely that there will be sufficient antigen on the surface to cause a response even in one highly allergic.

Classic *Toxicodendron* dermatitis is characterized by scattered linear groups of papules, vesicles, and bullae, but diagnosis of connubial *Toxicodendron* dermatitis can sometimes be sherlockian. However, management is little different from other forms of *Toxicodendron* dermatitis.

The best method of prevention is recognition and avoidance of the plant. Ordinary laundering satisfactorily removes the allergic potential from oleoresin-contaminated clothing [26] unless the stain has turned black, in which case dry cleaning may be necessary [28]. The antigen is rapidly degraded in the presence of water [26], which explains the value of soaking with cool water as prophylaxis immediately after suspected exposure [31]. Washing with soap must be done promptly after exposure and as early as 5 minutes in those highly allergic [26]. Usually that opportunity has been lost by the time the person can bathe, and sometimes washing a limited area can transfer the antigen to other areas, seemingly "spreading the rash" [30].

## Reactions to Medications and Topicals

Transfer of antigens from one marital partner to the other occurs perhaps more typically than transfer from preparations used intravaginally or on the genitalia. Two of us recently saw a man who was allergic on patch testing to multiple ingredients in Mycolog cream, but he was certain that he had never used the product. His wife, however, had been using that product for some time for a vulvar dermatitis.

Fisher [15] described a 55-year-old man, allergic to propylene glycol, who experienced severe allergic contact dermatitis of the penis and scrotum from lubricating jelly that his wife had used as a lubricant in sexual intercourse. He also saw an 80-year-old woman with a nummular eczema-like eruption, caused by allergy to Cetaphil lotion used by her husband [15]. Wilkinson [32] found connubial photodermatitis in a man who crushed phenothiazine tablets for his wife, and in a physician's wife who contacted the allergens (promethazine and chlorpromazine) in her husband's car.

## Reactions to Acne Products

Acne treatments tolerated by one partner may not be tolerated by the other. Caro [13] described connubial contact dermatitis in a male physician who had prescribed a topical benzoyl peroxide preparation for his wife's back and broke out after his clothing touched her. Fisher [15] had a similar case in a woman with dermatitis of the face, neck, and sometimes arms after sexual intercourse with a paramour who used an acne preparation containing 5% benzoyl peroxide. Avoidance by the partner cured the problem in both cases. Problems from such exposure are not limited to contact dermatitis or urticaria: one of us had a female patient whose husband developed diarrhea following her use of topical clindamycin for acne.

## Reactions to Vaginal and Vulvar Products

Contact dermatitis can occur to many chemicals found in spermicides and chemical contraceptive products, including phenylmercuric acetate, oxyquinoline sulfate, quinine HCl, and hexylresorcinol [23]. However, we have been unable to find published examples of allergic contact dermatitis due to these agents when used for these purposes. Irritation from such products is considered to be a common complaint. Reactions to vaginal antibacterial and antifungal products is well known [33,34].

Feminine hygiene sprays may cause vulvar and inguinal dermatitis as well as connubial contact dermatitis [35]. Causative ingredients include quaternary ammonium products (benzethonium and benzalkonium), isopropyl myristate, chlorhexidine, and fragrance ingredients. Such products also cause irritant dermatitis when the spray is applied too closely, and this type of reaction is said to be more common than the allergic one [35].

Systemic contact dermatitis and photocontact dermatitis may be caused by vaginal creams and suppositories [33]. Systemic reactions may be accompanied by a local reaction as well, and photocontact dermatitis may be accompanied by ordinary allergic contact dermatitis, making the clinical picture somewhat complex.

## Perfume Reactions

Mathias et al [12] saw a man who had chronic, recurrent dermatitis for 20 years before careful investigation found the underlying cause to be hydroxycitronellal, a fragrance ingredient in multiple products used by his wife, including cosmetics and a room deodorizer.

Swinyer [14] described a perfume (cinnamic alcohol)-allergic man who also reacted on patch testing to tincture of benzoin and balsam of Peru. Two nights after his wife used perfume, an eruption developed on his face where he had touched her. Since eruptions on the face often occur more rapidly, he probably was exposed some time after she applied the perfume.

## Reactions to Devices

Rubber condoms (or diaphragms) can cause reactions in either partner [22]. Leider et al [36] found 6 of 125 cases of rubber dermatitis, and 1 case of leukoderma due to monobenzyl ether of hydroquinone, were caused by condoms. In Hindson's report of condom dermatitis, 2 of 35 cases were women who presented with pruritus vulvae [20]. The 33 men experienced pruritus and edema following intercourse. As in most cases of rubber dermatitis, the causative allergen usually is an accelerator or an antioxidant. Nine of nine persons in one series [21] were reactive to dipentamethylene thiuram disulfide. Fisher described cheilitis and stomatitis in women from fellatio following contact with rubber condoms [22], and proctitis with gluteal and perianal dermatitis in homosexual males [22].

Less commonly, spermicides or preservatives may be the underlying cause in condom dermatitis. Sensitivity to the lubricant can sometimes be determined by a positive patch-test reaction to the outside of a condom with a negative response to the inside surface [22].

Once the cause is suspected, use of nonrubber condoms eliminates the problem. Fisher predicted that connubial contact dermatitis from rubber condoms will increase because of their recommended use for prevention of HIV (human immunodeficiency virus) infection [22].

Contraceptive devices are also known to cause and precipitate problems. Barranco [37] described a women who had a resistant eczematous eruption of the anus with scattered areas of involvement over the trunk that proved to be systemic contact dermatitis. She had a 4+ patch-test reaction to copper, but no source could be found until the patient remembered an intrauterine contraceptive device that had been inserted shortly before onset of the eruption. Removal of the IUD promptly cured the problem.

However, metal sensitivity in this region may not necessarily be induced by a device. Gochfield and Burger [18] reported a young woman who presented with a dermatitis of the pubic area who was patch-test reactive to 2.5% nickel sulfate. The husband was employed in a metal factory and was exposed to metallic nickel, which was carried home in his underwear. The husband was persuaded to shower and change clothes after work, which led to improvement of her condition.

### Reactions to Para-Amino Compounds

Dooms-Goossens et al [15] described a woman with contact dermatitis of the ears, neck, and eyelids from procaine in her husband's hair growth lotion. There are several reports of allergy to dyed hair [19,38,39], despite the dogma that the finished product does not cause allergy [40–42]. Mitchell [38], Cronin [39], and Warin [19] all described connubial contact dermatitis to hair dye. That reaction is possible after the dye has ostensibly been oxidized has been confirmed by Foussereau et al [43]. The variance from accepted principles has been explained as due to improper methodology in the dyeing procedure [41,44].

### Irritant Reactions

Irritant reactions are most likely common but usually do not reach the attention of a physician. Caustic agents can be transferred from the hands (Fig. 17.1) leaving a hand print of irritation. Fomites may also transfer nonallergic reactions.

Fiberglass dermatitis may occur in a husband and wife from contaminated work clothing [45], and the irritant material may be spread in the washing machine, causing a problem in other family members [41, p. 63]. Connubial chloracne has been described on the forearms of a 40-year-old woman whose husband delivered fuel oil and had "widespread chloracne" [14]. The reaction subsided 3 weeks after she started using forceps to put his clothing in the machine. Irritant dermatitis can be caused by a number of agents including soap, detergents, solvents, and fabric softeners. For example, quaternary ammonium compounds may cause both vulvar and penile irritation, fissuring, and dermatitis [46].

## Connubial Contact Urticaria

Contact urticarial reactions may be immunologic or nonimmunologic, or, when the mechanism is in doubt, "uncertain" [47]. The number of reported causative agents grows with each day's mail, but recent lists have been published by Guin [48] and by Von Krogh and Maibach [49].

Individual case histories can be fascinating. van Ketel [50] described a housewife who, according to history, developed flushing, swelling, and itching of the face 1 to 2 minutes after entering a bar. She tolerated kissing her husband after he drank most alcoholic beverages, but kissing him after he drank beer caused erythema and pruritus.

There are also reports of filial contact urticaria. One of us saw a case of chronic urticaria in a toddler that proved to be aggravated by exposure to her mother when the mother wore perfume. Patch testing produced both local and systemic symptoms and the generalized eruption persisted 48 hours. Avoidance of flavors and fragrances controlled the chronic urticaria. Camarasa et al [51] saw another case of filial exposure when the mother of a posttonsillectomy patient developed contact urticaria on exposure to the patient. The causative medication, aminophenazone, reproduced the eruption on testing.

Traumatic events can cause many types of cutaneous change, including factitial dermatitis; purpura from orogenital contact; "irritant" dermatitis; swelling, abrasions, and lacerations from sadomasochistic maneuvers and certain homosexual practices. These are beyond the scope of this article. We refer interested readers to the recent third edition of *Contact Dermatitis*, where the subject is covered in some detail by Fisher [41, pp. 64–69].

## References

1. Halpern BN, Ky T, Robert B: Clinical and immunological study of an exceptional case of reaginic type sensitization to human seminal fluid. *Immunology* **12**:247–1258, 1967.
2. Bernstein LI, Englander BE, Gallagher JS, et al: Localized and systemic hypersensitivity reactions to human seminal fluid. *Ann Intern Med* **94** (Part 1):459–465, 1981.
3. Kroon S: Allergy to human seminal plasma: A presentation of six cases. *Acta Derm Venereol* (Stockh) **60**:436–439, 1980.
4. Chang TW: Familial allergic seminal vulvovaginitis. *Am J Obstet Gynecol* **126**:442–444, 1976.
5. Shulman S, Jackson H, Stone ML: Antibodies to spermatozoa. VI. Comparative studies of sperm-agglutinating activity in groups of infertile and fertile women. *Am J Obstet Gynecol* **123**:139–144, 1975.
6. Levine BB, Siraganian RP, Schenkian I: Allergy to human seminal plasma. *N Engl J Med* **288**:894–896, 1973.
7. Mathias CG, Frick OL, Caldwell TM, et al: Immediate hypersensitivity to seminal fluid and atopic dermatitis. *Arch Dermatol* **116**:209–212, 1980.
8. Mumford DM, Haywood TJ, Daily LJ, et al: Female allergy to seminal plasma: A case report. *Ann Allergy* **40**:40–43, 1978.
9. Mikkelsen EJ, Henderson LL, Leiferman KM, et al: Allergy to human seminal fluid. *Ann Allergy* **34**:239–243, 1975.
10. Green RL, Green MA: Postcoital urticaria in a penicillin-sensitive patient. *JAMA* **254**:531, 1985.
11. Haddad ZH: Clearer picture of food allergens is still needed. *Perspect Allergy* **1**:2–3, 1978.
12. Mathias CG, Cram D, Ragsdale J, et al: Contact dermatitis caused by spouse's perfume and cologne. *Canad Med Assoc J* **119**:257–258, 1978.
13. Caro I: Connubial contact dermatitis to benzoyl peroxide. *Contact Dermatitis* **2**:362, 1976.
14. Swinyer LJ: Connubial contact dermatitis from perfumes. *Contact Dermatitis* **6**:226, 1980.
15. Fisher AA: Consort contact dermatitis. *Cutis* **24**:595–596, 668, 1979.
16. Dooms-Goossens A, Swinnen E, Vandermaesen J, et al: Connubial dermatitis from a hair lotion. *Contact Dermatitis* **16**:41–42, 1987.
17. Newton JA, White I: Connubial dermatitis from Morantel. *Contact Dermatitis* **16**:38–39, 1987.
18. Gochfield M, Burger J: Sexual transmission of nickel and poison oak contact dermatitis. *Lancet* **1**:589, 1983.

19. Warin AP: Contact dermatitis to partner's hair dye. *Clin Exper Dermatol* **1**:283–284, 1976.
20. Hindson TC: Studies in contact dermatitis. XVI. Contraceptives. *Trans St Johns Hosp Dermatol Soc* **52**:1, 1966.
21. Wilson HT: Rubber dermatitis. *Br J Dermatol* **81**:175–179, 1969.
22. Fisher AA: Condom dermatitis in either partner. *Cutis* **39**:281–285, 1987.
23. Fischer AA: Allergic reactions to contraceptives. *Cutis* **13**:337, 1974.
24. Fischer AA: Practical management of allergic contact dermatitis due to rubber in manufactured articles. *Dermatol Digest* **2**:23, 1986.
25. Rietschel RL, Lewis CW: Contact dermatitis to homomenthyl salicylate. *Arch Dermatol* **114**:442–443, 1978.
26. Kligman AM: Poison ivy (*Rhus*) dermatitis, an experimental study. AMA *Arch Dermatol* **77**:149–180, 1958.
27. Guin JD, Reynolds R: Jewelweed treatment of poison ivy dermatitis. *Contact Dermatitis* **6**:287–288, 1980.
28. Shelmire B: The poison ivy plant and its oleoresin. *J Invest Dermatol* **4**:337–348, 1941.
29. Guin JD: Clinical notes: Poison ivy in winter with an example of filial contact dermatitis. *J Ind State Med Assoc* **76**:184, 1983.
30. Resnick SD: Poison-ivy and poison-oak dermatitis. *Clin Dermatol* **4**:208–212, 1986.
31. Guin JD: Reaction time in experimental poison ivy dermatitis. *Contact Dermatitis* **6**:289–290, 1980.
32. Wilkinson DS: Connubial photodermatitis. *Contact Dermatitis* **1**:58, 1975.
33. Goette DK, Odom RB: Vaginal medications as a cause for varied widespread dermatitides. *Cutis* **26**:406–409, 1980.
34. Helander I, Hollmen A, Hopsu-Havu VK: Allergic contact dermatitis to chlordantoin. *Contact Dermatitis* **5**:54–55, 1979.
35. Fisher AA: Allergic reactions to feminine hygiene sprays. *Arch Dermatol* **108**:801–802, 1973.
36. Leider M, Furman D, Fisher AA: Sensitivity to rubber materials. AMA *Arch Dermatol Syphild* **65**:587–595, 1952.
37. Barranco VP: Eczematous dermatitis caused by internal exposure to copper. *Arch Dermatol* **106**:386–387, 1972.
38. Mitchell JC: Allergic contact dermatitis from paraphenylenediamine presenting as "nummular eczema." *Contact Dermatitis Newslet* **11**:270, 1972.
39. Cronin E: Dermatitis from wife's dyed hair. *Contact Dermatitis Newslet* **13**:363, 1973.
40. Reiss F, Fisher AA: Is hair dyed with para-phenylenediamine allergenic? *Arch Dermatol* **109**:221–222, 1974.
41. Fischer AA: *Contact Dermatitis*. 3rd ed. Philadelphia: Lea & Febiger, 1986, p. 381.
42. Fisher AA: Is hair dyed with para-phenylenediamine allergenic? *Contact Dermatitis* **1**:266, 1975.
43. Foussereau J, Reuter G, Petitjean J: Is hair dyed with PPD-like dyes allergenic? *Contact Dermatitis* **6**:143, 1980.
44. Calnan CD: Comment. *Clin Exper Dermatol* **1**:284, 1976.
45. Fisher BK, Warkentin JP: Fiber glass dermatitis. *Arch Dermatol* **99**:717–719, 1969.
46. Maibach HI, Mathias CT: Vulvar dermatitis and fissures: Irritant dermatitis from methyl benzethonium chloride. *Contact Dermatitis* **13**:340, 1985.
47. Maibach HI, Johnson HL: Contact urticaria syndrome, contact urticaria to diethyltoluamide. *Arch Dermatol* **11**:26–30, 1975.

48. Guin JD: The evaluation of the patient with urticaria. *Dermatol Clin* **3**:29–49, 1985.
49. Von Krogh G, Maibach HI: The contact urticaria syndrome, an updated review. *J Am Acad Dermatol* **5**:328–342, 1981.
50. van Ketel WG: Immediate typeallergy to malt in beer. *Contact Dermatitis* **6**:297–298, 1980.
51. Camarasa JMG, Alomar A, Perez M: Contact urticaria and anaphylaxis from aminophenazone. *Contact Dermatitis* **4**:243–244, 1978.

CHAPTER 18

# Cytomegalovirus Infection

Blaise L. Congeni

## Overview

Cytomegalovirus (CMV), a member of the herpesvirus group, was initially cultured in 1956. Large cells with intranuclear inclusions had previously been noted in the salivary glands of asymptomatic children. The characteristics of disease produced in congenitally infected infants were initially described by Weller and Hanshaw in 1962 [1]. CMV remains a major cause of birth defects, hearing loss, and retardation in congenitally infected infants. It was subsequently appreciated that CMV is similar to the other herpesviruses in producing infections that are most often asymptomatic. A persistent latent infection is then established in the host. CMV is being increasingly recognized as a cause of morbidity and mortality in the immunosuppressed host. Unfortunately, efforts aimed at treatment and prevention through active immunization have met with very limited success.

## Clinical Findings and Natural History

Since CMV is a ubiquitous virus, few escape infection. In developing countries, antibody levels approach 100% during early childhood. In North America, antibody to CMV appears more gradually with increasing age. Vertical transmission from mother to infant appears to be common and has long been recognized. On the other hand, horizontal transmission, that is, person to person, is uncommon. For example, several surveys have failed to document significant transmission to health care workers caring for infected patients [2,3]. Venereal transmission of CMV has only rarely been documented [4]. Certain populations of otherwise normal children have an earlier acquisition of infection, for example, children in day care [5] and breast-fed infants of seropositive mothers [6]. The major clinical syndromes seen in association with CMV infection are listed in Table 18.1. Comprehension of the epidemiology and natural history of infection is crucial to understanding the different clinical syndromes.

TABLE 18.1. Clinical syndromes see in association with cytomegalovirus infection.

| | |
|---|---|
| Neonates | |
| | Congenital infection |
| | Perinatally acquired infection |
| Infants and adults | |
| | Hepatitis |
| | Mononucleosis |
| | Postperfusion infection |
| | Posttransplant infection |
| | Infection in immunosuppressed patients |

## CONGENITAL INFECTION

As previously noted, approximately half of middle-class women have antibody to CMV upon entering their childbearing years. Higher rates and earlier acquisition are seen in lower income groups. CMV can be recovered from approximately 10% of pregnant women [7]. Most of these infections represent reactivation of latent virus, that is, secondary infection. With a single exception in the literature, symptomatic infection in the neonate has only been reported following a primary infection in the mother [8]. Seronegative pregnant women experience a primary infection about 2% of the time [9]. In these infected mothers, in utero transmission occurs approximately one third of the time and appears unrelated to when during the pregnancy the infection occurs. Infants who develop significant handicaps in this setting are more likely to be born to mothers infected during the first half of pregnancy.

The clinical and laboratory findings of neonates symptomatically infected with CMV were initially described by Weller and Hanshaw in 1962 [1]. The major features of cytomegalic inclusion disease (CID) described therein include hepatomegaly, splenomegaly, microcephaly, mental retardation, motor disability, jaundice, and petechiae. Chorioretinitis and cerebral calcifications were seen less often. Subsequently investigators noted that most congenital infections are inapparent or asymptomatic [10].

The prognosis for subsequent development of infants who are symptomatic at birth remains extremely poor [11]. The prognosis for asymptomatic infants with congenital infection is more controversial. Reynolds et al [12] found hearing loss in 9 of 16 patients with inapparent congenital CMV infection. A trend toward subnormal intelligence was also noted. These neonates were screened for infection using elevated IgM levels in cord blood. This may overestimate the likelihood of a handicap. Hanshaw et al [13] also found a predicted school failure rate based on IQ of 2.7 times greater in such infants compared with controls. In two separate investigations, however, Kumar et al [14,15], using CMV infection of the cervix as a screen, failed to demonstrate any differences in asymptomatically infected newborns compared with controls.

## Perinatal Infections

Infants born through an infected cervix commonly acquired infection. Although some of these infants will have signs of infection, the vast majority will remain asymptomatic [7]. Infants who are perinatally infected and symptomatic generally present with interstitial pneumonia before 3 months of age. Other findings include rash or organomegaly. In one study, CMV was recovered from 20% of children less than 3 months of age with pneumonitis [16]. These children do not appear at risk for late neurologic or developmental sequelae [15].

## Infection in Normal Children and Adults

Less than 1% of children or adults infected with CMV will be symptomatic. The two major syndromes seen include hepatitis and mononucleosis.

Hanshaw et al [17] reported in 1965 the association of liver abnormalities with CMV infection. Of 20 children asymptomatically infected, 14 were noted to have hepatomegaly. Modest abnormalities of liver function were also noted. The mononucleosis syndrome seen in association with CMV infection has been well described [18]. Patients with CMV mononucleosis are slightly older than those with heterophil-positive mononucleosis. Pharyngitis and hepatosplenomegaly are less common, but headache and adenopathy are typically seen. Atypical lymphocytosis is common.

## Postperfusion Infection

Subsequent to its occurrence in the initial patients described in the 1960s, CMV infection has been recognized to occur commonly in transfusion recipients. This syndrome is usually seen 3 to 7 weeks after transfusion and is generally characterized by fever, splenomegaly, hepatitis, atypical lymphocytosis, and a negative heterophil agglutination test [19]. Seroconversion to CMV frequently occurs in this group of patients without evidence of symptomatology. The risk of infection following a transfusion is proportional to the number of units transfused [20]. Patients with the highest risk of infection are seronegative recipients of seropositive blood.

Blood transfusions have also been an important source of CMV infections in sick neonates. Twenty percent of newborn infants in one study had serologic evidence of infection following exchange transfusions [21]. Neonates with perinatal infection acquired from blood products frequently manifest respiratory distress, hepatitis, fever, anemia, and thrombocytopenia [22]. The ability to use only seronegative blood or frozen blood in the neonatal intensive care unit will significantly diminish this problem [23].

## Infection in the Immunosuppressed Host

The patient receiving an organ transplant may develop infection with CMV in either of two ways: (a) A primary infection may occur in the seronegative recipient receiving an allograft from a seropositive donor. (b) A secondary infection may develop in the seropositive recipient following reactivation of endogenous latent virus. The primary infection tends to be more severe [24,25]. Fever, pneumonitis, and hepatitis are the most common symptoms. In the patient receiving a renal transplant, renal dysfunction may also occur; distinguishing rejection from infection may be difficult. Infection in recipients of cardiac and bone marrow allografts is also common and well described. As in the other instances previously discussed, preexisting antibody status of the recipient and allograft are major determinants of risk.

Patients with primary or secondary defects in cell-mediate immunity (i.e., those with malignancy or AIDS) are frequently infected with CMV. The spectrum of disease is similar to that seen in transplant recipients.

## Differential Diagnosis

### Congenital Infection

The pathogens responsible for producing congenital infections similar to CMV have been grouped together as "TORCH" agents. Toxoplasmosis and rubella produce illnesses that most closely resemble CMV infection. All three agents most often result in asymptomatic infection. Physicians frequently test the serum for these agents (i.e., obtain TORCH titers) when confronted with a neonate with infection. The antibody levels thus obtained most often reflect maternal antibody and are of limited usefulness [26]. Since IgM antibody does not cross the placenta, IgM-specific titers for CMV may be more useful, but the test is available only on a limited basis [27]. The congenitally infected neonate sheds large quantities of virus in the urine and saliva, and culture remains the method of choice for definitive diagnosis.

### Perinatal Infections

The perinatally infected infant most often presents with pneumonitis. *Chlamydia* is the major pathogen that must be distinguished from CMV. *Ureaplasma*, other viruses including respiratory syncytial virus, and on rare occasions pertussis may present with similar findings. Infants with chlamydia infection are usually afebrile and frequently have cough as the presenting complaint. They often are noted to have modest eosinophilia and elevated levels of IgG, IgA, and IgM antibodies in addition to serologic findings specific for *C. trachomatis*. The method of choice for diagnosis of CMV infection in this age remains culture.

### Older Infants and Adults

In older patients, pathogens considered in the differential diagnosis depend on the organ system involved. Especially in the compromised host, the differential diagnosis is extensive, and methods useful in distinguishing between the different pathogens is beyond the scope of this presentation. Major considerations are listed here:

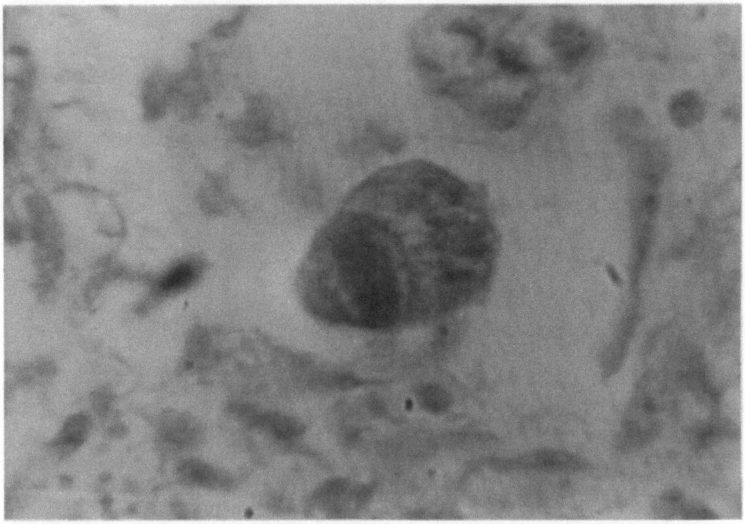

FIGURE 18.1. CMV infected fibroblasts showing typical cytopathic effects.

| Mononucleosis/Hepatitis | Pneumonitis |
|---|---|
| CMV | CMV |
| Epstein-Barr virus (EBV) | *Pneumocystis carinii* |
| *Toxoplasmosis* | Fungi, including *Candida* |
| Hepatitis A, hepatitis B, non-A non-B hepatitis | *Mycobacteria*, especially atypical strains |

## Histopathology

Morphologically, evidence of CMV infection may be found in most epithelial cells. The characteristic features include large cells, 20 to 35 μ in diameter (cytomegaly), with basophilia or amphophilia of the cytoplasm and the presence of prominent round or oval, basophilic intranuclear inclusions (5–10 μ) which are surrounded by a broad, clear halo between the inclusion and the marginated nuclear chromatin lying against the nuclear membrane. Cytoplasmic inclusions measuring 3 to 4 μ may also be seen (Fig. 18.1, 18.2).

## Management and Prevention

A variety of antivirals have been used in the treatment of CMV infections, with very limited success. Cytosine arabinoside was found to decrease renal excretion of the virus but had no visible clinical effect [28]. use of adenine arabinoside [29] and idox-

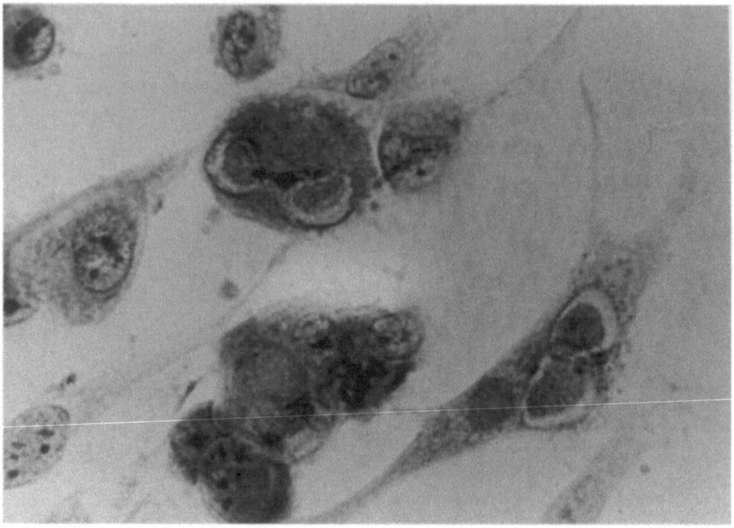

FIGURE 18.2. Intranuclear inclusion with CMV from infected lung.

uridine [30] has given similar disappointing results. Other modalities that have been tried include interferon and transfer factor, but neither was demonstrated to have clinical efficacy [31,32].

The only drug that has shown promise for the treatment of CMV infection is 9-(1,3-dihydroxy-2-propoxymethyl) guanine (ganciclovir). Although this drug is still investigational, trials with it have been conducted in a variety of clinical situations with immunosuppressed patients. Patients with CMV disease involving the retina, lungs, brain, liver, and gastrointestinal tract have all been treated [33]. In general, clinical improvement and lengthened survival were seen. The major toxicity encountered was hematologic.

Some progress has been made toward development of a live vaccine useful in the prevention of CMV infection. Because CMV is a member of the herpesvirus group, there are several theoretical concerns in this regard. This group of viruses has demonstrated oncogenic potential as well as latency. The possibility of different strains is also present. Nevertheless, at least two groups of investigators have developed candidate vaccines [34,35]. Unfortunately, following development of cellular and humeral immunity, recipients were found to lose compliment-fixing antibody within years of immunization.

## REFERENCES

1. Weller TH, Hanshaw JB: Virologic and clinical observations on cytomegalic inclusion disease. *N Engl J Med* **266**:1233–1244, 1962.
2. Dworsky ME, Welch K, Cassady G, et al: Occupational risk for primary cytomegalovirus infection among pediatric health-care workers. *N Engl J Med* **309**:950–953.

3. Balfour CL, Balfour HH: Cytomegalovirus is not an occupational risk for nurses in renal transplant and neonatal units. *JAMA* **256**:1909–1914, 1986.
4. Chretien JH, McGinniss CG, Muller A: Venereal causes of cytomegalovirus mononucleosis. *JAMA* **238**:1644–1645, 1977.
5. Pass RF, August AM, Dworsky ME, et al: Cytomegalovirus infection in a day-care center. *N Engl J Med* **307**:477–479, 1982.
6. Stagno S, Reynolds DW, Pass RF, et al: Breast milk and the risk of cytomegalovirus infection. *N Engl J Med* **302**:1073–1076, 1980.
7. Reynolds DW, Stagno S, Hosty TS, et al: Maternal cytomegalovirus excretion and perinatal infection. *N Engl J Med* **289**:1–5, 1973.
8. Stagno S, Pass RF, Dworsky ME, et al: Congenital cytomegalovirus infection: The relative importance of primary and recurrent maternal infection. *N Engl J Med* **306**:945–949, 1982.
9. Stagno S, Pass RF, Cloud G, et al: Primary cytomegalovirus infection in pregnancy. *JAMA* **256**:1904–1908, 1986.
10. Starr JG, Bart RD, Gold E: Inapparent congenital cytomegalovirus infection: Clinical and epidemiologic characteristics in early infancy. *N Engl J Med* **282**:1075–1078,
11. Pass RF, Stagno S, Myers GJ, et al: Outcome of symptomatic congenital cytomegalovirus infection: Results of long-term longitudinal follow-up. *Pediatrics* **66**:758–765, 1980.
12. Reynolds DW, Stagno S, Stubbs KG, et al: Inapparent congenital cytomegalovirus infection with elevated cord IgM levels. *N Engl J Med* **290**:291–296, 1974.
13. Hanshaw JB, Scheiner AP, Moxley AW, et al: School failure and deafness after "silent" congenital cytomegalovirus infection. *N Engl J Med* **295**:468–470, 1976.
14. Kumar ML, Nankervis GA, Gold E: Inapparent congenital cytomegalovirus infection: A follow-up study. *N Engl J Med* **288**:1370–1372, 1973.
15. Kumar ML, Nankervis GA, Jacobs IB, et al: Congenital and postnatally acquired cytomegalovirus infection: Long-term follow-up. *J Pediatr* **104**:674–679, 1984.
16. Dworsky ME, Stagno S: Newer agents causing pneumonitis in early infancy. *Pediatr Infect Dis* **1**:188–195, 1982.
17. Hanshaw JB, Betts RF, Simon G, et al: Acquired cytomegalovirus infection: Association with hepatomegaly and abnormal liver-function tests. *N Engl M Med* **272**:602–609, 1965.
18. Jordan MC, Rousseau WE, Stewart JA, et al: Spontaneous cytomegalovirus mononucleosis. *Ann Intern Med* **79**:153–160, 1973.
19. Lang DJ, Hanshaw JB; Cytomegalovirus infection and the postperfusion syndrome: Recognition of primary infections in four patients. *N Engl J Med* **280**:1145–1149, 1969.
20. Spector SA, Schmidt K, Ticknor W, et al: Cytomegaloviruria in older infants in intensive care nurseries. *J Pediatr* **95**:444–446, 1979.
21. Nankervis GA: Cytomegalovirus infections in the blood recipient. *Yale J Biol Med* **49**:13–15, 1976.
22. Ballard RA, Drew WL, Hufnagle KG, et al: Acquired cytomegalovirus infection in preterm infants. *Am J Dis Child* **133**:482–485, 1979.
23. Yeager AS, Grumet FC, Hafleigh EB, et al: Prevention of transfusion-acquired cytomegalovirus infections in newborn infants. *Fet Neonat Med* **98**:281–287, 1981.
24. National Institutes of Health: Summary of a workshop on cytomegalovirus infections during organ transplantation. *J Infect Dis* **139**:728–734, 1979.
25. Betts RF, Freeman RB, Douglas RG, et al: Clinical manifestations of renal allograft derived primary cytomegalovirus infection. *Am J Dis Child* **131**:759–763, 1978.
26. Leland D, French ML, Kleiman MB, et al: The use of TORCH titers. *Pediatrics* **72**:41–43, 1983.

27. Thomson RB, Benedict ML, Congeni BL: Laboratory diagnosis of neonatal cytomegalovirus infection using a commercially available CMV-IgM assay and viral culture. *Diag Microbiol Infec Dis* (in press).
28. McCracken GH, Luby JP: Cytosine arabinoside in the treatment of congenital cytomegalic inclusion disease. *J Pediatr* **80**:488–495, 1972.
29. Ch'ien LT, et al: Effect of adenine-arabinoside on cytomegalovirus infections. *J Infect Dis* **130**:32–39, 1974.
30. Barton BW, Tobin JO: The effect of idoxuridine on the excretion of cytomegalovirus in congenital infection. *Ann NY Acad Sci* **173**:90, 1970.
31. Emodi G, et al: Effect of human exogenous leukocyte interferon in cytomegalovirus infections. *J Infect Dis* **133**:199–204, 1976.
32. Thomas LT, et al: Transfer-factor treatment in congenital cytomegalovirus infection. *Lancet* **2**:10–56–57, 1977.
33. Chachoua A, et al: 9-(1,3-dihydroxy-2-propoxymethyl) guanine (Ganciclovir) in the treatment of cytomegalovirus gastrointestinal disease with the acquired immunodeficiency syndrome. *Ann Intern Med* **107**:133–137, 1987.
34. Plotkin SA, et al: Candidate cytomegalovirus strain for human vaccination. *Infect Immunol* **12**:521–527, 1975.
35. Elek SD, Stern H: Development of a vaccine against mental retardation caused by cytomegalovirus infection in utero. *Lancet* **1**:1–5, 1974.

CHAPTER 19

# Protozoa and Helminths: "The Gay Bowel Syndrome"

Louis Weinrauch and Joseph El-On

Sexual transmission of protozoal and helminthic diseases by orogenital or oroanal routes has become increasingly common during the last two decades, especially in young men. The outbreak of the acquired immunodeficiency syndrome (AIDS), and the medical and public campaign against it, seem to be changing sexual habits. Lately there has been a drop in the incidence of sexually transmitted enteric diseases.

There is no question about the fact that pathogenic and nonpathogenic intestinal parasites are also transmitted by ingestion of contaminated food or water that may contain cysts, ova, or live trophozoites. Nevertheless, in view of the multiplicity and versatility of sexual contacts among male homosexuals, it is not surprising that fecal oral transmission of a variety of infections including protozoa and helminths occurs more frequently in this group [1].

Amebiasis, for example, is a major cause of morbidity and mortality in tropical regions. Until recently in the Western world, this infection was diagnosed almost exclusively in tourists returning from endemic areas. Recent studies, however, have demonstrated that *Entamoeba histolytica* can be found in the stool of homosexual men with an estimated prevalence of 32%. Among homosexual men aged 20 to 39 years living in San Francisco, the incidence of reported systematic intestinal amebiasis jumped 8000% between the years 1973–1982 [2]. In the past this disease was usually foodborne or waterborne and occurred equally commonly in both sexes.

Sexual habits are a private matter for each mature individual, and the surrounding society has less and less influence on this behavior. Nevertheless, the physician is bound to advise and admonish patients regarding the risks associated with oroanal contact, fellatio, and cunnilingus. Anal sex can safely follow vaginal coitus, but the reverse must be avoided unless the penis, finger, or vibrator is carefully washed in between.

The clinician has an obligation to exclude pathogens in patients belonging to the particular risk group. Therefore, in men with promiscuous homosexual proclivities, a search for intestinal protozoa and helminths is indicated.

Table 19.1 summarizes drug treatment currently available for various protozoan and helminths infections.

TABLE 19.1. Treatment of sexually transmitted diseases caused by protozoa and helminths.

| Causative organism, degree of infection | Treatment | | |
|---|---|---|---|
| | Drug | Route | Adult dosage |
| *Entamoeba histolytica* | | | |
| Asymptomatic cyst carriers | Diloxanide furoate (Furamide) | Oral | 500 mg tid for 10 days |
| | Metronidazole (Flagyl) | Oral | 750 mg tid for 5–10 days |
| | Tinidazole (Fasigyn) | Oral | 2 g/day for 5 days |
| | Diiodohydroxyquine (iodoquinol) | Oral | 650 mg tid for 20 days |
| Mild to moderate infection | Metronidazole + | Oral | As above |
| | diiodohydroxyquine | Oral | As above |
| | Metronidazole + | Oral | As above |
| | diloxanide furoate | Oral | As above |
| Severe intestinal disease | Dehydroemetine | IM | 90 mg/day for 10 days |
| | + tetracycline (Achromycin) | Oral | 500 mg qid for 5 days |
| | Emetine hydrochloride + | IM | 60 mg/day for 10 days |
| | tetracycline | Oral | As above |
| Extraintestinal disease, amebic abscess | Metronidazole + | Oral | As above |
| | diloxanide furoate | Oral | As above |
| | Dehydroemetine or emetine hydrochloride | IM | As above |
| | + chloroquine (Aralen) | Oral | 300 mg bid for 1 day followed by 150 mg bid for 20 days |
| | Metronidazole + | Oral | As above |
| | dehydroemetine or emetine hydrochloride | IM | As above |
| *Dientamoeba fragilis* | Diiodohydroxyquine | Oral | As for *E. histolytica* |
| | Metronidazole | Oral | As for *E. histolytica* |
| | Tinidazole | Oral | 150 mg bid for 7 days |
| | Tetracycline | Oral | 500 mg qid for 10 days |
| *Giardia lamblia* | Quinacrine (Atabrine) | Oral | 100 mg tid for 5–10 days |
| | Metronidazole | Oral | 250–500 mg tid for 7 days or 2 g single dose daily for 3 days |

TABLE 19.1. *Continued.*

| Causative organism, degree of infection | Treatment | | |
|---|---|---|---|
| | Drug | Route | Adult dosage |
| *Giardia lamblia* (cont.) | Tinidazole | Oral | 150 mg bid for 10 days or 1.5–2 g single dose |
| *Cryptospordium spp.* | *No effective drug available* | | |
| *Isospora belli* | Trimethoprim + sulfamethoxazole (Bactrim) | Oral | 160 mg + 800 mg bid for 10 days |
| *Balantidium coli* | Tetracycline | Oral | 500 mg qid for 10 days |
| | Diiodohydroxyquine | Oral | 650 tid for 20 days |
| | Metronidazole | Oral | 750 mg tid for 5–10 days |
| *Enterobius vermicularis* | Pyrantel pamoate (Combantrin) | Oral | 11 mg/kg (max. 0.1 g) repeated after 2–3 weeks |
| | Mebendazole (Vermox) | Oral | 100 mg dose repeated after 2–3 weeks |
| | Pyrvinium pamoate (Poran) | Oral | 5 mg/kg (max. 350 mg) repeated after 2–3 weeks |
| | Piperazine citrate (Antepar) | Oral | 50–75 mg/kg/day (max. 3.5 g) for 3–5 days |

# Part 1. Protozoa

The following protozoa are parasites of the gastrointestinal system in humans:

Ameba: *Entamoeba histolyca*, *E. hartmani*, *E. coli*, *E. gingivalis*, *Dientamoeba fragilis*, *Endolimax nana*, and *Iodamoeba buetschlii*.
Flagellates: *Giardia lamblia*, *Trichomonas hominis*, and *T. tenax*.
Coccidia: *Cryptosporidium spp.* and *Isospora spp.*
Ciliate: *Balantidium coli*.

With the exception of *E. gingivalis*, which occurs in the mouth, the amebas are all intestinal. *E. histolytica* and *D. fragilis* are the only pathogenic amebas in humans, causing morbidity and mortality in almost 10% of the population, mainly in tropical areas.

*G. lamblia*, *Cryptosporidium spp.*, *Isospora spp.*, and *B. coli* are additional pathogenic intestinal protozoa of man.

## Entamoeba histolytica

*E. histolytica* is a cosmopolitan parasite of humans, occurring mainly in adults between 20 and 50 years of age. The parasite is located in the colon and cecum. It appears in two biologic forms, the trophozoite (10–20 μm) (Fig. 19.1), the mobile form, causing all the clinical manifestations, and the cyst (10 μm) (Fig. 19.2), which transfers the infection. The cysts are passed in the stool and may initiate new infection through ingestion of fecally contaminated food and water.

In developing countries, transmission of the parasite may occur mainly as a result of a low standard of hygiene, but in Western countries, where the incidence of amebiasis is low, transmission by oroanal sex is considerable. About 21 to 32% of homosexual men examined at sexually transmitted disease clinics in major cities in the United States [3] and 12% of those in the United Kingdom [4], were found to be infected with *E. histolytica*.

Trophozoite emerged from ingested cyst, on entry into the colon, may develop into either asymptomatic or symptomatic form. Race, sex, age, nutritional and immunologic conditions, and intestinal flora have been considered as factors affecting the virulence of the ameba. Considerable evidence suggests that a diet rich in carbohydrates and poor in protein supports infection. Recent studies [5] indicate that a specific mechanism based on carbohydrate recognition plays an important role in the interaction of the ameba with mammalian and bacterial cells and in the pathogenicity of this parasite. Interaction with specific bacteria is followed by the conversion of the ameba from a harmless parasite to a virulent state. The conversion has been shown in vitro to be associated with changes in the electrophoretic mobilities of the amebic enzymes [6,7]. Thus far no case of invasive amebiasis has been shown to have parasites with nonpathogenic enzymes. Recent data indicate that isoenzymes alone are not sufficient and are not completely reliable indicators of pathogenesis.

No correlation between pathogenicity and the number of secreted amebas has been described, and many parasites may be found in the stool of asymptomatic carriers. Intestinal mucosal invasion by the parasite leads to the formation of flask-shaped lesions with minimal tissue reaction. Granulomatous reaction may also develop and result in ameboma. The cecum and the rectosigmoid colon are the most common sites of amebic invasion, causing proctocolitis, but proctitis, enterocolitis, and enteritis may also occur. Amebic vaginitis; cutaneous amebiasis of the labia, prepuce, and glans penis of the sexual partner; and urethritis have also been described. The degree of tissue damage is variable. Most infections are either asymptomatic or cause only mild gastrointestinal disturbances. Occasionally the disease is accompanied by nausea, abdominal discomfort, and mild diarrhea. In severe cases, 10 to 20 stools a day containing blood and mucus are presented. This may be associated with sharp abdominal pain, vomiting, marked constipation, fever, and leukocytosis.

The major complication of invasive amebiasis is the development of tissue abscesses, mostly in the upper part of the right lobe of the liver. Extension of the abscesses to other organs, such as lungs, brain, and the skin, may also occur. Inva-

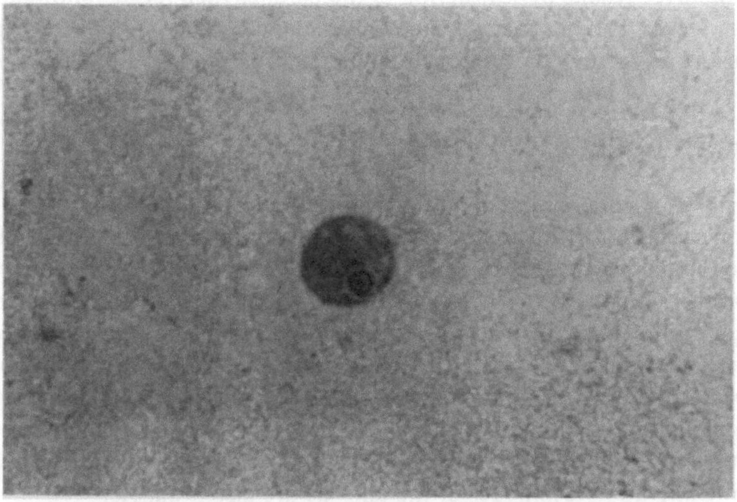

FIGURE 19.1. *Entamoeba histolytica* trophozoite in culture.

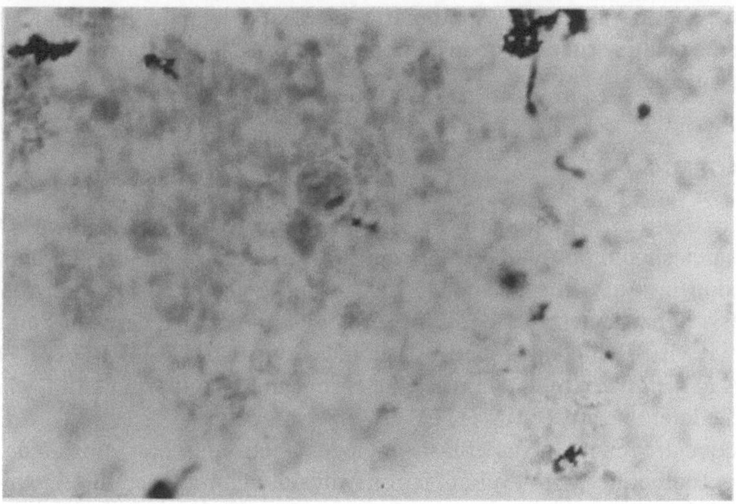

FIGURE 19.2. *Entamoeba histolytica* cysts in stool.

sion of the liver results in destruction of the parenchymal tissue followed by pain, chills, and fever. Patients may develop enlarged tender liver with functional abnormalities and an increased erythrocyte sedimentation rate.

## Clinical Findings

Diagnosis of amebiasis is made by detecting the trophozoites and/or the cysts in fresh or purged stool by direct microscopic examination. Fresh specimens should be examined immediately after submission to the laboratory. Several stool examinations are occasionally required to establish the diagnosis. Motility characteristics of the trophozoite, the number of nuclei, and the presence of organized chromatoid material in the cyst ar considered of diagnostic value. A mobile ameba containing erythrocytes is an indication for pathogenicity. Staining with Lugol solution or iron hematoxylin improves the diagnosis. The sensitivity of this test is increased by the concentration technique, either that of a saturated NaCl solution or a formalin-ether method. Cultivation techniques of the amebae are also available.

Serologic examination using passive hemagglutination, counterimmunoelectrophoresis, as well as bentonite agglutination and enzyme-linked immunoabsorbent assay (ELISA) are used for the diagnosis of invasive amebiasis. These tests have only little diagnostic value in asymptomatic cases and in mild intestinal amebiasis; however, a positive titer has been demonstrated in 60% of the invasive and in 95% of hepatic amebiasis.

## Management

Amebiasis, either symptomatic or asymptomatic, requires treatment. Asymptomatic cases should be treated to prevent transmission of the disease and possible conversion into a virulent state. It was recently suggested [3] that treatment of amebiasis is particularly essential in serologically positive cases of human T cell leukemia virus/lymphadenopathy-associated virus (HTLV-III/LAV). In these patients *E. histolytica* might increase the chronic mitogenic stimulation while shortening the latent period of the HTLV-III/LAV infection.

Effective treatment of amebiasis includes metronidazole, diloxanide furoate, 8-hydroxyquinolines, tetracycline, paromomycin, chloroquine, emetine hydrochloride, and dehydroemetine.

Diloxanide furoate, diiodohydroxyquine, and tetracycline have been successfully used to treat asymptomatic amebiasis. Tetracycline reduces the survival of the parasite by killing the bacteria necessary for its survival. Paromomycin, an aminoglycoside antibiotic, is an alternative luminal amebicide. The drug is not absorbed by the intestine and also kills most of the gram-positive and gram-negative bacteria. Occasionally the drug is given in combination with diiodohydroxyquine. The latter drug is not always available and, although it is generally well tolerated, in continuous use it may cause optic neuritis. It also may mimic amebiasis with bloating and colicky diarrhea.

Metronidazole is considered the drug of choice for the treatment of symptomatic intestinal and invasive amebiasis. This drug is highly absorbed and therefore not effective for totally eliminating the intestinal amebas. The drug is generally well tolerated although side effects, including nausea, fatigue, and depression as well as a metallic taste, may develop. In some people the urine becomes dark as a result of metabolic products of the drug. Metronidazole has also been shown to be mutagenic and carcinogenic in rodents and therefore is not allowed for use during pregnancy. Alcohol is interdicted during therapy.

Emetine hydrochloride and dehydroemetine are additional highly effective tissue amebicides. These drugs are used in cases with unsatisfactory reaction to metronidazole. Both drugs are generally associated with severe side effects. Chloroquine is effective only against hepatic amebiasis. Occasionally it is used in acute intestinal amebiasis as a prophylaxis against hepatic disease.

## Dientamoeba fragilis

*D. fragilis* is an additional intestinal ameba virulent to humans. This parasite 6–20 μm) is characterized by two nuclei connected to each other by a filament, and by the absence of a cyst stage. The parasite lives mainly in the cecum, but may also be found along the large intestine, living on the intestinal lumen debris. *D. fragilis* is asymptomatic in most individuals, but occasionally gastrointestinal disturbances such as nausea, vomiting, and diarrhea may occur. Anal pruritus is also a common sign. Diiodohydroxyquine and tetracycline are effective drugs against this disease [8–10].

## Prognosis

Both *E. histolytica* and *D. fragilis* respond completely to appropriate drugs. Relapses, if such occur, are usually a manifestation of reinfection. Unfortunately this is very common in promiscuous people. The fatality rate is less than 5%.

Community control of amebic diseases in selected population by periodic mass treatment with metronidazole and diloxanide furoate is worthwhile.

## *Giardia lamblia*

*G. lamblia* is a flagellated protozoan of the upper small intestine of humans. It has worldwide distribution, and is particularly prevalent in areas of low hygiene and of beaver contaminations. Children are the most susceptible to infection; adults develop resistance to the parasite, particularly to the local strain. Exposure to a new strain in a new geographic area may initiate new infection. Epidemics of *G. lamblia* infection have usually been associated with contaminated water supplies, although

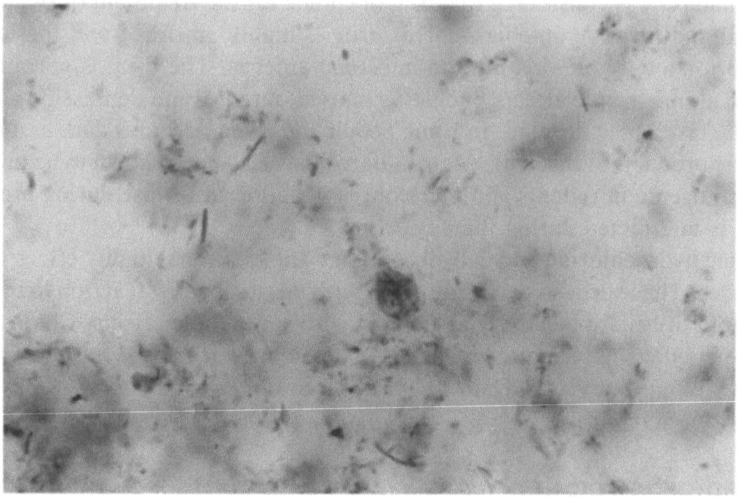

FIGURE 19.3. *Giardia lamblia* trophozoite in stool.

sexual transmission, by orogenital or oral anal routes, is now believed to be common in homosexuals [11].

The parasite, which is pear-shaped, appears in two forms: the trophozoite (10–18 μm) (Figs. 19.3, 19.4) and the cyst (10–14 μm) (Fig. 19.5). The mobile form, the trophozoite, causes the clinical symptoms and the cyst transmits the disease by contaminating food and water. Ten cysts are sufficient to cause infection. Most infections are asymptomatic, although they may be associated with gastrointestinal disturbance, low fat absorption (steatorrhea), weight loss, and chronic diarrhea. Most of the damage caused to the epithelial cells is mechanical as a result of attachment of the parasite to the intestinal villi, causing villous atrophy. In severe cases lactose intolerance develops and absorption of fat, D-xylose, and vitamin B-12 may be impaired.

## Diagnosis

Diagnosis of the disease is established by detecting the cyst and/or the trophozoite in a microscopic stool examination. Although the parasite can be cultivated in artificial media, this procedure is not useful in direct diagnosis. However, in suspected cases with cysts not detected in the stool, the string test (Enterotest) or duodenal aspiration is highly effective in detecting the trophozoite [12].

## Management

Treatment is recommended for both symptomatic and asymptomatic cases. Metronidazole and tinidazole are the drugs of choice against this disease. Both

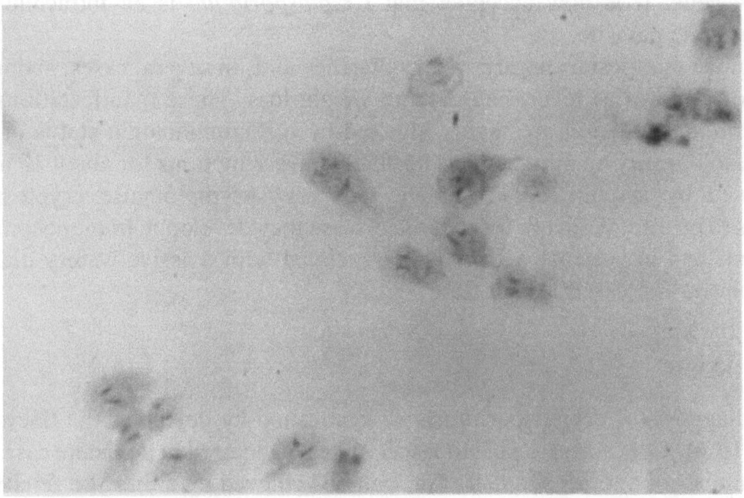

FIGURE 19.4. *Giardia lamblia* trophozoites in culture.

drugs, which are avoided during pregnancy, may be associated with nausea and metallic taste. Quinacrine and chloroquine are alternative drugs. In 90% of patients, radical clinical improvement is achieved within days, and normality is reached within an additional 4 to 6 weeks.

## *Cryptosporidium* spp.

The coccidian protozoan parasite *Cryptosporidium* was regarded as a rare opportunistic pathogen of the human being until recently, when it was found to be a relatively frequent intestinal pathogenic parasite [13]. Human infection with *Cryptosporidium* has been described in developed and less developed countries. People of all ages are susceptible to infection, although children are considered the most susceptible. The parasite is now recognized as an important microorganism causing gastrointestinal infection in both animals and humans and constitutes a public health problem of nearly global dimension.

*Cryptosporidium* was first described in mice in 1907 and only in 1976 in humans. Several species of *Cryptosporidium* exist in over 30 different hosts that have little or not host susceptibility. Zoonotic transmission is not significant, and person-to-person infection has been reported [14]. The disease is acquired by ingestion of fully sporolated oocyst from contaminated food and water. In the intestine, sporozoites excyst from the oocyst and parasitize epithelial cells. Asexual multiplication then occurs, followed by sexual multiplication. This results in the production of the oocyst, which is 4 to 6 μm in size. The parasites inhabit the microvilous region of the intestinal epithelial cells, where they are found mainly attached to the surface of the cells. It is now accepted that *Cryptosporidium* is an intracellular, extracytoplasmic parasite.

Clinical manifestations are watery diarrhea and, in several cases, abdominal discomfort, anorexia, fever, nausea, and weight loss. These manifestations of *Cryptosporidium* infection are highly affected by the immunologic status of the host. Immunologically healthy persons normally have symptoms for about 10 to 20 days, followed by spontaneous complete recovery. Asymptomatic cryptosporidiosis seems to be rare. A severe form of the disease may develop in immunocompromised patients and in patients with AIDS, associated with massive watery diarrhea and consequent increased loss of fluid.

### Diagnosis

The diagnosis of cryptosporidiosis is established by detecting the oocyst in stool (Fig. 19.6). Concentration of stool specimens is required in nonacute cases in which the number of oocysts is small. This can be achieved by either the flotation or the sedimentation technique. Fluorescent staining also has been used to detect *Cryptosporidium*, and specific anti-*Cryptosporidium* IgM and IgG may be detected in the sera of 95% of patients with cryptosporidiosis.

### Management

No effective treatment against the disease is yet available. The macrolide antibiotic, spiramycin, which was thought to be highly promising, has shown controversial results [15]. Supportive care with oral or intravenous hydration is the major therapeutic intervention today for human cryptosporidiosis.

## *Isospora* spp.

*Isospora*, like *Cryptosporidium*, is an intestinal small coccidian protozoan, 20 to 33 μm in size, causing diarrhea in domestic animals and humans. The genus *Isospora* contains three species, which all parasitize human beings: *I. belli*; *I. hominis*, and *I. natalensis*. Although the parasite is worldwide in distribution, particularly in the tropics and subtropics, it is considered an uncommon causative agent of diarrhea in humans. The parasites have asexual and sexual phases, which are completed in the same host.

The disease is acquired by ingestion of the oocyst with contaminated food and water. Each oocyst contains 4 to 8 sporozoites. These are liberated in the small intestine, where they invade the epithelial cells of the intestinal mucosa. The asexual multiplication of the parasite is followed by the sexual phase, which terminates in the production of oocysts. These are passed in the stool. The disease is generally asymptomatic and self-limited. The parasite may cause erosions of the intestinal wall, leading to abdominal disturbances and diarrhea. In immunocompromised patients, severe, chronic infection may develop, associated with watery diarrhea,

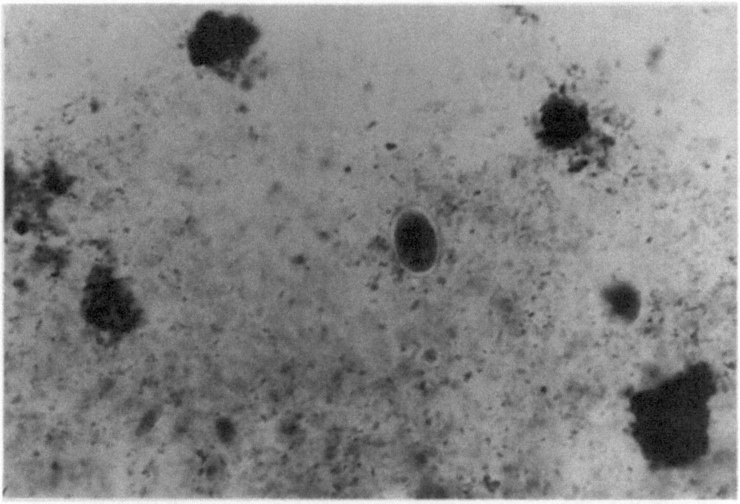

FIGURE 19.5. *Giardia lamblia* cysts in stool.

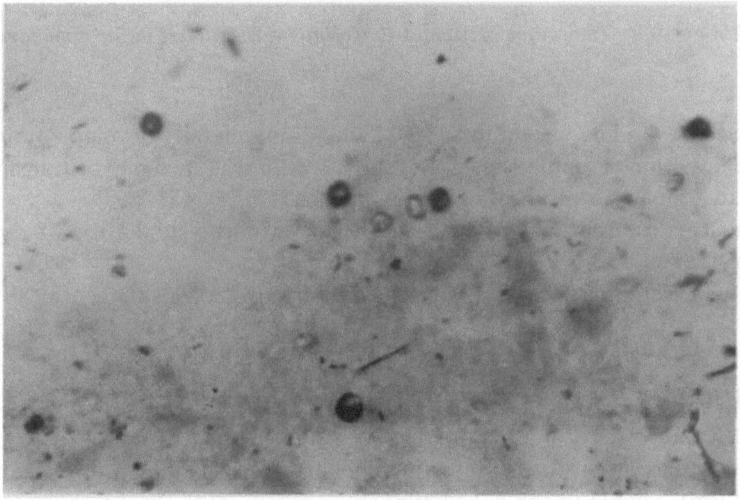

FIGURE 19.6. *Cryptosporidium* oocysts in stool.

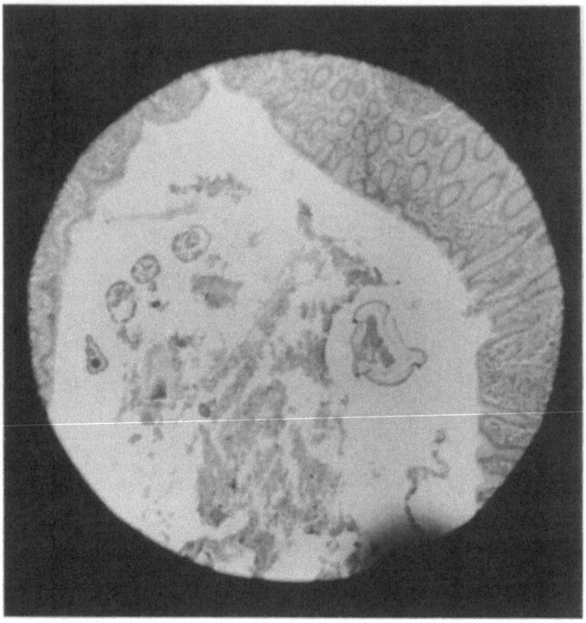

FIGURE 19.7. Transverse section of *Enterobius vermicularis* in the appendix.

steatorrhea, fever, and weight loss [16]. Symptoms generally develop within 8 days after the ingestion of viable oocyst. Recently, *I. belli* was shown to be transmitted in homosexual men as a result of oral-anal contact [17].

Diagnosis is established by detecting the oocyst in the stool 10 to 28 days after infection.

Treatment, seldom successful, consists of cotrimoxazole [18].

## *Balantidium coli*

*B. coli* is the largest protozoan infecting humans. It has a ciliated trophozoite stage (50–200 μm), visible to the naked eye, and a cystic stage. In diarrheic stools the trophozoite appears as a large ovoidal object covered with short cilia of uniform length, which propel the organism forward.

*B. coli* invades mainly the colon and appendix, where the trophozoite feeds on the cells of the intestinal wall or on bacteria as a lumen parasite. The rectosigmoid is the most involved region, with lesions appearing as small flask-shaped ulcers of a few millimeters in diameter, resembling the ulcerations of amebic colitis. The ulcers may be superficial, involving the mucosa and submucosa, or they may involve the entire thickness of the intestine, causing perforations. Although *B. coli* is a pathogen, it may live in the human bowel without producing symptoms. In most infected individuals, diarrhea is present and dysentery can also occur. Cases of urethritis, cystitis, pyelonephritis, and inflammatory vaginitis have also been reported. Clinical forms, complicated with perforations and peritonitis, have a poor prognosis with a mortality of up to 30% [12].

Diagnosis is made by the demonstration of mobile trophozoites in diarrheic stool or cysts in stool or semisolid feces.

Treatment of *B. coli* is urged in both carriers and symptomatic individuals. Tetracyclines, diiodohydroxyquine, and metronidazole are the drugs of choice.

# Part 2. Helminths

*Enterobius vermicularis* (pinworn, seatworm, threadworm, *Oxyuris*), a nematode primitive worm, is found in all climates and is probably the most common helminthic infection of humans (Fig. 19.7). The adult female pinworm is about 1 cm long, the male one fourth as large. They live attached to the mucosa of the cecum and distal colon. At night the female migrates through the anal canal, deposits about 10,000 eggs on the perianal skin, wanders for a short period, and dies. The eggs, containing embryos, may be transmitted by person-to-person contact, by bedclothes, or by the air.

## Clinical Findings

Pinworms are common in urban as well as rural populations in all climates, but are particularly common in group living situations and institutions [19]. The majority of infections are asymptomatic. The parasites in the intestine provoke minimal or no inflammation. The most common symptom is pruritus ani, especially at night, being related to the migration of the gravid female worms. Sleeplessness, irritability, enuresis, and scratching are secondary to the pruritus. Vaginal discharge and pruritus [20], salpingitis, endometritis, cystitis, balanitis, and urethritis have been reported.

## Diagnosis

Diagnosis may sometimes be made by seeing the 10-mm-long female worm on the perineal or perianal region at night, on toilet paper, or in the stool. The preferable method for detection of enterobiasis is the examination for ova of material obtained from the perianal skin by pressing to the area the gummed side of a cellophane tape. At least three to five tests, performed on consecutive mornings before the person bathes, are needed to make the diagnosis. Searching for ova in the feces is rarely helpful, but scrapings from under the nails may reveal ova. Eosinophilia is not common.

## Treatment

Since this parasite is easily transmitted from person to person, treatment should cover all the contacts of the infected individual. Pyrantel pamoate, mebendazole, pyrivinium pamoate, and piperazine citrate are the drugs of choice, and treatment should be repeated in 2 to 3 weeks. Risk population should be examined periodically to prevent enterobiasis.

## References

1. Markell EK, Havens RF, Kuritsubo RA, et al: Intestinal protozoa in homosexual men of the San Francisco Bay Area: Prevalence and correlates of infection. *Am J Trop Med Hyg* **33**:239–245, 1984.
2. Pearce RB: Intestinal protozoal infections and AIDS. *Lancet* **2**:51, 1983.
3. Petri WA, Ravdin JI: Treatment of homosexual men infected with *Entamoeba histolytica*. *N Engl J Med* **315**:393, 1986.
4. Allason-Jones E, Mindel A, Sargeaunt P, et al: *Entamoeba histolytica* as a commensal intestinal parasite in homosexual men. *N Engl J Med* **315**:356, 1986.
5. Mirelman D, Feingold C, Wexler A, et al: Interactions between *Entamoeba histolytica*, bacteria and intestinal cells. In: *Cytopathology of Parasitic Disease*. Ciba Foundation Symposium 99. Pitman, Bath, England. 1983; pp. 2–18.
6. Sargeaunt PG, Williams JE: Electrophoretic isoenzyme pattern of *Entamoeba histolytica* and *Entamoeba coli*: *Trans Roy Soc Trop Med Hyg* **72**:164–166, 1978.
7. Sargeaunt PG, Williams JE, Kumate J, et al: The epidemiology of *Entamoeba histolytica* in Mexico City: A pilot survey. I. *Trans Roy Soc Trop Med Hyg* **74**:653–656, 1980.
8. Shein R, Gelb A: Colitis due to *Dientamoeba fragilis*. *Am J Gastroenterol* **78**:634–636, 1983.
9. Spencer MJ, Chapin MR, Garcia LS: *Dientamoeba fragilis*: A gastrointestinal protozoan infection in adults. *Am J Gastroenterol* **77**:565–569, 1982.
10. Yang J, Scholten TH: *Dientamoeba fragiis*: A review with notes of its epidemiology, pathogenicity, mode of transmission, and diagnosis. *Am J Trop Med Hyg* **26**:16–22, 1977.
11. Kean BH, William DC, Luminais SK: Epidemic of amoebiasis and giardiasis in biased population. *Br J Vener Dis* **59**:375–378, 1979.
12. Knight R: Giardiasis, isosporiasis, and balantidiasis. *Clin Gastroenterol* **7**:31–47, 1978.
13. Tzipori S, Smith S, Birch C, et al: Cryptosporidiosis in hospital patients with gastroenteritis. *Am J Trop Med Hyg* **32**:931–934, 1983.
14. Barby D, Hart CA, Taylor C: Human cryptosporidiosis: A possible case of hospital cross infection. *Br Med J* **287**:1760–1761, 1983.
15. Anonymous. Update: Treatment of cryptosporidiosis in patients with acquired immunodeficiency syndrome (AIDS). *MMWR* **33**:117–119, 1984.
16. Hallak A, Yust L, Ratan Y, et al: Malabsorption syndrome, coccidiosis, combined immune deficiency and fulminant lymphoproliferative disease. *Arch Intern Med* **142**:196–197, 1982.

17. Forthal DN, Guest SS: *Isospora belli* enteritis in three homosexual men. *Am J Trop Med Hyg* **33**:1060–1064, 1984.
18. Westerman EL, Christensen RP: Chronic *Isospora belli* infection treated with cotrimoxazole. *Ann Intern Med* **91**:413–414, 1979.
19. World Health Organization: Intestinal protozoan and helminthic infections. *WHO Technical Report Series 1981*, No. 666. Geneva: WHO, 1981.
20. Pumpianski R, Sheskin J: Pruritus vulvae: A five year survey. *Dermatologica* **131**:446–451, 1965.

CHAPTER 20

# Chlamydia Trachomatis Infection

Angelika Stary, Peter Duschet, and Friedrich Gschnait

## Overview

*Chlamydia trachomatis* (*C. trachomatis*) is the most common agent eliciting sexually transmitted diseases [1–6], which in recent years have become an increasingly important problem of public health services in industrialized countries. More than 3 million new chlamydial infections, leading to infertility in more than 20,000 teenagers [7], are estimated to occur per year in the United States. The incidence of this disease is thus at least as great as that of diabetes mellitus.

The clinical picture, complications, and late sequelae of *C. trachomatis* infection closely resemble those of gonorrhea. In contrast to gonorrhea, however, *C. trachomatis* is often not detected clinically because the infection remains asymptomatic. Nevertheless, the pathologic processes proceed and may cause severe permanent damage. To prevent the often deleterious late sequelae, early diagnosis and treatment are of major importance not only for the affected patient but also for public health. Chlamydia screening programs thus will be of great importance in the future.

## Synonyms

Synonyms for *Chlamydia trachomatis* infection are miyagawanella, ehrlichia, chlamydozoon, *Rickettsia formis*, rakeia, chlamydia, bedsonia, colettsia, PLV (psittacosis lymphogranuloma venereum), POMP (psittacosis ornithosis mammalian pneumonitis), TRIC agent (trachoma inclusion conjunctivitis), and PLT (psittacosis lymphogranuloma trachoma).

## Historical Events

In 1907 Halberstaedter and von Prowazek [8] observed intraepithelial inclusions in conjunctival scrapings from experimentally infected orangutans. They suggested the name "chlamydozoa" (derived from Greek *chlamys*, which means a mantle, indicating the matrix around the elementary bodies in Giemsa's stain) and assumed the organism was a protozoan.

In 1909/1910, Lindner, Fritsch, and Hofstätter [9,10] established a pathogenic link between ocular and genital infections. Scrapings from the eyes of babies with ophthalmia neonatorum and from the cervix of mothers with cervical infections, and urethral secretions from men with nongonococcal urethritis (NGU), were inoculated on conjunctiva of monkeys, who developed inclusion conjunctivitis. This observation led to the discovery of an association between NGU and chlamydia, its sexual and perinatal transmission, and its involvement in ophthalmia neonatorum.

In 1934 Bedson and Bland [11] described similarities between the growth cycle of *C. trachomatis*, first isolated from patients with lymphogranuloma venereum, and *C. psittaci*, isolated during the psittacosis pandemic of 1929–1930.

In 1950 Harkness [12] claimed the existence of NGU as a new disease. T'ang et al [13] in 1957 described the isolation and demonstration of the trachoma agent by inoculation on yolk sacs of embryonated hens eggs. Jones, Collier, and Smith [14] in 1959 reported the first isolation of *C. trachomatis* from material recovered from the eyes of an infant with ophthalmia neonatorum and from the cervix of the infant's mother.

In 1965 Gordon and Quan [15] developed a tissue culture isolation procedure for *C. trachomatis*. In 1966 Page [16] reviewed the microbiology of *C. trachomatis* and classified them as bacteria. Since 1984 some rapid diagnostic techniques for *C. trachomatis* have become available, among them are a direct specimen test with monoclonal antibodies (immunofluorescence test, enzyme-linked immunoabsorbent assay [ELISA]) and a recombinant DNA technique [17].

## Microbiology

The order chlamydiae is a well-defined group of prokaryotic organisms. It is separated from other microbes by its distinctive mode of intracellular growth and by its biologic characteristics. Chlamydiae were first thought to be viruses because of their small size and their inability to survive on nonliving culture media. The presence of a cell wall, the inhibition of their growth by antibiotics, a carbohydrate metabolism, the presence of ribosomes of prokaryotic type, and the presence of DNA and RNA, however, are characteristics that bespeak their bacterial nature. *C. psittaci* and *C. trachomatis* share a common group antigen. This has been subdivided on the basis of type-specific antigens identified by a microimmunofluorescence test developed by Wang and Grayston [18].

Chlamydia possess a cell wall and cell membrane similar to those of gram-negative bacteria, but are devoid of muramic acid. There are no structural differences between the species. Chlamydia contain approximately 30 to 50% protein, and the common group antigen is composed of carbohydrates.

Two distinct forms of the organism exist, termed the elementary body and the initial or reticulate body. The elementary body represents the extracellular form and is a 300-nm round, metabolically inert coccus adapted to extracellular existence and the early events of host cell interactions. It is highly infectious. The outer envelope is a rigid trilaminar structure and surrounds a trilaminar cytoplasmic membrane. The cell wall contains lysine and D-alanine with linked peptidoglycans but is devoid of diaminopimelic acid and cholesterol. The DNA is compacted into the nucleoid as a double-stranded twisted circle with a genome size around $9.8 \times 10^8$ dalton and a guanine-cytosine percentage of about 45%.

After attachment to the cell, the elementary body actively penetrates the cell wall and remains within a phagocytic vesicle throughout the whole growth cycle. At this time the infectious particle differentiates into a metabolically active and larger coccoid form, the initial or reticulate body. This body is between 800 and 1200 nm in size and represents the intracellular reproductive form. Its cell wall is thinner and more fragile than that of elementary body. It replicates by binary fission within the inclusion vesicle, which contains large, small, and intermediate forms of the particle. Intracellular replication generally proceeds for 2 to 3 days. Gradually, the initial body is replaced by the elementary body, followed by the rupture and damage of the host cell.

## Infections of the Female Genital Tract

### Cervicitis

*C. trachomatis* is one of the most common pathogenic agents isolated from the cervix. Young, unmarried, sexually active women originating from socially poorer classes are most commonly affected. The prevalence within this epidemiologic group is reported to be 15 to 20%. Genital infections caused by *C. trachomatis* are thus even more frequent than gonorrhea.

Four to twenty-one percent of pregnant women harbor *C. trachomatis* within the cervical canal, and the newborn may be infected during passage through the birth canal. Such infection is followed by *C. trachomatis*-induced pneumonia, conjunctivitis, and pharyngitis.

Hormonal factors do not seem to be of importance in the pathogenesis of chlamydia-induced cervical infection, though the disease is more frequently observed in women using oral contraceptives. This may be explained by a higher promiscuity of this group compared with women not using oral contraceptive pills.

Cervicitis is the primary clinical manifestation of chlamydial infection in women. It leads first to a mucopurulent discharge [19] in about 40% of infected females. It is of the utmost importance that most women remain free of symptoms and thus are not aware of the infection but are at high risk for development of severe late complications such as adnexitis and infertility. They may also transmit the infection to their sexual partners.

Leukorrhea (mucopurulent cervical fluoror "mucopus") [20] is easily detected by the yellowish-purulent discoloration of a swab introduced into the cervical canal and rotated. The swab test, however, only proves the presence of mucopurulent inflammation. It does not allow the exact bacteriologic diagnosis, in particular the differential diagnosis between chlamydial and gonorrheal cervicitis. A suitable laboratory examination is mandatory, since deleterious complications of chlamydial cervicitis such as pelvic inflammatory disease (PID), infertility, and perihepatitis (Fitz-Hugh-Curtis syndrome) can only be avoided by effective and specific treatment based on the discovery of the eliciting organism.

## Cervical Ectopy

*C. trachomatis* exclusively affects high prismatic (cylindrical) and transitional epithelium. In cervical ectopy the squamous epithelium of the vaginal portion of the cervix is replaced by cylindrical epithelium. This region thus becomes susceptible for chlamydial infection [21]. At present there are no sufficient data to prove a causal role of *C. trachomatis* in the pathogenesis of cervical dysplasia. However, it has been demonstrated that serum antibodies directed against *C. trachomatis* are found in a higher percentage of women presenting with cervical dysplasia than in control groups [5,22].

## Urethritis

In women suffering from pollakiuria and dysuria, chlamydial urethritis should be taken into the differential diagnosis, in particular if routine bacterial cultures are negative [23]. Chlamydial urethritis, however, in most cases is associated with cervicitis and does not occur in isolation [24].

## Salpingitis (Pelvic Inflammatory Disease, PID)

*C. trachomatis* is responsible for approximately one third of all cases of acute salpingitis. This disease thus represents the most important complication of genital chlamydial infections [25]. In a great number of women who are infertile due to occlusion of the salpinx, high serum antibody titers against *C. trachomatis* are found [26–30].

Since clinical symptoms are usually mild (moderate abdominal pain), chlamydia-induced salpingitis may often be overlooked by the patient or the physician. Its diagnosis, however, is of tremendous importance, since, despite the absence of gross symptoms, tubal tissue is progressively destroyed, leading to occlusion and infertility [31]. There are no specific laboratory findings; in most cases a slightly elevated erythrocyte sedimentation rate is observed.

In only 5% of patients with *C. trachomatis*-induced salpingitis are chlamydial cultures from cervical smears found to be positive, even if antichlamydial antibody titers in the serum are high and chlamydia cultures from the endometrium are positive [32–34]. Chlamydial salpingitis thus should be diagnosed by examination of material aspirated from the tubes during laparoscopy and not only the basis of cervical smears [35]. "Blind" antibiotic treatment in a considerable number of cases masks the disease and gives rise to symptomless deleterious progression of the pathologic processes, which may lead to even more severe complications of chlamydial infection such as perihepatitis and infertility. If laparoscopy cannot be performed, a suitable combination of severl antibiotics should be used [36] for broad-spectrum treatment of possible infections with mycoplasms, other aerobic or anaerobic germs, and in particular *Neisseria gonorrhoeae*.

The pathologic processes involved in chlamydial salpingitis are not clearly understood. In vitro cell culture studies performed with *C. trachomatis* and *N. gonorrhoeae* indicate that *C. trachomatis* is less pathogenic than *N. gonorrhoeae* [37]. Therefore additional pathogenic factors such as different immunologic responses of the host to chlamydial and gonorrheal infection are discussed.

## Perihepatitis (Fitz-Hugh-Curtis Syndrome)

Perihepatitis (localized perihepatic peritonitis) is characterized by the development of acute pain in the right upper abdominal region that simulates acute cholecystolithiasis. The syndrome first was known as a complication of gonococcal infection, but more often may be caused by *C. trachomatis* [38]. Acute right-sided abdominal pain therefore may indicate advanced genital chlamydial infection.

## Endometritis

Isolated endometritis caused by *C. trachomatis* occurs rarely [39]. Within the course of an ascendant genital chlamydial infection, involvement of the endometrium seems to be common.

The role of *C. trachomatis* in the pathogenesis of cervical dysplasia and of complications during pregnancy is not yet fully established.

### Cervical Dysplasia

In women presenting with cervical dysplasia, higher titers of serum antibodies directed against *C. trachomatis* are found than in normal persons [5,22], indicating a possible causal relationship between cervical dysplasia and chlamydial infection. It is not yet clear, however, whether the epithelial repair processes following chlamydial infection may progress into cervical dysplasia and possibly carcinoma.

### Complications of Pregnancy

*C. trachomatis* has been reported to occur in the cervix of up to 26% of pregnant women [40]. It therefore has been argued that this organism may be associated with complications of pregnancy, in particular since in some animals *C. psittaci* causes abortion. No convincing data, however, exist concerning the role of *C. trachomatis* in abortion, fetal morbidity, or low birth weight [41,42]. Postabortion and postpartum endometritis are known complications of cervical chlamydial infection [43].

## Infections of the Male Genital Tract

### Nongonococcal Urethritis and Postgonococcal Urethritis

Nongonococcal urethritis (NGU) represents the most common manifestation of chlamydial infection in men [44]. At present, more than 50% of NGU cases are caused by *C. trachomatis*. In the United States, 20% of men suffering from gonococcal urethritis are simultaneously infected by *C. trachomatis*. In Europe this percentage is estimated to be even higher (40%) [2,45].

NGU is characterized clinically by a mucous to mucopurulent discharge that develops usually after an incubation period of approximately 1 to 3 weeks. Despite the fact that discharge in gonorrhea usually is creamlike and purulent, a differential diagnosis of NGU from gonorrhea on clinical grounds alone is not possible. Only laboratory examinations (see below) enable the physician to establish an exact diagnosis.

More than half of cases of NGU caused by *C. trachomatis* follow a mild and even asymptomatic course. Patients thus often do not seek medical care. Progression of the infection may lead to epididymitis and infertility, and untreated asymptomatic patients represent a source for uncontrolled spread of the disease.

Diagnosis of NGU is based on demonstration of an increased number of leukocytes in the urethral smear and/or in the centrifugate of the morning urine [19,46,47]. More than 15 leukocytes within the microscopic field (400-fold magnification) of the centrifugate of the morning urine or more than five leukocytes within the microscopic field (1000-fold magnification) of the urethral smear are diagnostic for NGU. After "establishment" of NGU the bacteriologic diagnosis should be made by demonstration of the infectious agent (see below).

Postgonococcal urethritis (PGU) develops 2 to 10 days after successful treatment of gonorrhea, due to simultaneous infection with *N. gonorrhoeae* and *C. trachomatis*. Since the incubation period of chlamydia-induced urethritis is longer than that of gonorrhea, clinical symptoms due to *C. trachomatis* occur usually after sufficient therapy of gonorrhea (symptomless interval). Twenty to forty percent of all men with gonorrhea are also infected by *C. trachomatis*, which is not identified by routine procedures for the diagnosis of gonorrhea (methylene blue stain, bacterial culture). Some authors recommend the administration of tetracyclines routinely after penicillin therapy for gonorrhea [5].

### Epididymitis

Epididymitis represents the most common complication of chlamydial infections of the male genital tract. About two thirds of all epididymitis cases are caused by *C. trachomatis*. Clinical examination in most patients reveals a tender epididymitis combined with symptoms of NGU, and *C. trachomatis* usually can be demonstrated in the urethral smear. However, the absence of urethritis and failure to culture *C. trachomatis* from the urethra do not exclude chlamydial etiology of the epididymitis.

In some instances, thus, bacteriologic investigations of aspirate obtained by the epididymis puncture should be performed.

### Proctitis

Twelve percent of proctitis cases in homosexual men are elicited by *C. trachomatis* and can be identified by a rectal smear [48]. Asymptomatic rectal infections are quite common: By rectal screening *C. trachomatis* could be demonstrated in 6% of asymptomatic homosexual men [48].

### Reiter's Disease

Recent observations suggest a causal relationship between *C. trachomatis* and Reiter's disease [49,50]. This is supported by several observations: Some patients report higher sexual promiscuity prior to the occurrence of Reiter's disease; *C. trachomatis* frequently has been identified in the urethral smear of such patients; and higher antichlamydial antibody titers in patients with Reiter's disease compared with patients with uncomplicated urethritis have been reported [49].

## Chlamydial Infections in the Newborn

### Pneumonia of the Newborn

In recent years atypical pneumonia in newborns caused by *C. trachomatis* has been observed in the United States and later in Europe [51–53]. Thirty to forty percent of pneumonia cases occurring within the first few months of life are now recognized to be due to *C. trachomatis* [52,54], and this organism thus is of major importance for perinatal morbidity. Affected children are afebrile but have a severe pertussislike cough. Laboratory examination reveals eosinophilia, hypergammaglobulinemia, and serum antichlamydial IgM antibodies [55].

### Inclusion Conjunctivitis

During the newborn's passage through the birth canal *C. trachomatis* can be transmitted from the infected mother to the infant. Inclusion conjunctivitis occurs in about 30% of such infants [52,53] after an incubation period of 6 to 19 days. In mild cases hyperemia and edema of the conjunctiva occur; rarely a severe course has been observed with mucopurulent conjunctivitis clinically indistinguishable from gonorrheal conjunctivitis. In contrast to gonorrheal conjunctivitis, inclusion conjunctivitis usually heals spontaneously. Blindness – a common complication of trachoma – is exceedingly rare.

### Nasopharyngeal Infection

Perinatally exposed infants may also develop extraocular chlamydial infections in the nasopharynx [51]. Colonization of this area is not necessarily associated with clinical symptoms but, by ascension, may cause secretory otitis media [56].

## Diagnosis

### Specimen Collection

The reliable identification of *C. trachomatis* from clinical materials requires carefully taken specimens. Cotton wool or calcium alginate-tipped wire swabs should be used to collect a sample from the involved site by vigorous rubbing against the tissue surface. Cervical discharge should be removed before specimen collection.

Different methods exist for diagnosing chlamydial infections including (a) isolation of the organism from clinical specimen in tissue culture, (b) diagnosis of elementary bodies in direct smears by ELISA technique or by visualization in the microimmunofluorescence test, and (c) serology.

No single laboratory test for identification of chlamydial infection is entirely satisfying and all methods have specific areas of usefulness. Currently, tissue culture techniques seem to be the most sensitive but are the most laborious and expensive methods.

### Nonculture Methods

Monoclonal antibodies allow direct demonstration of the infectious agent and offer a prompt, reliable, and economic diagnosis of chlamydial infection. Recently, two commercial tests seem to offer alternatives to tissue culture for detection of chlamydial infection. The microimmunofluorescence test is based on visualization of elementary bodies in the smear by a fluorescein-conjugated monoclonal antibody directed against the major outer membrane protein (Fig. 20.1). Evaluation of the elementary bodies is performed using a fluorescence microscope. Compared with the culture technique, the sensitivity of this method is approximately 90% and the specificity nearly 100%, provided the investigator is experienced in the evaluation of the test. In symptomatic persons, the sensitivity was found to be higher than in asymptomatic screening groups [17,57]. Since results are available within a few minutes, the method is particularly useful for screening. Chlamydiazyme, an enzyme-linked immunoassay, is easier to handle than the Micro Trak direct specimen test; chlamydial antigen obtained from a urogenital sample will be adsorbed to a polystyrene bead, coupled to *C. trachomatis* antibody, and then detected colorimetrically after reaction with horseradish-peroxidase-conjugated antibody and chromogen. Recent data indicate a good correlation between chlamydiazyme results and cell culture techniques [58].

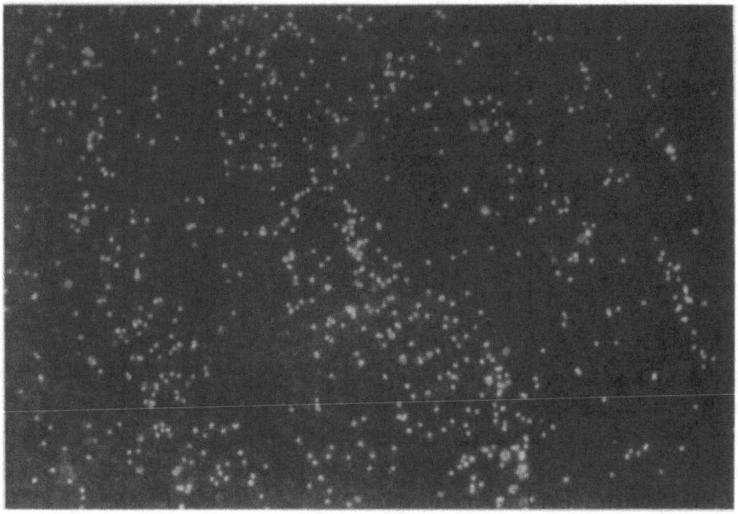

FIGURE 20.1. Direct specimen test: Apple-green fluorescing elementary bodies stained with fluorescein isothiocyanate (FITC)-conjugated monoclonal antibodies.

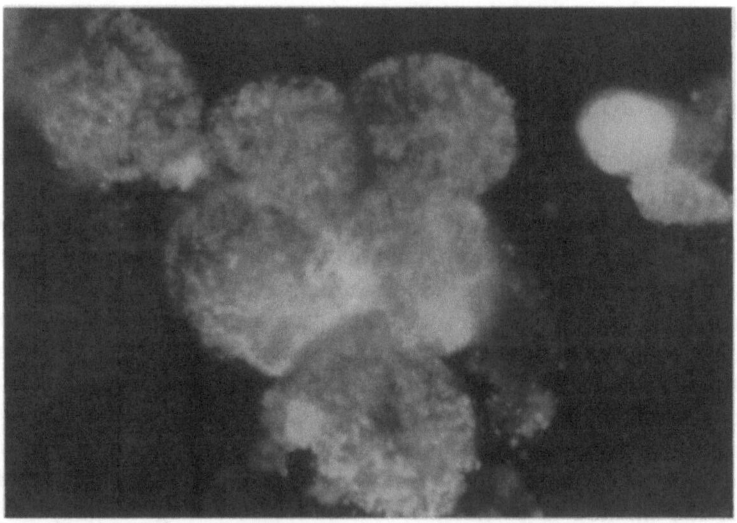

FIGURE 20.2. *C. trachomatis*-positive McCoy cell culture with inclusions containing reticulate bodies stained by FITC-conjugated monoclonal antibodies.

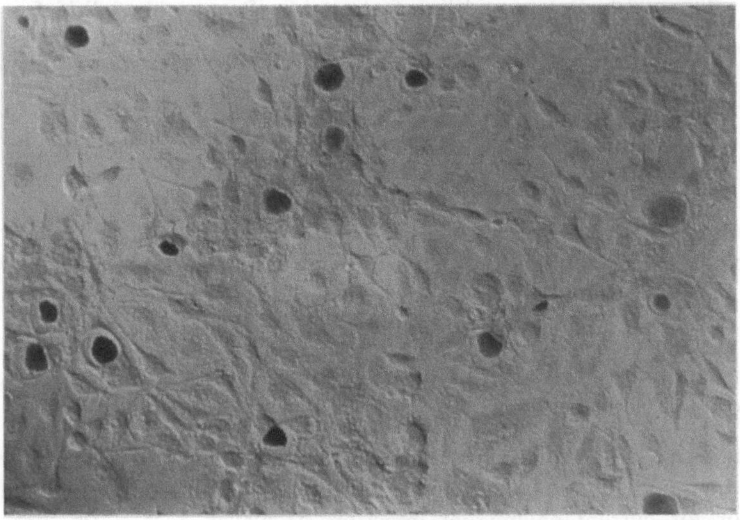

FIGURE 20.3. *C. trachomatis*-positive McCoy cell culture with iodine-stained inclusion bodies.

The sensitivity of direct cytology in the genital tract is low, and small numbers of inclusions are easily missed by an inexperienced observer.

## CELL CULTURE METHODS

The specimen is collected as described above, the swab immediately after collection being immersed in a special transport medium (2-SP) containing antibiotics. Refrigeration at 4°C is sufficient if the material is evaluated within 48 hours. Otherwise, it is recommended to cool the samples at −170°C. The obtained material is centrifugated onto McCoy cells at 3,000 G for 1 hour and subsequently incubated in a medium containing cycloheximide. After 48 to 72 hours, staining of the inclusion bodies is performed using immunofluorescence with monoclonal antibodies (Fig. 20.2). Other staining techniques (e.g., iodine staining, Giemsa's stain) are somewhat cheaper, but their sensitivity is much lower (Fig. 20.3). Negative cultures should be submitted to a second passage.

## SEROLOGY

Many different tests with varying antigens can be performed (Table 20.2) to discover systemic infection with chlamydiae and to measure genus-specific antibodies. They are not useful, however, to diagnose common genital tract infections [59–62].

The serologic response to chlamydial infection is of only limited use because there is a high prevalence of antibodies to *C. trachomatis* among the population. The presence of IgG antichlamydial antibodies therefore does not always indicate dis-

TABLE 20.1. Dosage guidelines for treatment of genital chlamydial infection.

| Preparation | Dosage | Duration of therapy |
|---|---|---|
| Oxytetracycline | 500 mg 4 times daily | 10 days |
| Doxycycline | 100 mg 2 times daily | 10 days |
| Erythromycin | 500 mg 4 times daily | 10 days |

ease and need for treatment. For diagnosis of a recent infection at least one of the following criteria should be fulfilled:

Seroconversion
Greater than fourfold rise in antibody titer to IgG.
Presence of IgM antibodies.

A fourfold rise in titer in paired sera is not particularly helpful for patient management because of the time factor. Demonstration of IgM antibodies might be a useful indicator for current chlamydial infection. However, IgM antibodies in STD patients are rarely found because of the short-living IgM and its lack in patients with recurrent infection.

Complications of lower genital tract infections such as acute salpingitis, the Fitz-Hugh-Curtis syndrome, or epididymitis may be more readily diagnosed by serology. Very high titers of IgG antichlamydial antibodies are seen in male and female patients with severe complications.

In neonatal chlamydial pneumonia, the detection of high levels (more than 1:32) of IgM antibody will support the clinical diagnosis of *C. trachomatis* infection and may be the only method available for diagnosis of *C. trachomatis* pneumonia.

## Therapy

The possibly deleterious late sequelae of genital chlamydial infections require effective treatment in both men and women as soon as possible. It is necessary to treat also asymptomatic partners, since transmission from men to women and vice versa occurs in more than 30% of cases [63]. At present, tetracyclines are regarded as the treatment of choice. Table 20.1 shows a routine regimen.

In pregnant women, success rates approximating 90% have been obtained with use of erythromycin ethylsuccinate, 1.6 g per day for 7 days, and stearate, 1 per day for 14 days [64; J. Schachter, unpublished data].

In PID it is useful to recommend antichlamydial drugs for at least 2 weeks (500 mg of tetracycline or erythromycin four times daily) combined with metronidazole (400 mg twice daily). Other suggested treatment regimens for in-patient therapy include combinations such as cefoxitin and a tetracycline or clindamycin and tobramycin [36].

Elimination of *C. trachomatis* can be achieved in more than 90% of cases. Treatment failures are rare and in most cases due to too short a duration of therapy, irregular administration of the drug, reinfection, or malabsorption of tetracyclines (the

TABLE 20.2. Serologic tests for chlamydial infection.

| |
|---|
| Complement fixation test (CFT) |
| Antibodies against group antigen, diagnosis of LGV* and Psittacosis |
| Microimmunofluorescence test (MIF) |
| Elementary body antigen (pooled) |
| Single-serotype elementary body antigen, LGV2 yolk-sac antigen, serotype specificity |
| Single-serotype inclusion body antigen, LGV2 tissue culture antigen, group specificity |
| Single-serotype reticulate body antigen, LGV2, group specificity, lower sensitivity than elementary body antigen |
| Enzyme-linked immunosorbent assay (ELISA) |
| LGV2 antigen, group specificity, high sensitivity |
| Radioimmunoassay (RIA) |
| LGV2 antigen, group specificity, high sensitivity |

*LGV, lymphogranuloma venereum.

simultaneous ingestion of milk and calcium preparations should be avoided). There is still much controversy about the ideal timing of bacteriologic treatment controls in NGU and chlamydial infection. It is known that some patients with initial resolution of symptoms and negative culture may relapse later after sexual abstinence or condom-protected intercourse. Clinical and laboratory controls 1 week after treatment seem suitable.

Rifampicin also is effective against *C. trachomatis*, whereas the penicillins fail. Studies with ofloxacin and thiamphenicol suggest that they are also effective in treating NGU, but their efficacy against *C. trachomatis* both in vitro and in vivo is modest [65]. Other quinolones such as ciprofloxacin and enoxacin appear to be promising oral agents.

Erythromycin represents the antibiotic of choice for pneumonia of the newborn. Inclusion conjunctivitis should be treated by systemically administered erythromycin (40 mg/kg of body weight). Topical therapy alone with drops or creams containing tetracyclines is not sufficient; treatment failures due to reinfection from the nasopharynx occur in more than 50% of these cases.

## References

1. Holmes KK: The chlamydia epidemic. *JAMA* **245**:428–435, 1981.
2. Oriel JD, Ridgway GL: Genital infection by *Chlamydia trachomatis*. London: Edwards Arnold, 1982, p. 144.
3. Schachter J, Hanna L, Hill EC, et al: Are chlamydial infections the most prevalent venereal disease? *JAMA* **231**:1252–1255, 1975.
4. Schachter J: Chlamydial infections. *N Engl J Med* **298**:428–435, 1978.
5. Schachter J, Dawson CR: *Human Chlamydial Infections*. PSG Publishing Co, Little, Massachusetts, 1978, p 144.
6. Taylor-Robinson D, Thomas BJ: The role of *Chlamydia trachomatis* in genital tract and associated diseases. *Clin Pathol* **33**:205–233, 1980.
7. Mardh PA, Luger A: Infektionen mit *Chlamydia trachomatis*. Kivik, Sweden: PAM, 1985.

8. Halberstaedter L, von Prowazek S: Über Zelleinschlüsse parasitärer Natur beim Trachom. *Arbeit kaiser Gesundheit* **26**:44–47, 1907.
9. Lindner K: Übertragungsversuche von gonokokkenfreier Blennorrhoea neonatorum auf Affen. *Wien Klin Wsch* **22**:1554–1659, 1909.
10. Fritsch HO, Hofstätter A, Lindner K: Experimentelle Studien zur Trachomfrage. *Graefe's Arch Ophthalmol* **76**:547, 1910.
11. Bedson SP, Bland JOW: The developmental forms of the psittacosis virus. *Br J Exp Pathol* **15**:243-247, 1934.
12. Harkness AH: Non-gonococcal urethritis. Edinburgh: Livingstone, 1950.
13. T'ang FF, Chang HL, Huan YT, et al: Studies on the aetiology of trachoma with special reference to isolation of the virus in chick embryo. *Chin Med J* **75**:429–447, 1957.
14. Jones BR, Collier LH, Smith CH: Isolation of virus from inclusion blennorrhoe. *Lancet* **1**:902–905, 1959.
15. Gordon F, Quan AL: Isolation of trachoma agent in cell culture. *Proc Soc Biol* (NY) **118**:354–359, 1965.
16. Page LA: Revision of the family Chlamydiaceae (Rake). *Int J Syst Bacteriol* **16**:223–252, 1966.
17. Stamm WE, Harrison HR, Alexander ER, et al: Diagnosis of *C. trachomatis* infections by direct immunofluorescence staining of genital secretions: A multicenter trial. *Ann Intern Med* **101**:638–641, 1984.
18. Wang SP, Grayston JT: Classification of TRIC and related strains with microimmunofluorescence. In RL Nichols (Ed): *Trachoma and Related Disorders Caused by Chlamydial Agents*. Princeton: Excerpta Medica, pp. 305–321, 1971
19. Arya OP, Mallinson H, Andrews BE, et al: Diagnosis of urethritis: Role of polymorphonuclear leukocyte counts in gram-stained urethral smears. *Sex Trans Dis* **11**:10–17, 1984.
20. Rees E, Davies JA, Bradley MG, et al: *Chlamydia trachomatis* in relation to postgonococcal cervicitis. In PA Mardh, KK Holmes, JD Oriel, et al (Eds): *Chlamydial Infections*. Amsterdam: Elsevier Biomedical Press, 1982, pp. 147–150.
21. Paavonen J, Vesterinen E, Meyer B: Genital *Chlamydia trachomatis* infections in patients with cervical atypia. *Obstet Gynecol* **54**:298–291, 1979.
22. Schachter J, Hill EC, King EB, et al: *Chlamydia trachomatis* and cervical neoplasia. *JAMA* **248**:2134–2138, 1982.
23. Stamm WE, Wagner KF, Amsel R, et al: Causes of the acute urethral syndrome in women. *N Engl J Med* **303**:409–415, 1980.
24. Paavonen J: Chlamydia trachomatis-induced urethritis in female partners of men with gonococcal urethritis. *Sex Trans Dis* **6**:69–71, 1979.
25. Westrom L: Incidence, prevalence and trends of acute pelvic inflammatory disease and its consequences in industrialized countries. *Am J Obstet Gynecol* **138**:880–892, 1980.
26. Gump DW, Gibson M, Ashikaga T: Evidence of prior pelvic inflammatory disease and its relationship to *Chlamydia trachomatis* antibody and intrauterine contraceptive device use in infertile women. *Am J Obstet Gynecol* **146**:153–158, 1983.
27. Henry-Suchet J, Catalan F, Loffredo V, et al: Microbiology of specimens obtained by laparoscopy from controls and from patients with pelvic inflammatory disease of infertility with tubal obstruction: *Chlamydia trachomatis* and *Ureaplasma urealyticum*. *Am J Obstet Gynecol* **138**:1022–1025, 1980.
28. Jones RB, Ardery BR, Hui SL, et al: Correlation between serum antichlamydial antibodies and tubal factor as a cause of infertility. *Fertil Steril* **38**:553–558, 1982.

29. Moore DE, Foy HM, Daling FR, et al: Increased frequency of serum antibodies to *Chlamydia trachomatis* in infertility due to distal tubal disease. *Lancet* **2**:574–577, 1982.
30. Punonen R, Terho P, Nikkanen V, et al: Chlamydial serology in infertile women by immunofluorescence. *Fertil Steril* **31**:656–659, 1979.
31. Svensson L, Westrom L, Mardh PA: Acute salpingitis with *Chlamydia trachomatis* isolated from the fallopian tube: Clinical, cultural and serological findings. *Sex Trans Dis* **8**:51–55, 1982.
32. Eschenbach DA, Buchanan TM, Pollock HM, et al: Polymicrobial etiology of acute pelvic inflammatory disease. *N Engl J Med* **293**:166–171, 1975.
33. Sweet R, Mills J, Hadley K, et al: Use of laparoscopy to determine the microbiologic etiology of acute salpingitis. *Am J Obstet Gynecol* **134**:68–74, 1979.
34. Thompson SE, Hager WD, Wong KH: The microbiology and therapy of acute pelvic inflammatory disease in hospitalized patients. *Am J Obstet Gynecol* **136**:1979–1986, 1980.
35. Mardh PA, Ripa T, Svennson L, et al: *Chlamydia trachomatis* infection in patients with acute salpingitis. *N Engl J Med* **296**:1377–1379.
36. Sexually transmitted diseases: Treatment guidelines 1982. *Rev Infect Dis* (Suppl):729–746, 1982.
37. Hutchinson GR, Taylor-Robinson D, Dourmashkin RR: Growth and effect of chlamydiae in human and bovine oviduct organ cultures. *Br J Vener Dis* **55**:194–202, 1979.
38. Müller-Schoop JW, Wang SP, Munzinger J, et al: *C. trachomatis* as a possible cause of peritonitis and perihepatitis in young women. *Br Med J* **1**:1022–1024, 1978.
39. Mardh PA, Moller BR, Ingerselv HJ, et al: Endometritis caused by *Chlamydia trachomatis*. *Br J Vener Dis* **57**:191–195, 1981.
40. Harrison HR, Boyce WT, Haffner WH, et al: The prevalence of genital *Chlamydia trachomatis* and mycoplasmal infections during pregnancy in an American Indian population. *Sex Trans Dis* **10**:184–186, 1983.
41. Martin DH, Koutsky L, Eschenbach DA, et al: Prematurity and perinatal morbidity in pregnancies complicated by maternal *Chlamydia trachomatis* infections. *JAMA* **247**:1585–1588, 1982.
42. Thompson SE, Lopez B, Wong KH, et al: A prospective study of *Chlamydia trachomatis* and mycoplasma infections and maternal morbidity. In PA Mardh, KK Holmes, JD Oriel, et al (Eds): *Chlamydial Infections*. Amsterdam: Elsevier Medical Press, 1982, pp. 155–158.
43. Wager GP, Martin DH, Koutsky L, et al: Puerperal infections morbidity: Relationship to route of delivery and to antepartum *Chlamydia trachomatis* infection. *Am J Obstet Gynecol* **138**:1028–1033, 1980.
44. Holmes KK, Handsfield HH, Wang SP, et al: Etiology of non-gonococcal urethritis. *N Engl J Med* **292**:1109–1205, 1975.
45. Stary A, Söltz-Szöts J, Kopp W, et al: Epidemiologic developments of *Chlamydia trachomatis* in different Viennese STD risk groups. *Eur J Sex Trans Dis* **3**:191–195, 1986.
46. Bowie WR: Comparison of Gram stain and first-voided urine sediment in the diagnosis of urethritis. *Sex Trans Dis* **5**:39–42, 1978.
47. Kraus SJ: Semiquantitation of urethral polymorphonuclear leukocytes as objective evidence of nongonococcal urethritis. *Sex Trans Dis* **11**:10–17, 1984.
48. Quinn TC, Goodell SE, Mkrtichian E, et al: *Chlamydia trachomatis* proctitis. *N Engl J Med* **305**:195–200, 1984.
49. Martin DH, Pollock S, Kuo CC, et al: *Chlamydia trachomatis* infections in men with Reiter's syndrome. *Ann Intern Med* **100**:217–213, 1984.

50. Is Reiter's syndrome caused by chlamydia? (Editorial) *Lancet* **1**:317–320, 1985.
51. Beem MO, Saxon EM: Respiratory tract colonization and a distinctive pneumonia syndrome in infants infected with antepartum *Chlamydia trachomatis* infection. *N Engl J Med* **296**:306–310, 1977.
52. Beem MO, Saxon OM: *Chlamydia trachomatis* infections in infants. In PA Mardh, KK Holmes, JD Oriel, et al (Eds): *Chlamydial Infections*. Amsterdam: Elsevier Biomedical Press, pp. 199–212, 1982.
53. Schachter J, Grossman M: Chlamydial infections. *Ann Rev Med* **32**:45–61, 1981.
54. Wang SP, Grayston JT: Microimmunofluorescence antibody responses in *Chlamydia trachomatis* infections: A review. In PA Mardh, KK Holmes, Oriel JD, et al (Eds): *Chlamydial Infections*. Amsterdam: Elsevier Biomedical Press, pp. 301–316, 1982.
55. Schachter J, Grossman M, Azimi PH: Serology of *Chlamydia trachomatis* in infants. *J Infect Dis* **146**:530–535, 1982.
56. Tipple MA, Beem MO, Saxon EM: Clinical characteristics of the afebrile pneumoniae associated with *C. trachomatis* infection in infants under 6 months old. *Pediatrics* **63**:192–197, 1979.
57. Stary A, Kopp W, Gebhart W, et al: Culture versus direct specimen test: Comparative study of infections with *Chlamydia trachomatis* in Viennese prostitutes. *Gentourin Dis* **61**:258–260, 1985.
58. Baselski V, McNeeley G, Ryan G, et al: A comparison of chlamydiazyme 6 cell culture isolation for the detection of *C. trachomatis* in cervical swab specimens. Abstracts of Annual American Society of Microbiology Meeting. St. Louis, Mo., C 108, 1984.
59. Schachter J, Cles L, Ray R, et al: Failure of serology in diagnosing chlamydial infections of the female genital tract. *J Clin Microbiol* **10**:647–649, 1979.
60. Wang SP, Grayston JT, Alexander ER, et al: Simplified microimmunofluorescence test with trachoma-lymphogranuloma venereum (*Chlamydia trachomatis*) antigens for use as a screening test for antibody. *J Clin Microbiol* **1**:250–255, 1975.
61. Levy NJ, Mundoz A, McCormack W: Enzyme linked immunoabsorbent assay for the detection of antibody to *Chlamydia trachomatis* and *Chlamydia psittacii*. *J Lab Clin Med* **102**:918–925, 1983.
62. Mahony JB, Schachter J, Chernesky MA: Detection of antichlamydial immunoglobulin G and M antibodies by enzyme linked immunosorbent assay. *J Clin Microbiol* **19**:270–275, 1983.
63. Oriel JD, Ridgway GL: Studies of epidemiology of chlamydial infection of the human genital tract. In PA Mardh, KK Holmes, JD Oriel, et al (Eds): *Chlamydial Infections*. Amsterdam: Elsevier Biomedical Press, pp. 425–428, 1982.
64. Podgore JK, Belts R, Alden E, et al: Effectiveness of maternal third term erythromycin in prevention of infant *Chlamydia trachomatis* infection. In *Programs and Abstracts of the 20th Interscience Conference on Antimicrobial Agents and Chemotherapy*. Washington, D.C.: American Society for Microbiology (abstract 524).
65. Fong IW, Hook EW, Stamm WE: Recent clinical trials in Chlamydial infections: The value of quinolones. Second World Congress on Sexually Transmitted Diseases, Paris, 1986.

CHAPTER 21

# The Acquired Immunodeficiency Syndrome

Anne G. Matlow and Benjamin K. Fisher

## Introduction

The acquired immunodeficiency syndrome (AIDS) was first identified in the United States in 1981. By April 1, 1987, a total of 45,608 cases had been reported to the World Health Organization Global Control Program on AIDS, with patients in the Americas accounting for 80% of all reported cases [1]. A concentrated research effort has identified the etiologic agent of this infection as a retrovirus, which has most recently been termed HIV (human immunodeficiency virus) [2]. The rapid emergence and spread of this disease represents an epidemic of major proportions. It is certainly apparent that with the protean manifestations of AIDS and the AIDS-related conditions, it behooves physicians in all disciplines of medicine to have a working knowledge of the etiology, clinical manifestations, natural history, and management of this newly described infectious disease.

## Definition

A strict definition of AIDS was proposed by the Centers for Disease Control (CDC) in Atlanta, Georgia, in 1982 [3] to ensure a standardized reporting system. To meet the definition of AIDS, adults had to have a disease of at least moderately predictive of underlying cellular immunodeficiency, in the absence of any other known cause for susceptibility to that disease. Diseases at least moderately predictive of underlying cellular immunodeficiency have been outlined by the CDC [4] [4a] (Table 21.1). It should be noted that these diseases fall into two basic categories: opportunistic infections, including *Pneumocystis carinii* pneumonia, and neoplasms, including Kaposi's sarcoma.

Although a number of classification systems have been proposed to facilitate further reporting and surveillance of HIV-related diseases [5–7], it is still useful to classify the other major clinical presentations of HIV infection into PGL (persistent generalized lymphadenopathy) and ARC (AIDS-related complex).

PGL is defined as lymphadenopathy (at least one node greater than or equal to 1 cm in diameter) of at least 3 months' duration involving two or more extrainguinal

TABLE 21.1. Diseases moderately predictive of underlying cellular immunodeficiency.

| |
|---|
| Opportunistic infections |
| Bacterial infections |
| Atypical mycobacteriosis, including *Mycobacterium avium* intracellulare causing pulmonary or disseminated infection |
| Extrapulmonary tuberculosis |
| Recurrent salmonella septicemia |
| Fungal Infections |
| *Candida esophagitis* or disseminated infection |
| Cryptococcal meningitis or disseminated infection |
| Disseminated histoplasmosis not confined to lung or lymph nodes |
| Disseminated coccidiomycosis |
| Viral infections |
| Cytomegalovirus infection—pulmonary, gastrointestinal, or CNS |
| Mucocutaneous herpes simplex infection (duration >1 month) or disseminated infection |
| Progressive multifocal leukoencephalopathy |
| Parasitic infections |
| *Pneumocystis carinii* pneumonia |
| Intestinal cryptosporidiosis or isosporiasis with diarrhea (duration >1 month) |
| Strongyloidiasis causing pneumonia, CNS, or disseminated infection |
| Toxoplasmosis causing CNS or disseminated infection |
| Cancers |
| Kaposi's sarcoma |
| Non-Hodgkin's lymphoma (diffuse undifferentiated, B cell, or unknown immunologic phenotype) —biopsy proven |
| Primary CNS lymphoma |

Adapted from Shepherd et al. [9].

sites, and confirmed on physical examination. There should be no concurrent illness or drug use known to cause lymphadenopathy, and lymph node biopsy, if done, should demonstrate reactive hyperplasia [8].

The term *ARC* is used in the presence of PGL, or when a patient presents with two clinical and two laboratory criteria as outlined in Table 21.2 [9].

Serologic testing for antibodies to HIV, where done, should be positive.

# Etiology

Initial case reports of AIDS were characterized by *P. carinii* pneumonia and Kaposi's sarcoma in homosexual men [10,11]. From early on, lymphopenia was noted to be a frequent laboratory concomitant to the clinical presentation [12,13], and further efforts were concentrated upon elucidating the nature of this lymphocyte defect. The recognition of a selective defect in the T4 subset (helper lymphocytes) of T cells, resulting in a reversed T4/T8 (helper/suppressor) ratio, raised the possibility that a human retrovirus that selectively infects T4 cells might be implicated in the pathogenesis of this disease. Precedent for this had previously been established by noting that HTLV-I (human T cell leukemia virus I) and HTLV-II, the only other known

TABLE 21.2. Criteria for diagnosis of AIDS-related complex (ARC).

| |
|---|
| Lymphadenopathy |
| At least one node ≥1 cm in diameter |
| At least 3 months' duration |
| Involving two or more extrainguinal sites |
| OR |
| Any two clinical criteria |
| Fever >38.5°C |
| Weight loss > 10% of body weight or 6.0 kg |
| Diarrhea: 3 or more unformed stools per day, no identifiable pathogen |
| Extreme fatigue |
| Night sweats |
| PLUS |
| Any two laboratory abnormalities |
| Anemia, leukopenia, thrombocytopenia |
| Low number of helper T cells (<400/mm) |
| Helper:suppressor T cell ratio <1.0 |
| Depressed blastogenesis |
| Elevated serum immunoglobulin level |
| Cutaneous anergy |

Adapted from Shepherd et al. [9].

human retroviruses, caused diseases of T4 lymphocytes and predominantly infected T4 lymphocytes in vitro [15]. It should be noted that in addition to the human retroviruses, other retroviruses with both oncogenic and nononcogenic potential, and with varying host specificities within the animal kingdom, have previously been described. These include avian leukemia virus (leukemia, birds), Rous sarcoma virus (sarcoma, birds), visna virus (encephalitis, sheep) and maedi virus (pneumonia, sheep).

Retroviruses are unique in that they contain an enzyme, reverse transcriptase, that synthesizes double-stranded DNA from viral RNA. This newly formed DNA enters the nucleus of the host cell where it integrates with host cell DNA. Once it is integrated, viral genes are duplicated along with host genes, so that all progeny of the original cell will contain viral genes and the potential for expression of this genetic material. The consequences of retroviral genomic integration into host chromosomal matter include malignant transformation of the original cell or premature cell death [15]. Figure 21.1 illustrates viral replication of retroviruses, and contrasts this with replication of DNA and RNA viruses.

Identification of the causal agent in AIDS was accomplished almost concurrently by two groups of investigators, one headed by Montagnier in France and the other by Gallo in the United States. They termed their isolates LAV (lymphadenopathy-associated virus [16] and HTLV-III (human T cell leukemia virus III) [17], respectively. Sophisticated techniques have shown these retroviruses to be identical, and the new terminology proposed for the agent is HIV (human immunodeficiency virus) [2]. Two human retroviruses, HIV-1 and HIV-2, have been implicated in AIDS to date, the latter accounting for a few cases of ARC and AIDS in West Africa [18].

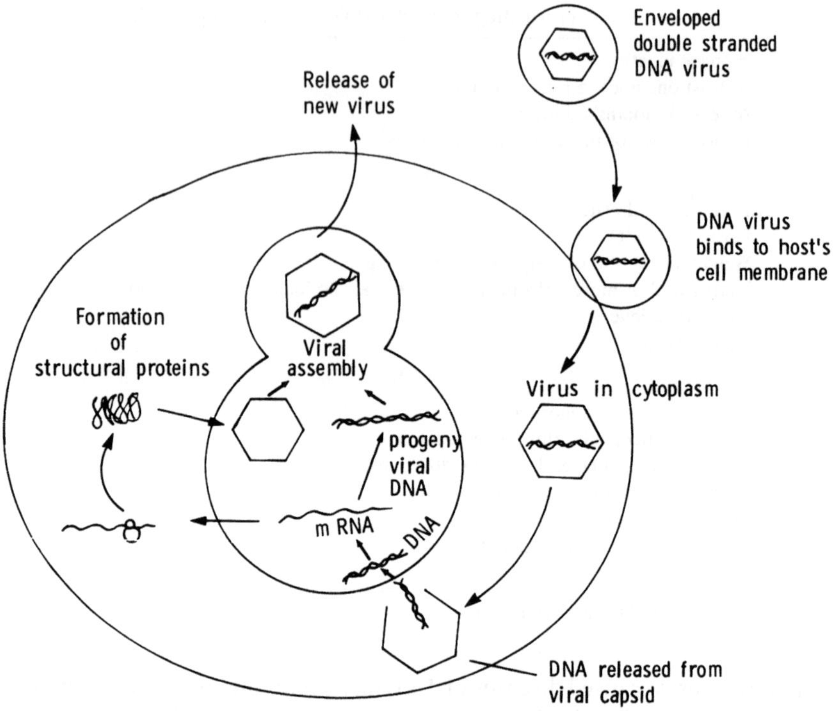
Enveloped double stranded DNA virus
Release of new virus
DNA virus binds to host's cell membrane
Formation of structural proteins
Viral assembly
Virus in cytoplasm
progeny viral DNA
m RNA
DNA
DNA released from viral capsid

a

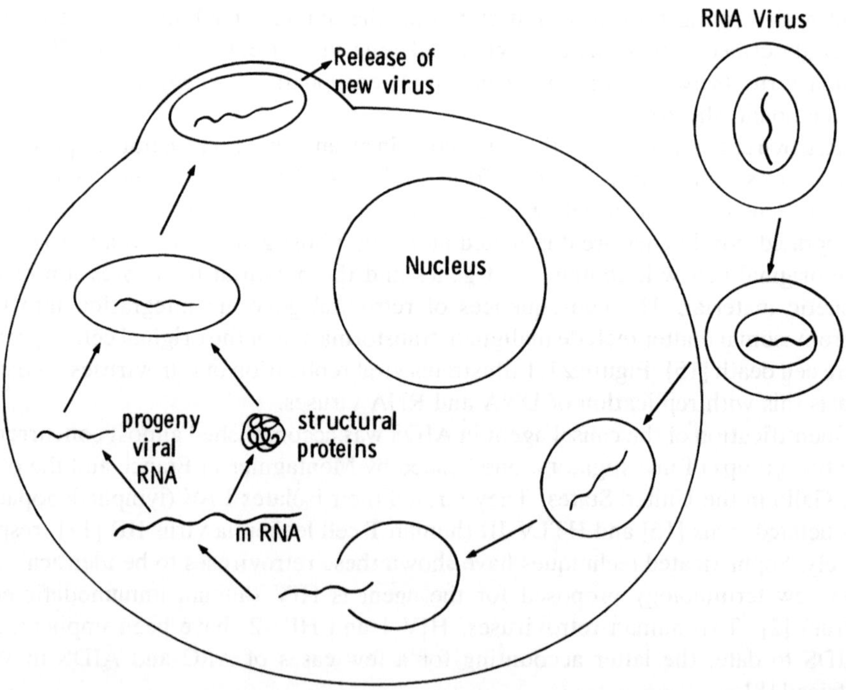
RNA Virus
Release of new virus
Nucleus
progeny viral RNA
structural proteins
m RNA

b

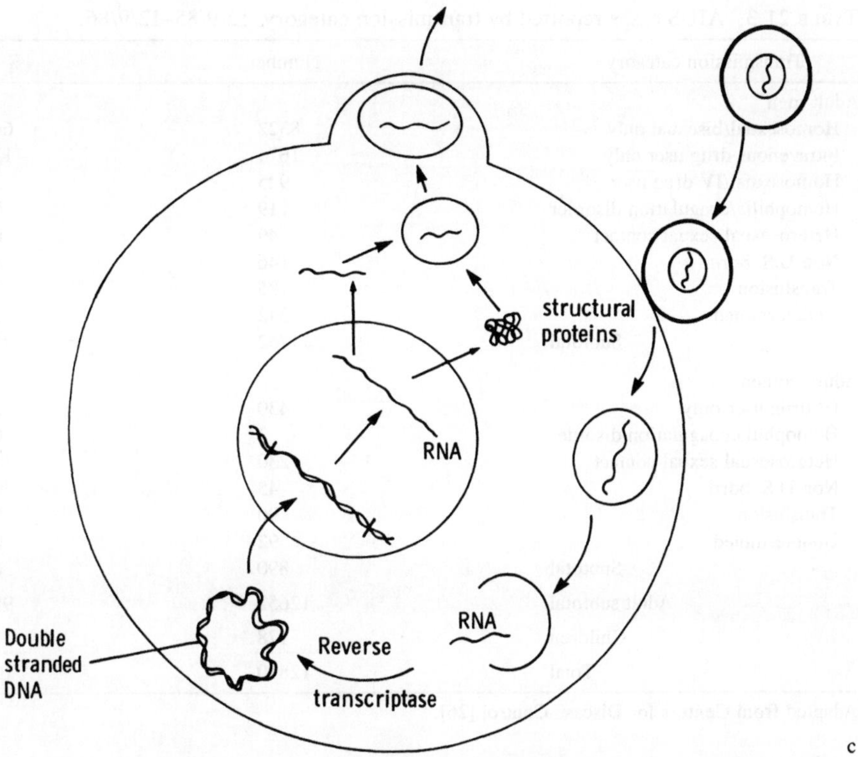


FIGURE 21.1. Viral replication of retroviruses compared with that of DNA and RNA viruses. (a) DNA virus replication. Upon entering the host cell, the DNA of this double-stranded DNA virus is released from the virion, penetrating the cell nucleus. Inside the nucleus, viral RNA is formed, ultimately leading to the synthesis of structural proteins (intracytoplasmically) and nucleic acid (intranuclearly). The complete new virion is then assembled. (b) RNA virus replication (nonretrovirus). Although there are numerous different types of RNA viruses, basic viral replication consists of release of viral RNA into the host cell cytoplasm. If of the proper polarity, this RNA can act as its own messenger RNA, to be transcribed into viral nucleic acid and structural proteins, which are assembled into new virions and released from the cell. (c) Retrovirus replication. Unique to the retroviruses is the enzyme *reverse transcriptase*. This enzyme leads to the formation of double-stranded DNA from viral RNA in the cytoplasm. This DNA then enters the nucleus and becomes incorporated into host DNA, which leads to the transcription of RNA. New viral RNA and structural proteins become assembled into new virions.

TABLE 21.3. AIDS cases reported by transmission category, 12/9/85–12/9/86.

| Transmission category | Number | % Total |
|---|---|---|
| Adult men | | |
| Homosexual/bisexual only | 8322 | 64.9 |
| Intravenous drug user only | 1674 | 13.0 |
| Homosexual/IV drug user | 925 | 7.2 |
| Hemophilia/coagulation disorder | 119 | 0.9 |
| Heterosexual sexual contact | 49 | 0.4 |
| Non-U.S. born | 146 | 1.1 |
| Transfusion | 185 | 1.4 |
| Undetermined | 342 | 2.7 |
| Subtotal | 11762 | 91.7 |
| Adult women | | |
| IV drug user only | 430 | 3.4 |
| Hemophilia/coagulation disorder | 3 | 0.02 |
| Heterosexual sexual contact | 230 | 1.8 |
| Non-U.S. born | 45 | 0.4 |
| Transfusion | 90 | 0.7 |
| Undetermined | 92 | 0.7 |
| Subtotal | 890 | 6.94 |
| Adult subtotal | 12652 | 98.6 |
| Children | 178 | 1.4 |
| Total | 12830 | 100% |

Adapted from Centers for Disease Control [26].

## Origin of the Virus

Available evidence suggests that AIDS has been present in Central Africa since the late 1970s [19–22]. Retrospective analysis of stored serum from patients in Uganda has shown a high degree of seropositivity as far back as 1970 [23], and a single plasma sample from Zaire in 1959 has also tested positive to HIV [24]. This evidence, as well as the isolation of a related virus from the African green monkey [25], has led to the hypothesis that HIV originated in Africa. It is apparent, however, that AIDS is now an epidemic of global proportions, with numerous countries worldwide reporting cases to the World Health Organization.

## Epidemiology and Pathogenesis

The most recent statistics published by the CDC highlight the epidemiologic distribution of AIDS in the United States (Table 21.3) [26]. These numbers bring to 28,098 the total of AIDS cases in the United States as of December 8, 1986. The 1985–1986 statistics in the table are clearly representative of the distribution of all AIDS cases reported in the United States to date, about two thirds of all cases being accounted for by homosexual/bisexual adult men. Of note, the ratio of men to women in the American statistics is about 14:1, clearly different from the 1:1 [20] male/female ratio described in AIDS cases reported from Africa. The reasons for this difference will be described below.

A knowledge of which tissues and body fluids contain the virus allows one to appreciate the epidemiology of this disease. HIV has been isolated from human blood, semen, bone marrow, tears, saliva, urine, cerebrospinal fluid, lymph nodes, feces, and brain tissue [27], as well as from cervical and vaginal secretions [28,29]; however, evidence to date suggests that the disease can only be transmitted by (a) close sexual contact, (b) sharing of contaminated needles, (c) injection of infected blood or blood products, and by (d) transplacental transfer of the virus from mother to child [27]. A probable case of transmission of the virus to a newborn through breast milk has also been described [30]. Although there are obvious marked epidemiologic similarities between disease due to HIV and that due to hepatitis B (HBV), it should be noted that the risk of acquiring HBV after a needlestick exposure ranges from 6 to 30%, much higher than the quoted risk of acquiring HIV after a similar exposure ($<1\%$ [31]). In addition, there appears to be minimal risk of transmission of HIV to casual household contacts [32].

A recent study has shed light on the epidemiology of AIDS in Africa [33]. Investigation of HIV antibody status in prostitutes in Nairobi revealed a seropositivity of 66% in prostitutes of low socioeconomic status and of 31% in prostitutes of higher socioeconomic status. This information has emphasized the role played by heterosexual transmission in the spread of this disease, and partly explains the high female/male ratio of AIDS in Africa, where homosexuality and intravenous drug use do not appear to play a role [20]. Scarification techniques and reuse of disposable medical materials may also be risk factors in Africa [21].

Risk factors for seropositivity to HIV in homosexual patients have included number of partners and numerous exposures through receptive anal intercourse [34]. Some work suggests that it is more the number of sexual partners from high-risk areas, along with certain sexual practices, rather than the total number of partners that constitutes the major risk factor for seropositivity [35]. The major risk factor for virus acquisition in hemophiliacs has been the use of factor concentrates [34].

## Natural History of HIV Infection

The number of patients who have evidence of viral exposure as judged by seropositivity is substantial. It has been difficult, however, to exactly define which proportion of seropositive patients will go on to develop AIDS or AIDS-related disorders. Part of the reason for this appears to be the long incubation period from exposure to clinical illness, which may be at least 5 years [36,37]. A median incubation period of 52 months has been quoted for transfusion-associated AIDS [38].

One group of studies has reported that between 4 and 19% of seropositive patients have developed AIDS during 1 to 4 years of follow-up, with another 25% developing symptoms suggestive of AIDS-related conditions [39–41]. A recent study reported that 34% of seropositive patients progressed to AIDS in 3 years [42].

It is not known which patients will progress from the asymptomatic seropositive state to the symptomatic phase of ARC or AIDS. A recent analysis of HIV-seropositive homosexual men with PGL noted that patients with constitutional symptoms and a low T helper cell count at their first visit were at higher risk for AIDS than other PGL patients [43]. Another study reported a multivariate analysis done on seropositive homosexual men, noting that a decreased number of T helper lymphocytes, an increased number of T suppressor lymphocytes, a low level of antibody to HIV, a high titer of cytomegalovirus antibody, and a history of sex with someone in whom AIDS developed, were independently associated with the subsequent development of AIDS [44]. Whether these are markers or determinants of progression of HIV-induced disease must await further study. More recently, a falling p24 antibody level, HIV antigemia and HIV viremia have been noted to be indicators of disease progression in HIV infected patients [44a,b,c].

## Testing for Human Immunodeficiency Virus

Seroconversion to HIV occurs from 8 to 12 weeks after exposure to the virus [45]. Serologic testing for HIV currently involves a screening test followed by a confirmatory test for all positives. At present the enzyme-linked immunoabsorbent assay (ELISA test) is the screening test most commonly used, with a sensitivity of 97% and a specificity of 99.8%. Western blot testing is the most widely used confirmatory test, with a positive predictive value of 99% in high prevalence groups [46].

HIV culture can be performed but requires high-level containment facilities. The incidence of virus recovery is approximately 50% for patients with AIDS, 80% for patients with ARC, and 30% for healthy high risk people [47].

Newer assays being developed include ones designed to detect HIV antigens and neutralizing antibodies [11]. A recent survey of serologic markers to HIV in hemophiliac patients noted that HIV antigen appeared first, then antibody to envelope, followed by antibody to core antigens [48]. It is thus apparent that more sensitive techniques can detect exposure to HIV earlier than presently available tests, with implications for earlier diagnosis and possible prevention.

## Clinical Manifestations of AIDS

The clinical manifestations of AIDS are protean and affect virtually every organ in the body. Symptoms are often subtle and insidious in onset, and without careful questioning may easily go undetected. Any new symptom or change in symptoms in a known HIV antibody-positive patient, in a patient in a high-risk group, or in a patient with documented AIDS must be taken seriously and investigations instituted to discern its etiology. Cutaneous manifestations are numerous and will be dealt with in the subsequent chapter. In this chapter, the major noncutaneous clinical manifestations of AIDS will be described and classified according to organ system and their differential diagnosis and treatment will be discussed.

## Pulmonary Manifestations

The chief complaints of pulmonary manifestations of AIDS are fever, malaise, dyspnea, and cough. The types and frequency of pulmonary disorders in 441 patients with AIDs have been reviewed [49]. Of 502 pulmonary disorders, 93% were infectious in origin and 7% were due to Kaposi's sarcoma (KS). *P. carinii* pneumonia (PCP) accounted for 80% of infectious etiologies, and was found along with a coexisting infection (often of questionable clinical significance) in 30% of these patients. The pulmonary pathogens found along with *P. carinii* or on their own included cytomegalovirus, *M. avium*-intracellulare, *M. tuberculosis*, *Cryptococcus neoformans*, herpes simplex virus, and legionella. Because of its predominance as the main pulmonary complication in AIDS patients, this chapter will focus on PCP, with mention also of pulmonary Kaposi's sarcoma.

### *Pneumocystis carinii Pneumonia* (PCP)

*P. carinii* is a ubiquitous protozoan organism. Evidence suggests that the infection is acquired early in childhood and remains in a latent stage until reactivated by some immunosuppressive condition. PCP is part of the presenting clinical picture in about 60% of AIDS patients, and may occur in up to 85% of patients at some time during their lifetime [50].

Malaise, fever, nonproductive cough, and dyspnea are the usual presenting symptoms [51]. Nonspecific symptoms not referable to the pulmonary system may predominate; physical signs in the chest are often absent. The classic radiographic appearance is that of diffuse pulmonary infiltrates (Fig. 21.2), although the infiltrates may be unilateral or concentrated in the upper or lower lung zones. In 5% of patients the chest x-ray may be clear. Usually diagnostic bronchoscopy is performed once an abnormal chest radiograph is documented. However, in patients whose initial chest radiograph is normal, the diffusing capacity for carbon monoxide as well as a gallium scan of the lungs (each with a sensitivity for PCP of 90% and a negative predictive value of 60%) [2] should be performed prior to contemplating the more invasive procedure.

In early studies, bronchoscopy with bronchial washings or bronchoalveolar lavage offered a 79% [1] to 89% [52,53] yield for confirming a diagnosis of PCP. With the addition of transbronchial biopsy, the sensitivity of the procedure for PCP has been increased to 100% [53]. A false-negative rate of about 10% may occur when either procedure is used alone and may be corrected by a repeat bronchoscopy. The need for open-lung biopsy should be considered in less than 5% of patients. Recent evidence suggests that examination of saline-induced sputum for pneumocysts may obviate the need for bronchoscopy in some patients [54].

Gomori's methenamine silver stain can be done on bronchoalveolar lavage specimens or on fixed tissue, and demonstrates the typical pneumocysts (Fig. 21.3). Giemsa's and Gram-Weigert stains may be used to identify sporozoites and trophozoites, while Gram's stain may be of use in some situations to identify the cyst wall

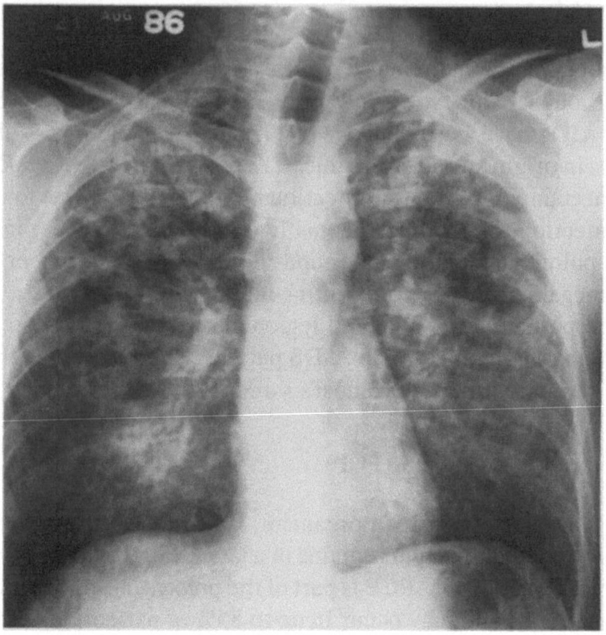


FIGURE 21.2. Chest radiograph showing diffuse pulmonary infiltrates typical of *Pneumocystis carinii* pneumonia.

and internal sporozoites [51]. Histopathology of fixed tissue reveals a marked desquamative alveolitis, with numerous cysts filling the alveolar spaces.

The treatment recommended for PCP in patients with AIDS is a 21-day course of either trimethoprim-sulfamethoxazole (TMP-SMX) intravenously or orally (20 mg/kg of trimethoprim daily in four divided doses) or pentamidine isethionate (4 mg/kg/day) intravenously. Neither regimen, when studied prospectively, has been shown to have a statistically significant difference in efficacy or in the frequency of side effects [55]. This contrasts with previously reported cases of a higher incidence of adverse reactions to TMP-SMX than to pentamidine in AIDS patients with PCP [56,57]. The main side effects from TMP-SMX include rash, fever, leukopenia, thrombocytopenia, and hepatitis, while those from pentamidine include azotemia, leukopenia, hypoglycemia, rash, fever, and thrombocytopenia [57]. Drug toxicity is usually apparent during the second week of therapy. Discontinuation of therapy due to toxicity may be necessary in 50% of patients on either regimen [58], and in such a situation the other regimen should be substituted. Patients who switch regimens due to drug toxicity have a more favorable outcome than those who switch due to clinical failure [49]. Further regimens that may prove useful in some patients with AIDS and PCP include dapsone-trimethoprim [58], difluoromethylornithine [59] and trimetrexate.

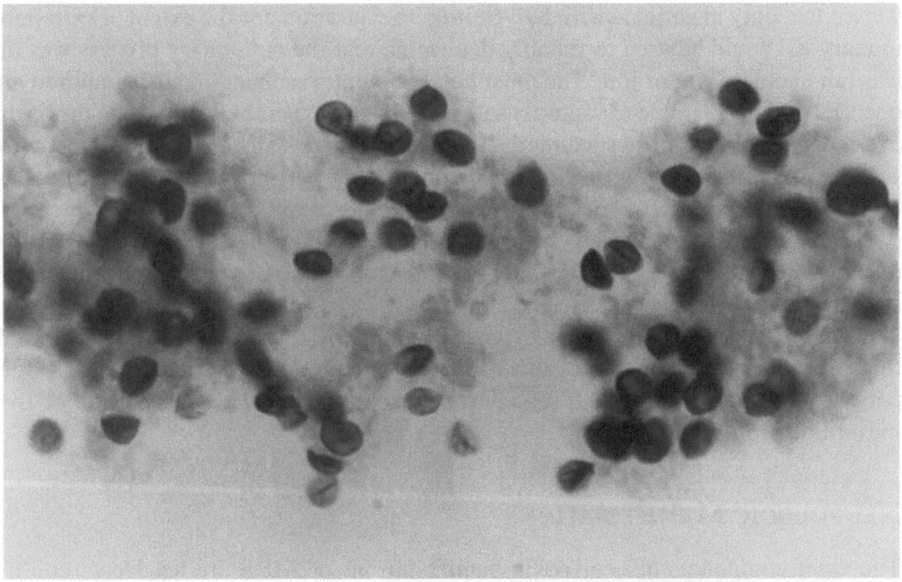

FIGURE 21.3. Gomori's methenamine silver stain of fluid obtained by bronchoalveolar lavage. Cysts magnification × 1,000.

Successful treatment of PCP in AIDS patients ranges from 57 [60] to 75% [61]. A 26% recurrence rate has been quoted, and the results of therapy of second episodes of PCP may be equally as successful as treatment of the initial episodes [61]. Of patients who require mechanical ventilation, however, only 14% may survive [62]. Of those who survive, prophylaxis with oral TMP-SMX, where tolerated, may be advantageous [63]. Secondary prophylaxis with pyrimethamine-sulfadoxine has not been as successful [64].

## Pulmonary Kaposi's Sarcoma

In the review of pulmonary complications cited previously, pulmonary Kaposi's sarcoma accounted for 7% of pulmonary conditions in AIDS patients [49]. All of these patients, however, had an associated pulmonary infection, and thus one could not easily discern the contribution of the pulmonary KS to the pulmonary picture. A more recent review has focused upon KS as a cause of severe respiratory disease in patients with AIDS [65].

Thirty patients with biopsy-proven mucocutaneous or lymphadenopathic KS had a diagnostic lung biopsy performed for suspicion of pulmonary disease. Twelve of the 30 had pulmonary KS; half of these patients had pulmonary KS alone and the other half had a concurrent pulmonary infection. Patients presented with a combination of fever, cough, and dyspnea. Interstitial or alveolar infiltrates could not differentiate pulmonary infection from pulmonary KS, although pleural effusions were noted only in patients with KS. Neither the duration nor the extent of extrapulmonary KS could be used to reliably determine that the pulmonary process was or was not neoplastic in origin. The most notable point was that diagnosis required an open-lung biopsy sample (or autopsy sample); diagnosis was never made on the basis of a transbronchial biopsy specimen. Histopathology revealed vascular lumina with swollen endothelial cells, or lumina surrounded by perithelial (adventitial) cells. Spindle cells, extravasated erythrocytes, and hemosiderin deposits were typical.

Combination chemotherapy with adriamycin, vinblastine, bleomycin, dactinomycin, vincristine, and dacarbazine, or whole lung irradiation, provided temporary symptomatic relief in three patients.

Because open-lung biopsy was essential to diagnosis, the authors recommended this procedure when initial bronchoscopic investigation was negative or if the patient failed to improve in spite of bronchoscopic evidence of resolution of the initial infection [65].

## Neurologic Manifestations

The chief complaints of neurologic manifestations of AIDS are headache, confusion, change in personality, focal deficits, and seizures. Neurological manifestations are numerous, and may be referable to both the central nervous system (CNS) and peripheral nervous system. A review of 31% of patients in San Francisco with AIDS or generalized lymphadenopathy noted that 10% of all patients had neurologic symptoms at the time of presentation, with 39% of all AIDS patients being neurologically symptomatic [66]. The discovery of the neurotropism of HIV-I [67–69] has expanded our appreciation of the neurologic complications of AIDS, and has allowed us to understand symptoms that were previously unexplained. Table 21.4 lists the more common neurologic manifestations of AIDS as collated from the San Francisco Review [66]. It is of interest to note that the "subacute encephalitis" cases may in fact have been cases of encephalitis due to the HIV itself (see below). One can again appreciate that infectious causes of neurologic disease far outnumber neoplastic causes. This section will concentrate on the two most common neurologic complications of AIDS, cerebral toxoplasmosis (CTg) and HIV-induced neurologic disease.

### Cerebral Toxoplasmosis (CTg)

*Toxoplasma gondii* (Tg) is a ubiquitous protozoan organism. Up to 50% of the U.S. population may be infected by 12 years of age [50], and in these hosts the parasite exists in a latent cyst phase in many organs, including the brain, eye, and heart muscle. Clinical infection in the immunocompromised host is usually a result of reactivation of this latent infection.

The clinical presentation of CTg in AIDS patients is usually that of focal deficits and altered level of consciousness [66,70]; about 15% of patients present with seizures. Cerebrospinal fluid (CSF) findings are nonspecific, often being characterized

TABLE 21.4. Neurologic manifestations of AIDS.

| |
|---|
| Central nervous system |
| Viral syndromes |
| Subacute encephalitis |
| Atypical aseptic meningitis |
| Herpes simplex encephalitis |
| Progressive multifocal leukoencephalopathy |
| Nonviral infections |
| *Toxoplasma gondii* |
| *Cryptococcus neoformans* |
| *Candida albicans* |
| Atypical mycobacteria |
| Neoplasms |
| Primary CNS lymphoma |
| Systemic lymphoma with CNS involvement |
| Kaposi's sarcoma |
| Cranial nerve syndromes |
| Multiple neuropathies due to chronic inflammatory polyneuropathy |
| Multiple neuropathies due to lymphoma |
| Bell's palsy |
| Peripheral nervous system |
| Chronic inflammatory polyneuropathy |
| Distal symmetrical neuropathy |
| Herpes zoster radiculitis |

Adapted from Levy et al. [66].

by an elevated protein level and lymphocytic pleocytosis of varying degree. CSF antibody levels to *T. gondii* are also not diagnostically helpful [66].

Contrast-enhanced computerized tomography (CT) scan is the most helpful diagnostic aid for CTg, and it is also the pivot of diagnosis of CNS disease in AIDS patients. Single or multiple ring-enhancing lesions with surrounding low density and slight or disproportionately small mass effect are typical of CTg [71] (Fig. 21.4), although no enhancement may be seen [72]. MRI scanning may be a useful adjunct in the rare case with a negative CT scan. Other causes of focal CT findings include lymphoma, herpes simplex encephalitis, tuberculosis, and nocardiosis. CNS lymphoma does not usually enhance with contrast. Cryptococcal meningitis, which may present as headache, confusion, or seizures, does not usually have focal findings.

Because of the severe immunocompromised status of AIDS patients, serologic studies are of limited usefulness in diagnosing acute CTg in these patients. Although IgM antibody against *T. gondii* and a rising titer of IgG against this organism are not commonly seen [72], the presence of any IgG antibody to *T. gondii* has been so consistently found that its absence is said to effectively rule out a diagnosis of CTg. However, a definitive diagnosis can only be established on the basis of brain biopsy of a radiologically delineated abnormality.

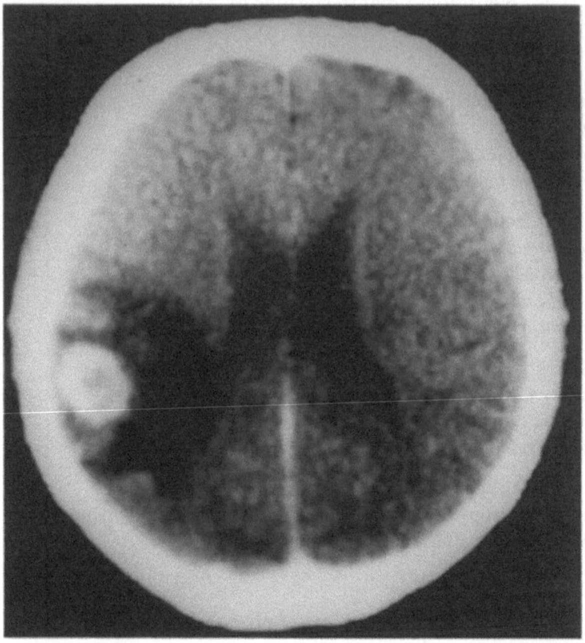

FIGURE 21.4. Computerized tomographic scan showing an oval-shaped enhancing lesion in the left parietal lobe with edema. *Toxoplasma gondii* was identified in the specimen at brain biopsy.

Treatment of CTg with pyrimethamine and a sulfonamide is reserved for AIDS patients with biopsy-proven CTg, or patients with a high likelihood of CTg, for example, with a positive serum IgG test and ring-enhancing lesions on CT scan. In the latter situation, failure to improve clinically or radiologically after 2 to 3 weeks necessitates a biopsy if the diagnosis was not biopsy proven. Because relapses occur when treatment is discontinued, lifelong therapy is advocated.

## HIV-Induced Neurologic Disease

A subacute encephalitis with progressive dementia of uncertain etiology was noted in an early review of the neurologic complications of AIDS [73]. CSF findings were nonspecific, and CT scan was remarkable for demonstrating advanced cerebral atrophy. No infectious etiology could be demonstrated conclusively to be responsible for these findings.

The finding of HIV DNA in the brains of five patients with AIDS [67], as well as the finding of viral-specific RNA in the brains of four of these patients, raised the possibility that HIV itself could easily cause neurologic disease. Of note, it has been appreciated in the past that T lymphocytes and brain cells share common cell surface antigens [67], and thus both the lymphotropism and neurotropism of this virus could be explained.

HIV has been isolated from the CSF and/or brain tissue of patients with acute aseptic meningitis associated with HIV seroconversion, chronic meningitis, and AIDS-associated dementia. In addition it has been cultured from the spinal cord of an AIDS patient with myelopathy and from the sural nerve of an AIDS patient with a peripheral neuropathy [68]. HIV-specific antibodies have been found in the CSF of the majority of AIDS or ARC patients with neurologic symptoms [69], and where tested the CSF antibody titer to HIV was higher than that in the serum, indicating local production. It is apparent that HIV is potentially responsible for a wide variety of central and peripheral nervous system manifestations.

## Gastrointestinal Manifestations

Diarrhea and weight loss are a prominent part of the symptomatology in both ARC and AIDS. In a review of 22 AIDS patients, 96% had weight loss and 55% had diarrhea [74]. Gastrointestinal infections were found in 45% of patients, with diarrhea and malabsorption more common in the infected group. Some patients had a nonspecific enteropathy characterized by mononuclear cell infiltration of the lamina propria. Two patients had intestinal Kaposi's sarcoma. The infections reported in this study included those due to *M. avium*-intracellulare, cryptosporidiosis, giardiasis, *Campylobacter*, *Candida* (esophagitis), herpes (esophagitis), and *Salmonella*. Interestingly, cytomegalovirus (CMV) was not found in this study. It was suggested that gastrointestinal involvement in AIDS may be limited in the main to homosexual patients [74].

Infection due to *Isospora belli* or *Cryptosporidium* typically causes a high-volume diarrhea with malabsorption and weight loss [75]. Cytomegalovirus colitis may present as diarrhea, abdominal pain, hematochezia, or intestinal necrosis [76]. *M. avium*-intracellulare infection may present as chronic diarrhea, extrabiliary obstructive jaundice due to intraperitoneal adenopathy, or malabsorption with a Whipple's diseaselike picture on biopsy [77].

Clinically the various diarrhea/weight loss syndromes cannot be differentiated with certainty. The following diagnostic approach should be undertaken. Stools should be submitted and examined for bacteria, mycobacteria, viruses, fungi, ova, and parasites, including *Cryptosporidium* and *Isospora*. If lower gastrointestinal symptoms predominate, sigmoidoscopy with possible colonoscopy should be performed in a search for intestinal KS or CMV colitis. Either may have hemorrhagic lesions on colonoscopy, and therefore histopathologic differentiation is essential [75]. If the diarrhea remains unexplained, upper endoscopy and small-bowel biopsy may provide a diagnosis of M. avium-intracellulare or the nonspecific AIDS enteropathy as described above.

Table 21.5 outlines recommended treatment for the more common gastrointestinal infections.

TABLE 21.5. Treatment recommendations for common gastrointestinal infections in AIDS.

| Infection | Treatment |
|---|---|
| Cryptosporidiosis | Spiramycin, 1 g tid (investigational in some countries); not always effective |
| Isosporiasis | Trimethoprim (160 mg) and sulfamethoxazole (800 mg), qid for 1–2 weeks, then prophylaxis |
| Cytomegalovirus colitis | 9-(2-hydroxy-1 [hydroxymethyl] ethoxymethyl) guanine (investigational) |
| *Mycobacterium avium*-intracellulare | Combination that may include 4 to 6 of following: isoniazid (300 mg/day), rifampin (600 mg/day), or ansamycin (150–300 mg/day); clofazimine (100 mg tid), ethambutol (25 mg/kg/day for 6 weeks, then 15/mg/kg/day), ethionamide (500–1,000 mg/day) and streptomycin (15 mg/kg IM daily × 60 days). Therapy not consistently effective; some investigators opt to withhold specific antimycobacterial therapy |

## Treatment and Prevention of Infection With HIV

A number of issues seem apparent at this stage of our consideration of therapeutic options in HIV disease [78]. It appears as though therapy given to recently infected patients, before severe immunologic compromise takes place, might be optimal. The ideal drug should cross the blood-brain barrier to eliminate the CNS reservoir of the virus. Furthermore, the drug should be relatively safe with high specificity to HIV.

Most of the antiviral agents available for this infection inhibit the reverse transcriptase enzyme that makes double-stranded DNA from the viral genomic RNA, which then integrates into host cell DNA. Such drugs include suramin, antimoniotungstate (HPA-23), phosphonoformate, and azidothymidine (AZT) [78]. Unacceptable side effects or limited results of therapy have limited the use of suramin and HPA-23. Of the above, AZT has currently been released for treatment of some patients with AIDS and other HIV-related syndromes.

An initial uncontrolled study using AZT in patients with AIDS or ARC showed both immunologic and clinical improvement in many [79]. A further controlled study of AZT versus placebo in patients with ARC, or with AIDS within 120 days after a first episode of PCP, revealed a reduction in both morbidity and mortality in the patients on the study drug at 3 to 6 months of follow-up [80]. Recent information has shown improvement in HIV-related neurologic disease in patients on AZT [81]. The drug, however, is not without side effects: Significant bone marrow suppression may occur [80]. Further studies will be important to delineate the optimal dose and duration of therapy, as well as the group of patients who might benefit most from its use.

Numerous other antiviral agents are being studied in this disease, as are various immunomodulators including interleukin-2, interferon, and isoprinosine [78]. The most useful regimen, however, is yet to be defined.

Further efforts are being geared toward preventive strategies in HIV disease. The first is that of immunization, the second of education.

The recent development of a vaccine against another retrovirus, the feline leukemia virus, lends optimism to the development of a vaccine against HIV [82]. A possible stumbling block is that related to phenotypic variations of the virus, particularly in the envelope region [82], in addition to the suggestion of genetic variation in HIV isolates in a single individual over time [83]. The degree of protective immunity as well as the safety of any candidate vaccine will have to be assessed in both animals and high-risk seronegative populations [78]. Certainly we should await the development of such a vaccine with hope and with optimism.

The educational component of prevention of HIV disease includes behavior modification in high-risk groups and targeting of relevant facts to young people even before they are involved in sexual encounters. The physician can play a big part in community education. The use of condoms should be condoned in both the homosexual and even the young heterosexual population [84]. A strong effort toward education can greatly facilitate any strategy based on immunization, and might ultimately diminish the importance of the availability of therapeutic drugs.

## Conclusion

A large reservoir of HIV seropositive individuals exists globally, particularly in the United States and in Africa, and the short-term forecasts include a burgeoning number of AIDS and ARC cases in coming years. Patients present in many ways. We have tried to outline some of the more common noncutaneous clinical manifestations of AIDS in this chapter. Since the identification of HIV as the causative agent in AIDS, major strides have been made in the development of both therapeutic and preventive approaches to this disease. Early identification of symptomatic disease may at some point in the future enable early administration of drugs and alteration if not cure of the disease. For this reason we feel that all physicians require a basic understanding of AIDS, including background, clinical presentation, and knowledge of therapeutic and preventive strategies.

### References


1. LCDC. AIDS surveillance. *CDWR* **73**:13–16, 1987.
2. Coffin J, Haase A, Levy JA, et al: Human immunodeficiency viruses. (Letter). *Science* **232**:697, 1986.
3. Centers for Disease Control: Update on acquired immunodeficiency syndrome (AIDS)—United States. *MMWR* **31**:507–514, 1982.
4. Centers for Disease Control: Revision of the case definition of acquired immunodeficiency for national reporting— United States. *MMWR* **34**:373, 1985.

4a. Centers for Disease Control: Revision of the CDC. Surveillance case definition for Acquired Immunodeficiency Syndrome. *MMWR* **36**:1–155, 1987.

5. Haverkos HW, Gotlieb MS, Killen JY, et al. Classification of HTLV III/LAV-related diseases. *J Infect Dis* **151**:1095, 1985.
6. Redfield RR, Wright DC, Tramont EC: The Walter-Reed staging classification for HTLV-III/LAV infection. *N Engl J Med* **314**:131–132, 1986.

7. Centers for Disease Control: Classification system for human T-lymphotropic virus type III/lymphadenopathy-associated virus infection. *MMWR* **35**:334–339, 1986.
8. Centers for Disease Control: Persistent generalized lymphadenopathy among homosexual males. *MMWR* **31**:249–241, 1982.
9. Shepherd FA, Fanning MM, Duperval R, et al: A guide to the investigation and treatment of patients with AIDS and AIDS-related disorders. CMAJ **134**:999–1008, 1986.
10. Centers for Disease Control: Pneumocystis pneumonia-Los Angeles. *MMWR* **30**:250–252, 1981.
11. Centers for Disease Control: Kaposi's sarcoma and pneumocystis pneumonia among homosexual men—New York City and California. *MMWR* **30**:305–308, 1981.
12. Siegal FP, Lopez E, Hammer GS, et al: Severe acquired immunodeficiency in male homosexuals, manifested by chronic perianal ulcerative herpes simplex lesions. *N Engl J Med* **305**:1439–1444, 1981.
13. Gottlieb MS, Schroff R, Schanker HM, et al: *Pneumocystis carinii* pneumonia and mucosal candidiasis in previously healthy homosexual men: Evidence of a new acquired cellular immunodeficiency. *N Engl J Med* **305**:1425–1431, 1981.
14. Fauci AS, Macher AM, Longo DL, et al: Acquired immunodeficiency syndrome: Epidemiologic, clinical, immunologic, and therapeutic considerations. *Ann Intern Med* **100**:92–106, 1984.
15. Gallo RC, Wong-Staal F: A human T-lymphotropic retrovirus (HTLV-III) as the cause of the acquired immunodeficiency syndrome. *Ann Intern Med* **103**:679–689, 1985.
16. Barre-Sinoussi F, Chermann JC, Rey F, et al: Isolation of a T-lymphotropic retrovirus from a patient at risk for acquired immunodeficiency syndrome (AIDS). *Science* **220**:868–871, 1983.
17. Popovich M, Sarngadharan MG, Reed E, et al: Detection, isolation and continuous production of cytopathic retroviruses (HTLV-III) from patients with AIDS and pre-AIDS. *Science* **224**:497–500, 1984.
18. Clavel F, Guetard D, Brun-Vezinett, et al: Isolation of a new human retrovirus from West African patients with AIDS. *Science* **233**:343–346, 1986.
19. Clumeck N, Sonnet J, Tallman H, et al: Acquired immunodeficiency syndrome in African patients. *N Engl J Med* **310**:492–497, 1984.
20. Piot P, Quinn TC, Taelman H, et al: Acquired immunodeficiency syndrome in a heterosexual population in Zaire. *Lancet* **2**:65–69, 1984.
21. Van de Perre P, Rouvroy D, Lepage P, et al: Acquired immunodeficiency syndrome in Rwanda. *Lancet* **2**:62–65, 1984.
22. Brun-Vezinet F, Rouzioux C, Montagnier L, et al: Prevalence of antibodies to lymphadenopathy-associated retrovirus in African patients with AIDS. *Science* **226**:453–456, 1984.
23. Saxinger WC, Levine PH, Dean AG, et al: Evidence for exposure to HTLV-III in Uganda before 1973. *Science* **227**:1036–1038, 1985.
24. Nahmias AJ, Weiss J, Yao X, et al: Evidence for human infection with an HTLV-III/LAV like virus in central Africa. *Lancet* **1**:1279–1280, 1986.
25. Kanki PJ, Alroy J, Essex M, et al: Isolation of T-lymphotropic retrovirus related to HTLV-III/LAV from wild-caught African green monkeys. *Science* **230**:951–954, 1985.
26. Centers for Disease Control: Update: acquired immunodeficiency syndrome—United States. *MMWR* **35**:758–766, 1986.
27. Infectious Diseases Society of America: Acquired immunodeficiency syndrome. *J Infect Dis* **154**:1–9, 1986.
28. Vogt MW, Craven DE, Crawford DF, et al: Isolation of HTLV-III/LAV from cervical secretions of women at risk for AIDS. *Lancet* **1**:525–527, 1986.

29. Wofsy CB, Hauer LB, Michaelis BA, et al: Isolation of AIDS-related retrovirus from genital secretions of women with antibodies to the virus. *Lancet* **1**:527–529, 1986.
30. Ziegler JB, Johnson RO, Cooper DA, et al: Postnatal transmission of AIDS-associated retrovirus from mother to infant. *Lancet* **1**:896–898, 1985.
31. Centers for Disease Control: Recommendations for preventing transmission of infection with human T-lymphotropic virus type III/lymphadenopathy-associated virus in the workplace. *MMWR* **34**:682–695, 1985.
32. Friedland GH, Saltzman BR, Rogers MF, et al: Lack of transmission of HTLV-III/LAV infection to household contacts of patients with AIDS or AIDS-related complex with oral candidiasis. *N Engl J Med* **314**:344–349, 1986.
33. Kreiss JK, Koech D, Plummer FA, et al: AIDS virus infection in Nairobi prostitutes: Spread of the epidemic to East Africa. *N Engl J Med* **314**:414–418, 1986.
34. Blattner WA, Biggar RJ, Weiss SH, et al: Epidemiology of human T-lymphotropic virus type III and the risk of the acquired immunodeficiency syndrome. *Ann Intern Med* **103**:665–670, 1985.
35. DeGruttora V, Mayer K, Bennett W: AIDS: Has the problem been adequately assessed? *Rev Infect Dis* **8**:295–305, 1986.
36. Feorino PM, Jaffe HW, Palmer E, et al: Transfusion-associated acquired immunodeficiency syndrome: Evidence for persistent infection in blood donors. *N Engl J Med* **312**:1293–1296, 1985.
37. Maloney MJ, Cox F, Wray BB, et al: AIDS in a child 5 ½ years after a transfusion. (Letter) *N Engl J Med* **312**:1256, 1985.
38. Luik J, Lawrence DN, Morgan WM, et al: A model-based approach for estimating the mean incubation period of transfusion-associated acquired immunodeficiency syndrome. *Proc Natl Acad Sci (USA)* **83**:3051–3055, 1986.
39. Landesman SH, Ginzburg HM, Weiss SH: The AIDS epidemic. *N Engl J Med* **312**: 521–525, 1985.
40. Curran JW, Morgan WM, Hardy AM, et al: The epidemiology of AIDS: Current status and future prospects. *Science* **229**:1352–1357, 1985.
41. Francis DL, Jaffe HW, Fultz PN, et al: The natural history of infection with the lymphadenopathy-associated virus human T-lymphotropic virus type III. *Ann Intern Med* **103**:719–722, 1985.
42. Goedert JJ, Biggar RJ, Weiss SH, et al: Three year incidence of AIDS in five cohorts of HTLV-III infected risk group members. *Science* **231**:992–995, 1986.
43. Kaplan JE, Spira JJ, Fishbein DB, et al: Lymphadenopathy syndrome in homosexual men: Evidence for continuing risk of developing the acquired immunodeficiency syndrome. *JAMA* **257**:335–337, 1987.
44. Polk BF, Fox R, Brookmeyer R, et al: Predictors of the acquired immunodeficiency syndrome developing in a cohort of seropositive homosexual men. *N Engl J Med* **316**: 61–66, 1987.
44a. Allain J-P, Laurian Y, Paul DA, et al: Long-term evaluation of HIV antigen and antibodies to p24 and gp41 in patients with hemophilia: potential clinical importance. *N Engl J Med* **317**:1114–1121, 1987.
44b. Wittek AE, Phelan MA, Wells MA, et al: Detection of Human immunodeficiency virus core protein in plasma by enzyme immunoassay: association of antigenemia with symptomatic disease and T-helper cell depletion. *Ann Int Med* **107**:286–292, 1987.
44c. Spira TJ, Kaplan JL, Feorino PM, et al: Human immunodeficiency virus viremia as a prognostic indicator in homosexual men with lymphadenopathy syndrome. *N Engl J Med* **317**:1093–1094, 1987.

45. Ho DD, Sarngadharan MG, Resnick L, et al: Primary human T-lymphotropic virus type III infection. *Ann Intern Med* **103**:880–883, 1985.
46. Goedert JJ: Testing for human immunodeficiency virus. *Ann Intern Med* **105**:609–610, 1986.
47. Markham PD: Biological properties and isolation of HTLV-III. *Ann Intern Med* **102**:800–813, 1985.
48. Allain JP, Paul DA, Laurian Y, et al: Serological markers in early stages of human immunodeficiency virus infection in hemophiliacs. *Lancet* **2**:1233–1236, 1986.
49. Murray JF, Felton CP, Garay S, et al: Pulmonary complications of the acquired immunodeficiency syndrome: Report of the National Heart, Lung and Blood Institute workshop. *N Engl J Med* **310**:1681–1688, 1984.
50. Mills J: *Pneumocystis carinii* and *Toxoplasma gondii* infections in patients with AIDS. *Rev Infect Dis* **6**:1001–1011, 1986.
51. Catterall JR, Potasman I, Remington JS: *Pneumocystis carinii* pneumonia in the patient with AIDS. *Chest* **88**:758–762, 1985.
52. Ognibene FP, Shelhamer J, Gill V, et al: The diagnosis of *Pneumocystis carinii* pneumonia in patients with the acquired immunodeficiency syndrome using subsegmental bronchoalveolar lavage. *Am Rev Resp Dis* **129**:929–932, 1984.
53. Broaddus C, Dake MD, Stulbarg MS, et al: Bronchoalveolar lavage and transbronchial biopsy for the diagnosis of pulmonary infections in the acquired immunodeficiency syndrome. *Ann Intern Med* **102**:747–752, 1985.
54. Bigby T, Margolskee D, Curtis J, et al: The usefulness of induced sputum in the diagnosis of *Pneumocystis carinii* pneumonia in patients with the acquired immunodeficiency syndrome. *Am Rev Resp Dis* **133**:515–518, 1986.
55. Wharton JM, Coleman DL, Wofsy CB, et al: Trimethoprim-sulfamethoxazole or pentamidine for *Pneumocystis carinii* pneumonia in the acquired immunodeficiency syndrome: A prospective randomized trial. *Ann Intern Med* **105**:37–44, 1986.
56. Kovacs JA, Hiemenz JW, Macher AM, et al: *Pneumocystis carinii* pneumonia: A comparison between patients with the acquired immunodeficiency syndrome and patients with other immunodeficiencies. *Ann Intern Med* **100**:663–671, 1984.
57. Gordin FM, Simon GL, Wofsy CB, et al: Adverse reactions to trimethoprim-sulfamethoxasole in patients with the acquired immunodeficiency syndrome. *Ann Intern Med* **100**:495–499, 1984.
58. Leoung GS, Mills J, Hopewell PC, et al: Dapsone-trimethoprim for *Pneumocystis carinii* pneumonia in the acquired immunodeficiency syndrome. *Ann Intern Med* **105**:45–48, 1986.
59. Golden JA, Sjoerdsma A, Santi DV: *Pneumocystis carinii* pneumonia treated with difluoromethylornithine. *West J Med* **141**:613–623, 1984.
60. Haverkos HW: Assessment of therapy for *Pneumocystis carinii* pneumonia. *Am J Med* **76**:501–508, 1984.
61. Small CB, Harris CA, Friedland GH, et al: The treatment of *Pneumocystis carinii* pneumonia in the acquired immunodeficiency syndrome. *Arch Intern Med* **145**:837–840, 1985.
62. Steinbrook R, Lo B, Moulton J, et al: Preferences of homosexual men with AIDS for life-sustaining treatment. *N Engl J Med* **314**:457–460, 1986.
63. Hughes WT, Kuhn S, Chaudhary S, et al: Successful chemoprophylaxis for *Pneumocystis carinii* pneumonitis. *N Engl J Med* **297**:1419–1426, 1986.
64. Fischl MA, Dickinson MA: Fansidar prophylaxis of *Pneumocystis pneumonia* in the acquired immunodeficiency syndrome. *Ann Intern Med* **105**:629, 1986.

65. Ognibene FP, Steis RG, Macher AM: Kaposi's sarcoma causing pulmonary infiltrates and respiratory failure in the acquired immunodeficiency syndrome. *Ann Intern Med* **102**:471–475, 1985.
66. Levy RM, Bredesen DE, Rosenblum ML: Neurological manifestations of the acquired immunodeficiency syndrome (AIDS): Experience at UCSF and review of the literature. *J Neurosurg* **62**:475–495, 1985.
67. Shaw GM, Harper ME, Hahn BH, et al: HTLV III infection in brains of children and adults with AIDS encephalopathy. *Science* **227**:177–182, 1985.
68. Ho DD, Rota JR, Schooley RT: Isolation of HTLV-III from cerebrospinal fluid and neural tissues of patients with neurologic symptoms related to the acquired immunodeficiency syndrome. *N Engl J Med* **313**:1493–1497, 1985.
69. Resnick L, diMarzo-Veronese F, Schupbach J, et al: Intrablood-brain-barrier synthesis of HTLV-III specific IgG in patients with neurologic symptoms associated with AIDS or AIDS-related complex. *N Engl J Med* **313**:1498–1504, 1985.
70. Wong B, Gold JWM, Brown AE: Central-nervous-system toxoplasmosis in homosexual men and parenteral drug abusers. *Ann Intern Med* **100**:36–42, 1984.
71. Bursztyn EM, Lee BCP, Bauman J: CT of acquired immunodeficiency syndrome. Am J **5**:711–714, 1984.
72. Navia BA, Petito CK, Gold JWM, et al: Cerebral toxoplasmosis complicating the acquired immune deficiency syndrome: Clinical and neuropathological findings in 27 patients. *Ann Neurol* **19**:224–238, 1986.
73. Snider WD, Simpson DM, Nielsen S, et al: Neurological complications of acquired immunodeficiency syndrome: Analysis of 50 patients. *Ann Neurol* **14**:403–418, 1983.
74. Dworkin B, Wormser GP, Rosenthal WS, et al: Gastrointestinal manifestations of the acquired immunodeficiency syndrome: A review of 22 cases. *Am J Gastroenterol* **80**:774–778, 1985.
75. Payne P, Lancaster LA, Heinzmann M, et al: Identification of cryptosporidium in patients with the acquired immunodeficiency syndrome. *N Engl J Med* **309**:613–614, 1983.
76. Meiselman MS, Cello JP, Margaretten W: Cytomegalovirus colitis: Report of the clinical, endoscopic, and pathological findings in two patients with the acquired immune deficiency syndrome. *Gastroenterology* **88**:171–175, 1985.
77. Grant IH, Armstrong D: Management of infectious complications in acquired immunodeficiency syndrome. *Am J Med* **81** (Suppl 1A):59–72, 1986.
78. Vogt M, Hirsch MS: Prospects for the prevention and therapy of infections with the human immunodeficiency virus. *Rev Infect Dis* **8**:991–1000, 1986.
79. Yarchoan R, Klecker RW, Weinhold, et al: Administration of 3'-azido-3' deoxythymidine, an inhibitor of HTLV-III/LAV replication, to patients with AIDS or AIDS-related complex. *Lancet* **1**:575–580, 1986.
80. Azidothymidine for AIDS. *Med Lett* **28**:107–109, 1986.
81. Yarchoan R, Berg G, Brouwers P: Response of human-immunodeficiency-virus-associated neurological disease to 3'-azido-3' deoxythymidine. *Lancet* **1**:132–135, 1987.
82. Francis DP, Petriccipani JC: The prospects for and pathways toward a vaccine for AIDS. *N Engl J Med* **313**:1586–1590, 1985.
83. Hahn BH, Shaw GM, Taylor ME, et al: Genetic variation in HTLV-III/LAV over time in patients with AIDS or at risk for AIDS. *Science* **232**:1548–1553, 1986.
84. DeGruttola V, Mayer K, Bennett W: AIDS: Has the problem been adequately assessed? *Rev Infect Dis* **8**:295–305, 1986.

CHAPTER 22

# Cutaneous Manifestations of the Acquired Immunodeficiency Syndrome

Benjamin K. Fisher, Leonard C. Warner, and Anne G. Matlow

Numerous skin lesions and skin diseases are associated with the acquired immunodeficiency syndrome (AIDS), and it is expected that more lesions will be reported in the future [1,2]. We shall attempt to summarize the skin lesions reported in the literature to mid-year 1987. (Table 22.1) [2]. Some of these lesions may be the first sign of AIDS at any of its stages. It is important, therefore, that the family physician or consulting dermatologist be acquainted with them so that early diagnosis can be achieved.

The cutaneous manifestations of AIDS may be divided for convenience into three large categories:

1. Neoplastic.
2. Infectious.
3. Other.

A few neoplastic and infectious manifestations are practically unique to patients with AIDS, for example, Kaposi's sarcoma in a young homosexual male or oral hairy leukoplakia of the tongue. Other conditions, such as molluscum contagiosum, syphilis, scabies, psoriasis, and hair thinning, are not specific to AIDS but may present in atypical or exaggerated forms because of the underlying immunosuppression.

## Neoplastic Diseases

### Kaposi's Sarcoma

Kaposi's sarcoma is the most common neoplasm associated with AIDS. The origin of this tumor is unknown [3], although its cells are believed to derive either from the endothelium of the blood microvasculature [4] or from lymphatic vessels [5]. AIDS-associated Kaposi's sarcoma frequently disseminates to involve lymph nodes, liver, lung, and the gastrointestinal system [6], thus pursuing a rapidly fatal course.

Clinically, Kaposi's sarcoma in AIDS may look like a red, violaceous, bluish or brownish macule, papule, small plaque, or smooth raised tumor [3] (Fig. 22.1). The lesion may initially appear inconspicuous and benign and may easily be misdiag-

TABLE 22.1. Cutaneous manifestations associated with acquired immunodeficiency syndromes reported to 1987

*Neoplastic*
- Kaposi's sarcoma
- Lymphoma (B cell usually)
- Squamous cell carcinoma
- Basal cell carcinoma
- Melanoma

*Bacterial infections*
- Abscesses
- Folliculitis
- Impetigo
- Ecthyma
- Cellulitis
- Ulcers (*Pseudomonas* and polymicrobial)
- Mycobacterial infection
- Actinomycosis
- Atypical syphilis
- Scalded-skin syndrome

*Fungal and yeast infections*
- Candidosis
- Dermatophytosis
- Tinea versicolor
- Alterniosis
- Cryptococcosis
- Histoplasmosis
- Sporotrichosis
- Scopulariopsis

*Viral infections*
- Molluscum contagiosum infection
- Herpes simplex infection
- Herpes zoster infection
- Chickenpox
- Epstein-Barr virus exanthemata
- Oral hairy leukoplakia
- Condylomata acuminata

*Protozoal infections*
- *Amoebiasis cutis*

*Arthropod infections*
- Scabies
- Crusted scabies

*Mixed infections*
- Viral, bacterial, and fungal

*Vascular lesions*
- Vasculitis
- Thrombocytopenic purpura
- Telangiecasia
- Splinter hemorrhages
- Hyperalgesic pseudothrombophlebitis syndrome
- Cutis marmorata

*Papulosquamous disorders*
- Seborrheic dermatitis
- Psoriasis
- Pityriasis rosea

*Oral*
- Angular stomatitis
- Aphthosis
- Gingivitis (simple and necrotizing)

*Miscellaneous*
- Xerosis and ichtyosis
- Nutritional deficiencies
- Eosinophilic pustular folliculitis
- Exanthemata and erythroderma
- Papular and lichenoid eruptions (some with atypical infiltrate)
- Atopic dermatitis
- Pseudolymphoma cutis
- Granuloma annulare
- Pyoderma gangrenosum
- Premature aging of skin
- Bullous pemphigoid
- Erythema elevatum diutinum
- Transient acantholytic dermatosis (Grover's disease)
- Drug reactions
- Urticaria and pruritus

*Hair and nails changes*
- Alopecia areata
- Thinning of hair
- Premature graying
- Telogen effluvium
- Nail deformities
- Nail color changes

*Exaggeration of:*
- Infections (e.g., syphilis)
- Infestations (e.g., scabies)
- Dermatoses (e.g., psoriasis)

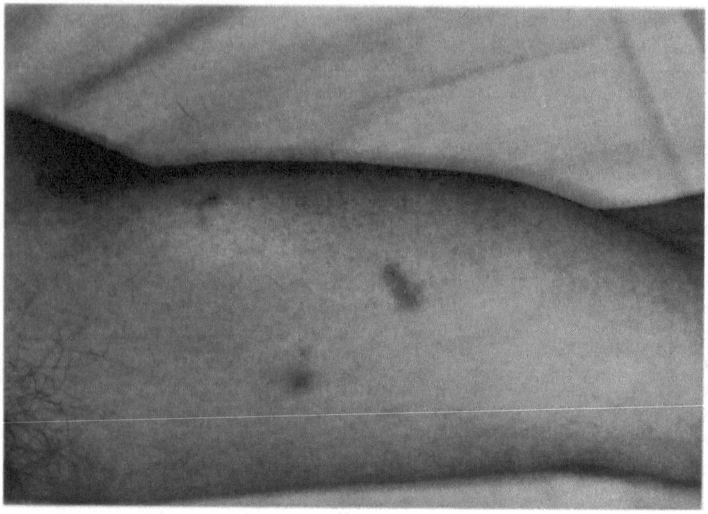

FIGURE 22.1. Kaposi's sarcoma in AIDS. These early lesions consist of red and violaceous macules, papules, and patches. Notice linear borders of the largest lesion.

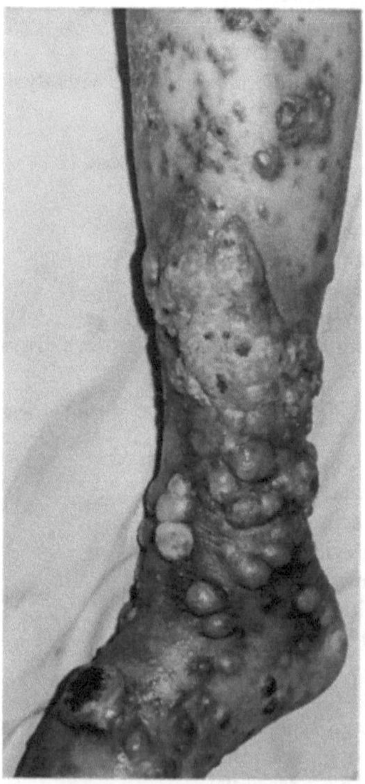

FIGURE 22.2. Kaposi's sarcoma in AIDS. Late lesions on the lower extremity consist of numerous nodules and tumors. This patient was preterminal.

nosed as a small hemangioma, pyogenic granuloma, dermatofibroma, flat nevus, malignant melanoma, molluscum contagiosum, bruise, or patch of lichen planus [7,8]. Early lesions are frequently bright red or purplish in color, while late lesions assume a violaceous or brownish hue. Lesions frequently have linear borders (Fig. 22.1). Older lesions may become large and ulcerated (Fig. 22.2).

The lesions may appear anywhere on the skin including palms, soles, body folds, ears, scalp, and mucosal surfaces, particularly on the hard palate. Usually the lesions progress to purpuric plaques and nodules, which tend to follow the tension lines of the skin. Any red or hyperpigmented macule, papule, patch, or plaque in an individual who might have been exposed to the AIDS virus should be considered as Kaposi's sarcoma and biopsied [1]. The clinical presentation of Kaposi's sarcoma may be very atypical, and therefore a high index of suspicion is necessary. Kaposi's sarcoma may even mimic chronic paronychia [9]. Even in the absence of cutaneous involvement, Kaposi's sarcoma may involve lymph nodes, lungs, and the gastrointestinal tract. A recent review of postmortem findings found no correlation between the degree of cutaneous involvement and visceral involvement [10].

Treatment of Kaposi's sarcoma is unsatisfactory. Small solitary lesions may be left untreated [5]. Superficial lesions may be treated with radiotherapy or excision. Intralesional treatment with high concentration of vinblastine or bleomycin has been used. Single-agent and combination chemotherapy occasionally induces remissions, as do electron beam therapy and alpha interferon [8]. Unfortunately, chemotherapeutic agents aggravate the patient's already profound immunosuppression [11]. Most AIDS patients with Kaposi's sarcoma die of opportunistic infections [11].

## Lymphomas

Several types of lymphoma may develop in AIDS patients. Both Hodgkin's [12] and more commonly non-Hodgkin's B cell lymphoma [13,14] may involve the skin. The lesions may present as nodules or papules.

## Squamous and Basal Cell Carcinomas

Oral [15] and anorectal [16] squamous cell carcinomas have been reported in AIDS patients. Basal cell carcinoma has been reported in such patients on several occasions [17,18]. At this time it is not certain whether the incidence of basal cell carcinomas is increased in AIDS. Basal cell carcinoma generally metastasizes only very rarely. When this happens patients often show a defect in their cell-mediated immunity [19]. There has been a recent report of a metastatic basal cell carcinoma in a patient with AIDS-related complex (ARC) [20]. Therefore, any basal cell carcinoma in a human immunodeficiency virus (HIV)-infected individual should be completely excised without delay.

### Malignant Melanoma

There is a report of rapid growth of an invasive malignant melanoma in a patient with AIDS and Hodgkin's lymphoma [21]. Another patient infected with HIV developed a malignant melanoma [22]. At present it is impossible to say whether there is an increased incidence of melanoma in patients with AIDS.

## Infections

### Bacterial Infections

Bacterial infections are commonly seen in AIDS patients [22]. Both staphylococcal and streptococcal cutaneous infections occur. Ecthymatous lesions caused by *Staphylococcus aureus* have been observed [22]. Other staphylococcal skin infections reported are cellulitis, abscesses, pyomyositis, impetigo, and folliculitus [22,23]. Sterile folliculitis also occurs [7]. In this culture-negative folliculitis, skin scrapings often are positive for *Pityrosporum orbiculare* [8]. These lesions may be intensely pruritic. Treatment includes topical corticosteroids and antifungals as well as antihistamines [8].

Staphylococcal scalded-skin syndrome clinically, similar to toxic epidermal necrolysis, is caused by group 2, phage type 71 *Staph. aureus*. There is a report [24] of a homosexual man who developed staphylococcal scalded-skin syndrome associated with a *Staph. aureus* septicemia. The patient had polyadenopathy and an immunologic profile consistent with ARC. The patient's HIV status was unfortunately not reported.

The following bacterial infections have been described in HIV-infected individuals [22]: severe cellulitis of the soft tissue of the neck secondary to *Hemophilus influenzae*, an abscess secondary to *Rhodococcus equi*, polymicrobial ulceration of the entire rectal area secondary to cryptosporidial diarrhea, and *Pseudomonas* skin ulcers. There is a report of a bisexual man with HIV infection who developed right facial and parotid swelling, pain, and trismus after extraction of a right maxillary molar tooth. Fluid aspirated from a fluctuant mass in the right parotid region grew *Actinomyces israelii*. The patient responded well to oral penicillin [25].

Syphilis is common in HIV-infected patients, especially homosexuals [22]. The clinical presentation of secondary syphilis may be atypical. Generalized papulosquamous lesions, hyperpigmented macules in the axillae, and scaling hyperpigmented macules of the palms have all been reported as manifestations of secondary syphilis in AIDS patients. The skin lesions disappeared with penicillin therapy [22].

A serious problem that has emerged recently is the apparent failure of benzathine penicillin given in the usual doses for treatment of early syphilis in a small number of AIDS cases. This has been followed by confirmed neurosyphilis within a few months.

The question arises whether syphilis should be treated differently in AIDS patients, that is, in which cases early syphilis should be treated like neurosyphilis.

It is obvious, however, that syphilis in HIV-infected individuals must be monitored carefully to prevent the irreversible damage that neurosyphilis may inflict [26–28].

## Myobacterial Infections

Disseminated tuberculosis has been frequently described in patients with AIDS, especially Haitians [29,30]. Both typical and atypical mycobacteria have been isolated. Scrofuloderma has been reported in AIDS [31]. One patient with systemic *Mycobacterium avium*-intracellulare infection had ill-defined macular, discolored lesions on the forearms [32]. Biopsy demonstrated numerous acid-fast organisms within histiocytes, a typical finding in *M. avium*-intracellulare infection. Another patient who had a *M. marinum* skin infection presented with ecthymatous lesions [22].

## Fungal Infections

### Candidosis

Oral candidisis may be the initial manifestation of AIDS [33]. It is relatively uncommon in previously healthy persons who have not been treated with antibiotics or corticosteroids. One prospective study showed that the presence of unexplained oral candidisis in patients at high risk for AIDS predicted the development of serious opportunistic infections more than 50% of the time [33].

Clinically, the presence of white patches in the oral mucosa is characteristic. There may be only tiny dotlike white lesions on the tongue or uvula, several white patches may occur anywhere in the oral mucosa, or the entire oral mucosa may be covered with white patches with a cheesy exudate over an inflamed mucosa [33]. White patches may be seen in the pharynx (Fig. 22.3). KOH-treated scrapings always show pseudohyphae and budding yeast when examined microscopically. The infection may progress and cause painful esophagitis [34]; small-bowel, large-bowel, and anal candidisis [6]; and occasionally brain and liver abscesses [34]. Topical therapy with nystatin (mouthwash or tablets held in the mouth to dissolve) or clotrimazole tablets used similarly is effective in controlling most lesions [34]. Refractory cases should be treated systemically with ketoconazole, which is also the drug of choice for esophagitis in AIDS [34]. Candidal nail dystrophies are quite common and frequently resistant to topical and systemic antifungals [22].

### Superficial Fungal Infections

Tinea cruris, tinea pedis, and tinea versicolor occur frequently in AIDS patients [7] (Fig. 22.4). Tinea versicolor may occur both early and late in HIV infections [22,35]. The lesions may be widespread and may show areas of thickened skin. The condition is often refractory to selenium sulfide, miconazole, or clotrimazole. Systemic ketoconazole is useful, but relapses occur [22]. Superficial fungal infections may present in atypical clinical patterns. Tinea faciale may mimic erythema mul-

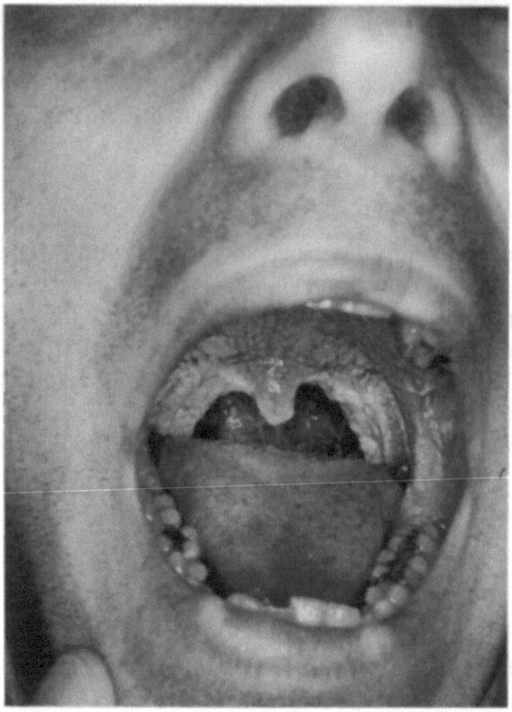

FIGURE 22.3. Widespread oral candidiasis in AIDS. The oral mucosa and pharynx show white patches.

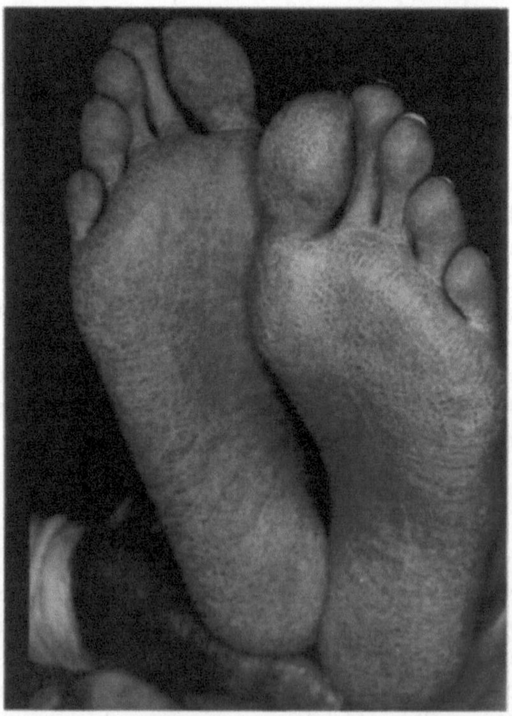

FIGURE 22.4. Tinea pedis in AIDS. Entire soles show diffuse scaling.

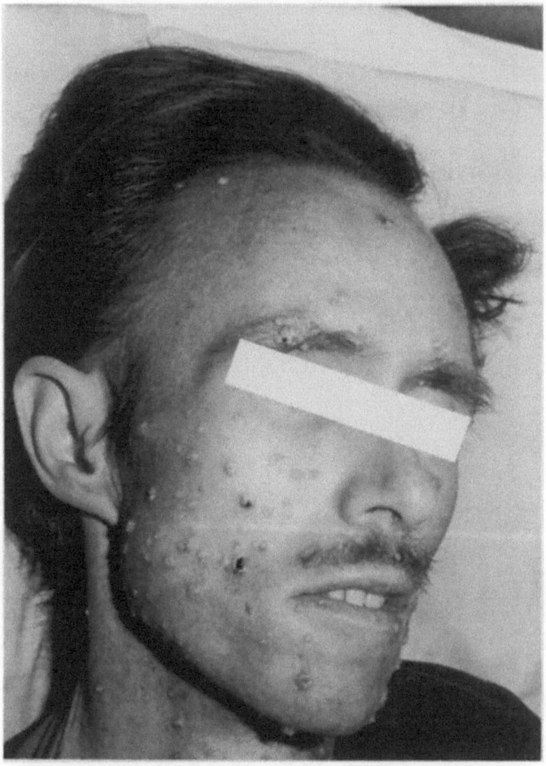

FIGURE 22.5. Molluscum contagiosum in moribund AIDS patient. Numerous umbilicated small and large papules are seen on the face and neck.

tiforme [32] or seborrheic dermatitis [36]. Tinea of the neck may present as flat-topped papules [33]. *Tricophyton rubrum* infection may present as keratoderma blenorrhagica or palmoplantar keratoderma [22]. Onychomycoses may occur frequently, independently or in association with palmoplantar hyperkeratosis. *Trich. rubrum* is the most commonly isolated organism. The paronychium is frequently involved [22]. Proximal white subungual onychomycosis has been described in a patient with AIDS [37].

## Cryptococcosis

Disseminated cryptococcosis has been reported as presenting with herpetiform lesions or as an ulcer in homosexual men with AIDS [38,39]. Cryptococcal lesions may resemble those of molluscum contagiosum [40]. Once a diagnosis of cutaneous cryptococcosis has been made, a thorough investigation for systemic involvement should be carried out including the appropriate studies of cerebrospinal fluid, serum, urine, sputum, and prostatic secretions. Thus, a systemic and life-threatening infection may be discovered and treated rapidly with the indicated antibiotics [38].

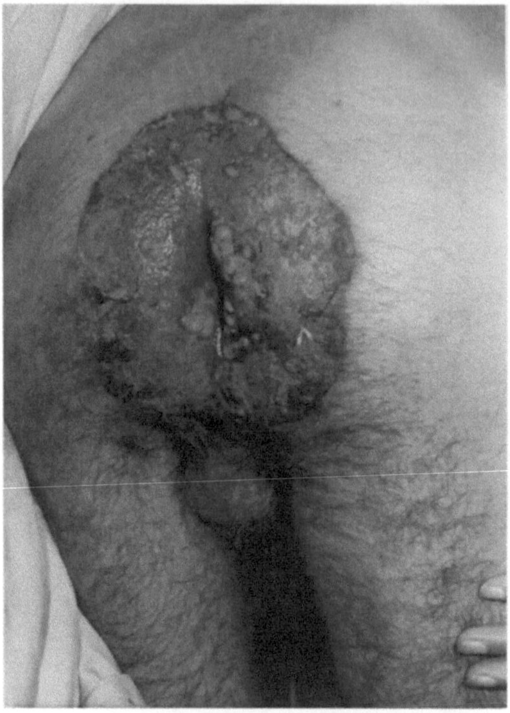

a

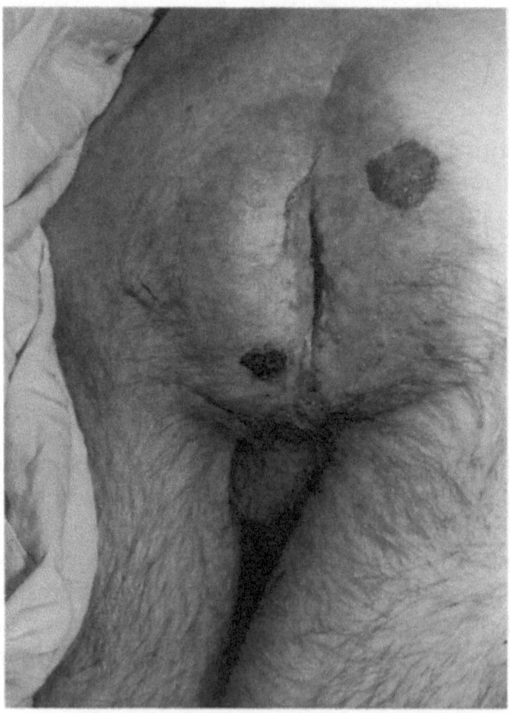

b

FIGURE 22.6. Herpes simplex in AIDS. (a) Non-healing painful large perianal ulcer. Viral cultures were negative. (b) Almost complete healing after 3 weeks of systemic acyclovir therapy. The two erosions on the periphery are traumatic.

### Histoplasmosis

Disseminated histoplasmosis is not unusual in AIDS patients [41–43]. The skin manifestations of histoplasmosis are very nonspecific. They may resemble molluscum contagiosum [44], may present with papules having a central keratotic plug [45], or may present a picture of folliculitis, pustules, and perianal ulcers [46]. One case presented as a maculopapular exanthema with slight scaling [42].

### Sporotrichosis

Systemic sporotrichosis has been described in patients with HIV infection [47,48]. In contrast to typical lymphocutaneous sporotrichosis, a history of exposure to soil or plants is uncommon. The portal of entry of the organism is presumed to be the lungs, with secondary hematogenous dissemination. The disease begins with the insidious onset of fatigue, weight loss, and low-grade fever. The skin lesions are widespread enlarging red papules and nodules that ulcerate with the formation of crusted necrotic centers. Chronic erosive arthritis and osteomyelitis are common [47]. Lungs, lymph nodes, and meninges may become involved. The diagnosis is established by skin biopsy and cultures. Numerous organisms are seen in skin biopsy, in contrast to the finding of hardly any in biopsies from non-AIDS patients. Potassium iodide treatment is not effective in AIDS-associated disseminated sporotrichosis. Amphotericin B seems to be the treatment of choice [48].

### Scopulariopsis

Scopulariopsis infection has been seen in a patient who subsequently developed AIDS. The lesions consisted of patchy alopecia with fungal elements present at the base of the hair [22].

## Viral Infections

### Molluscum Contagiosum

Molluscum contagiosum, a poxvirus, commonly infects children and adults. In children lesions may occur anywhere, and face lesions are common. In healthy adults the anogenital area and trunk are commonly affected [49,50]. Lesions consist typically of shiny, waxy, and umbilicated papules [49–52]. In patients with AIDS, molluscum contagiosum often appears as facial papules. Over a period of several months the papules increase both in number and size and spread to the scalp, forehead, and nose (Fig. 22.5). Treatment is most frustrating in AIDS cases and recurrences are common, regardless of the type of treatment used [22].

### Herpes Simplex

There is an increased incidence of herpes simplex infections in patients with AIDS [53,54]. The lesions may present as severe chronic perianal ulcerations with circinate borders. Nonhealing ulcers in the perianal area in a homosexual man must be

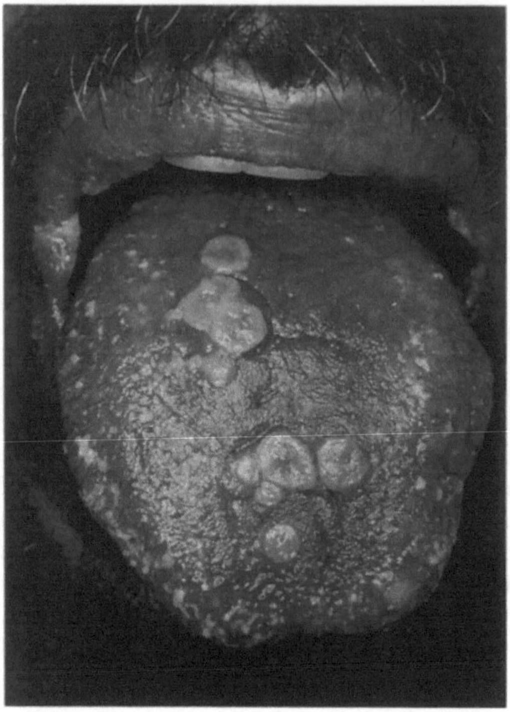

FIGURE 22.7. Herpes simplex on the dorsum of the tongue in AIDS. Lesions are painful yellowish flat papules with central depression. This picture is also seen in primary herpes in healthy adults. Notice blisters in the angles of the mouth and pinpoint white candidal lesions on the tongue.

thought to be caused by herpes simplex until proven otherwise, even if biopsies, smears, and cultures are negative (Fig. 22.6). Herpes proctitis, an excruciatingly painful condition, may show only slight edema and redness in the perianal area. A careful examination may at times show small herpes vesicles. Both conditions respond rapidly to intravenous acyclovir treatment [2]. In AIDS patients herpes simplex infection may assume a variety of clinical patterns: vesicular eruption of the hands, chronic "leg ulcers" [32], or a varicelliform eruption [22]. Oral recurrences commonly result in nonhealing erosions and scabs about the mouth rather than the classic vesicles on an erythematous base [1,22]. Lesions on the tongue may show depressed whitish tender papules (Fig. 22.7). Scabby nonhealing lesions may be confused with impetigo. In addition to nasolabial herpes [55], digital lesions may be seen [29]. Digital lesions may present as ulcers [2]. The esophagus and tracheobronchial mucosa may be infected with the virus [56], which may also infect the spinal cord [53]. Continuous oral acyclovir may be necessary to control recurrent mucocutaneous herpes infections [1].

## Herpes Zoster and Chickenpox

Primary chickenpox can be very severe in the HIV-infected individual [22]. Patients may require intravenous acyclovir and intravenous gamma globulin. There is a report of a child with AIDS who developed primary chickenpox, which was rapidly

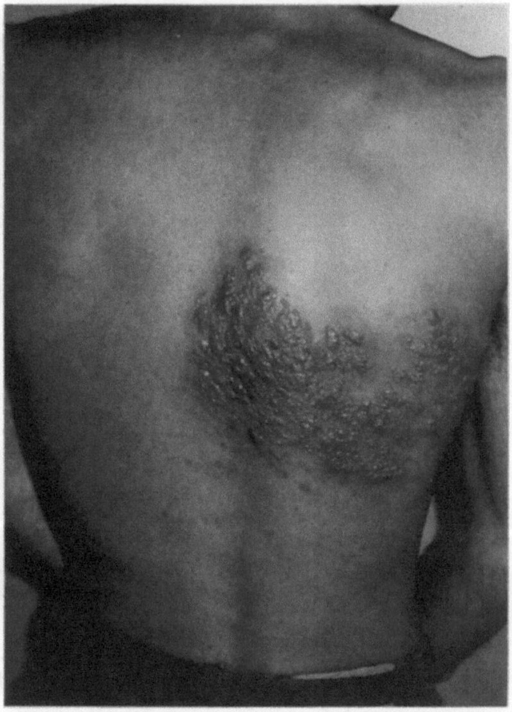

FIGURE 22.8. Herpes zoster in a 23-year-old previously healthy male homosexual. There was severe involvement of dermatomes, $T_4$ and $T_5$. A test for HIV antibodies was positive.

followed by herpes zoster infection [22]. Another child had chickenpox complicated by varicella pneumonia.

The appearance of herpes zoster in a young homosexual man is very suggestive of immunologic compromise that could ultimately evolve into AIDS [57] (Fig. 22.8). HIV antibody testing should be carried out in all these cases. Herpes zoster in AIDS is usually localized to the involved dermatome but disseminated lesions do occur [58]. Frequently, two or three adjacent dermatomes may be involved. The eruption may be quite severe with many necrotic lesions.

## Epstein-Barr Virus

An HIV-infected individual developed primary infectious mononucleosis. Extensive macular rash was present on his chest and extremities [22].

## Oral Hairy Leukoplakia

Oral hairy leukoplakia (oral viral leukoplakia) was first described in 1984 by Greenspan et al [59,60]. These lesions seem to be unique to HIV-infected individuals. They consist of abnormal white thickening anywhere in the oral mucosa but most commonly on one or both lateral margins of the tongue (Fig. 22.9). The lesions are slightly raised and poorly demarcated with a corrugated or "hairy" surface. They

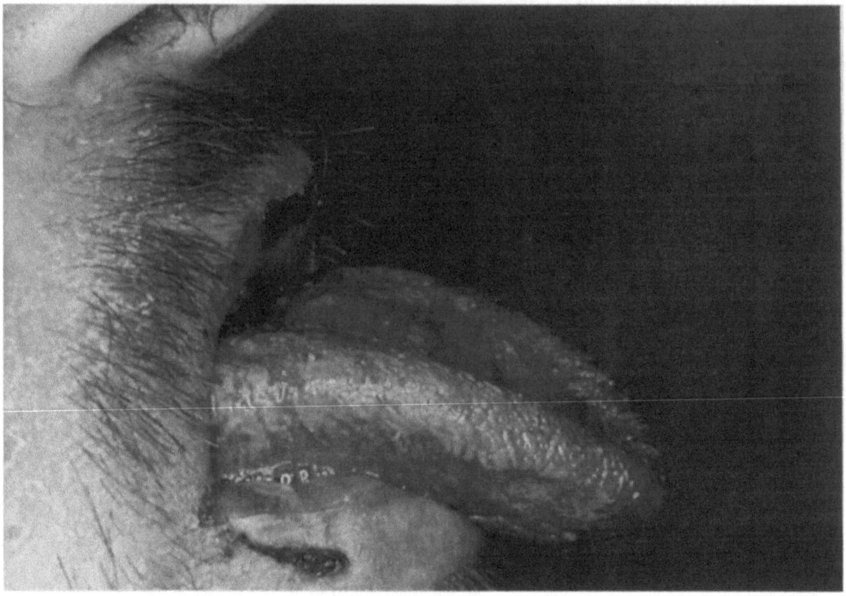

FIGURE 22.9. Oral hairy leukoplakia. White, linear, corrugated patches are seen along the lateral border of the tongue. Whitish lesions extend to dorsal and ventral surfaces of the tongue.

measure from a few millimeters to 3 cm. They are usually asymptomatic but sometimes may be sore. Histologically the epithelium shows acanthosis, parakeratosis, and fine keratotic projections resembling hair. In the upper stratum malpighi there are "balloon cells" with pyknotic nuclei similar to koilocytes seen in cervical condylomata [61]. Oral hairy leukoplakia is believed to be caused by the symbiotic action of two viruses, which have been identified by electron microscopy as the Epstein-Barr virus and a papilloma virus. Candidal organisms are frequently present in lesions of oral hairy leukoplakia [61]. Conant [62] has reported that topical tretinoin (Retin-A) solution is effective for this condition, but repeated treatments are necessary for recurrences. Greenspan [63] found that descyclovir by mouth can eliminate or reduce the size of these oral lesions. In our experience, a 100-mg tablet of clotrimazole sucked once a day over a period of several days caused the reduction or elimination of oral hairy leukoplakia [2]. It is likely, therefore, that *Candida* contributes to the development of these lesions in synergy with the two viruses mentioned above.

## Common Warts and Condylomata Acuminata

Common warts occur frequently in HIV-infected individuals, often on the face, hands, and feet. Recurrences after treatment are common [22]. Homosexuals with AIDS are prone to develop large perianal condylomata acuminata [64]. These lesions may be difficult to treat and may require surgical or laser treatment.

### Protozoal Infections

Amebiasis cutis has been described in a homosexual man with disseminated acanthamoeba castellani infection. A nonspecific papule was present on the thigh. Biopsy showed amebic trophozoites within an inflammatory infiltrate.

### Arthropodal Infestations

#### Scabies

Scabies has been reported in HIV-infected patients [22,65]. Pruritic generalized papulosquamous lesions appeared beyond the characteristically affected body areas in this disease. The face and scalp may be involved. The diagnosis was often missed initially. Patients responded to topical application of gamma-benzene-hexachloride [22].

Crusted (Norwegian) scabies is an uncommon and unusual form of scabies. It usually occurs in people with immunologic suppression or neurologic impairment. Hundreds to thousands of adult *Sarcoptes scabiei* infest the body. Clinically, this highly contagious disease is characterized by hyperkeratotic scaly plaques. Lesions may be generalized but usually are prominent on the neck, scalp, and trunk. Norwegian scabies has been seen in several AIDS patients [66]. We found that post-scabies dermatitis after successful treatment of scabies may be a problem in AIDS patients. Severe itching and dermatitic patches may last for months with no evidence of mites. Treatment may be difficult and frustrating [2].

### Mixed Infections

Viral, bacterial, and fungal organisms may coexist in the same lesion in AIDS patients [67–69]. Lesions may present as necrotic ulcers [67], lesions mimicking molluscum contagiosum [68], or keratotic vegetating plaques [69]. The profound immunosuppression in AIDS evidently may create a situation where different pathogens interact to create new and unfamiliar clinical entities.

## Vascular Lesions

### Vasculitis

Several AIDS patients have developed purpura secondary to biopsy-proven leukocytoclastic vasculitis. Indirect immunofluorescence using a high-titer anti-HIV serum against frozen postmortem tissue showed bright fluorescence in the vessels in one patient [7].

### Thrombocytopenic Purpura

Patients with AIDS are prone to develop petechiae secondary to idiopathic thrombocytopenic purpura (ITP). This form of ITP is clinically indistinguishable from

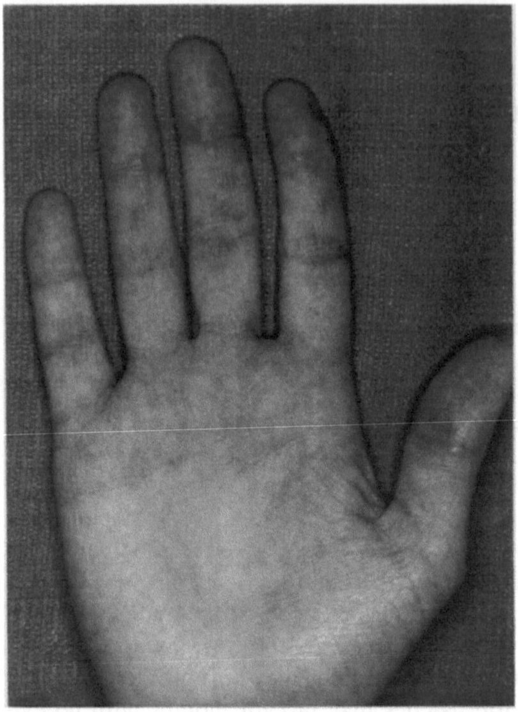

FIGURE 22.10. Telangiectasia in AIDS. Several telangiectatic patches are seen on the volar aspect of all fingers. Although the patches are clinically suggestive of vasculitis, biopsy showed enlarged capillaries with perivascular lymphocytic infiltrate.

classic ITP [70]. Cytomegalovirus is also capable of causing thromobocytopenic purpura as well as maculopapular rashes [32]. It is presumed that, in patients with ITP, immune complexes coat platelets and are subsequently consumed by phagocytic cells, leading to thrombocytopenia [70].

## Telangiectasia

Telangiectasia is associated with the complete spectrum of HIV disease [71]. Telangiectases characteristically appear across the chest in a crescent-shaped distribution from shoulder to shoulder with extension above the clavicles. Lesions may also appear on the ears, palms, and fingers [1,22] (Fig. 22.10). The telangiectases are often associated with a mild diffuse erythema in the same distribution. Biopsy shows dilated blood vessels and small-cell perivascular infiltrates [71].

## Hyperalgesic Pseudothrombophlebitis Syndrome

Several AIDS patients with Kaposi's sarcoma have developed swelling of a lower extremity associated with erythematous and exquisitely tender overlying skin [72]. Most of the patients had fever greater than 39.5°C and tender, erythematous cords overlying superficial veins of the affected extremity. Deep-vein thrombosis was ruled out by venography. This syndrome was thought to be of unknown etiology. However, recently two patients with a clinical picture consistent with hyperalgesic pseudothrombophlebitis syndrome were found to have Kaposi's sarcoma in the lymph nodes adjacent to phlebitic veins in the leg [22]. Possibly this syndrome is just a complication of Kaposi's sarcoma with secondary phlebitis.

### Cutis Marmorata

Several pediatric patients with AIDS have been reported with a generalized reticulate pattern of the skin resembling cutis marmorata [73].

## Papulosquamous Disorders

### Seborrheic Dermatitis

Seborrheic dermatitis is a common papulosquamous disorder that potentially may involve any or all of the following areas: scalp, face, axillae, chest, groin, and genitals. It usually presents as a moderate scaling of the scalp and eyebrows with a scaling erythema in the ears and in the perinasal and infraorbital areas. The lesions may vary from a dry, flaky, branny desquamation to a greasy, yellowish-red patch with indistinct borders. Eisenstat and Wormser [74] found a 46% prevalence of seborrheic dermatitis in AIDS patients, versus a 5% incidence in non-AIDS patients.

In AIDS, seborrheic dermatitis often presents acutely and severely. The center of the face is very commonly involved (Fig. 22.11). Lesions on the face may be confused with a lupus erythematosus rash [74].

A recent clinicopathologic study compared patients with seborrheic dermatitis associated with AIDS and patients with seborrheic dermatitis who had neither AIDS nor its risk factors [75]. It was found that the seborrheic-like dermatitis associated with AIDS differed from classic seborrheic dermatitis in the greater severity of the former, its occurrence in younger populations, and the involvement of areas such as the trunk and extremities, not typically involved in seborrheic dermatitis. Histologically, AIDS-associated seborrheiclike dermatitis was distinct because microscopic lesions showed spotty keratinocytic necrosis, leukoexocytosis, a perivascular infiltrate of plasma cells in the dermis, a few neutrophils with focal leukocytoclasis, and hyperkeratosis in long-standing lesions [75].

Seborrheic dermatitis has been reported up to 2 years before the onset of AIDS [74] and may be the initial manifestation [10]. The severity of the seborrheic dermatitis may have prognostic significance [76].

It has been suggested that the yeast *Pityrosporum ovale* is important in the etiology of seborrheic dermatitis [77]. This theory is supported by the finding that seborrheic dermatitis responds to oral and topical ketoconazole [78,79].

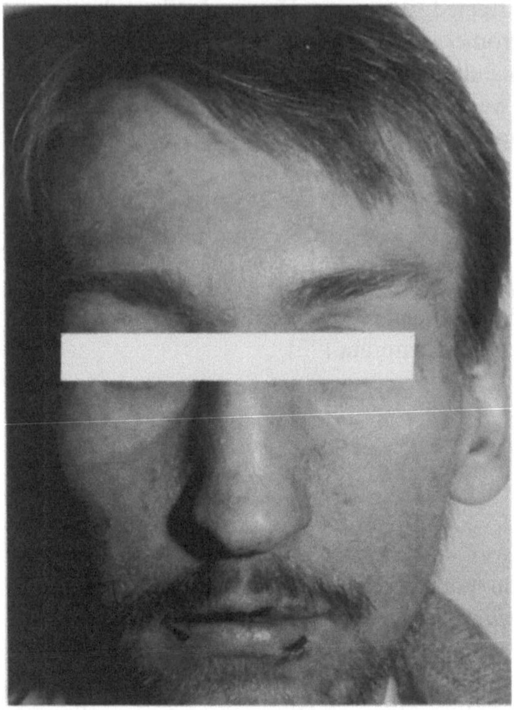

FIGURE 22.11. Seborrheic dermatitis in AIDS. Erythema and scaling on face, chin, eyebrows, and hairline. Notice crusts of herpes simplex on both lips.

## Psoriasis

There are reports of patients who developed AIDS and psoriasis simultaneously. Other patients with a history of mild psoriasis for years suddenly developed extensive erythrodermic psoriasis in the same month in which they were diagnosed as having AIDS [80].

AIDS-associated psoriasis is often atypical in distribution [81]. Prominent involvement of the groin, axilla, and scalp may occur. The lesions may be guttate or pustular. Reiter's syndrome consisting of the triad of urethritis, conjunctivitis, and arthritis may develop together with the onset of new psoriasis or the exacerbation of preexisting psoriasis. Keratotic papules and pustules may arise on the palms and soles (keratoderma blennorhagicum). Circinate balanitis may develop on the penis. Onychodystrophy of the nails with paronychia occurs. This severe form of psoriasis is often resistent to treatment. Methotrexate, which is often used in cases of severe psoriasis, is contraindicated in AIDS patients: It may cause leukopenia, encephalopathy, infection, and death. Ultraviolet light therapy is also immunosuppressive and has been associated with exacerbation of or appearance of new Kaposi's sarcoma lesions.

Some AIDS patients with psoriasis have responded to etretinate. Unfortunately, side effects from this drug such as arthralgias, headaches, and liver function abnormalities are difficult to distinguish from manifestations of ARC and AIDS [81].

Psoriasis may be the first manifestation of HIV infection and in general suggests a poor prognosis [81]. The development of explosive psoriasis or a sudden flare of preexisting psoriasis in potential AIDS candidates should raise the possibility of underlying HIV infection. Testing for HIV should be done prior to initiation of antipsoriatic immunosuppressive therapy.

Interestingly, AIDS patients may have improvement or resolution of severe psoriasis and seborrheic dermatitis as their overall clinical course deteriorates and their immune system fails altogether [81,82]. It seems, therefore, that the existence of psoriasis requires that at least part of the immune system be functional, albeit defectively.

### Pityriasis Rosea

There is a recent report of a pityriasis rosea-like eruption in an AIDS patient that persisted for 12 months until the patient died. The histology was consistent with pityriasis rosea [22].

## Oral Disorders

### Aphthosis and Gingivitis

Gingivitis is almost universal in ARC or AIDS patients; it responds well to penicillin or metronidazole [8]. Tooth extraction is often required. Recently in San Francisco, an acute necrotizing ulcerative gingivitis-like lesion has been described characterized by rapid loss of periodontal bone attachment [82]. No associated organism was isolated. Very severe aphthous ulceration occurs in a minority of patients with AIDS or ARC [8].

### Angular Cheilitis (Perlèche)

Angular cheilitis is common in patients with HIV disease [7]. It is usually associated with oral candidisis [8]. Angular cheilitis responds well to local application of antifungal/hydrocortisone combination creams [8].

## Miscellaneous Disorders

### Ichthyosis, Xerosis, and Erythroderma

Erythroderma [22], xerosis [7], asteatolic eczema [7] of the lower legs, and acquired ichthyosis have been described in AIDS patients [7,22]. It is interesting to note that acquired ichthyosis is known to occur in Hodgkin's lymphoma, lepromatous leprosy, and sarcoidosis, all conditions with immune deficiencies. Kaplan et al [22] noted a frequent association of erythroderma, xerosis, and seborrheic dermatitis with the development of dementia and spinal cord disease in AIDS patients.

## Nutritional Deficiencies

Nutritional disease is common in children with AIDS. In one child, verrucous hyperpigmented lesions appeared on the legs. A skin biopsy specimen showed changes consistent with pellagra, zinc deficiency, or acquired acrodermatitis enteropathica. A second child developed a follicular petechial eruption on the legs and bleeding of the gums, a clinical picture compatible with scurvy [32].

One pediatric AIDS patient with dermatitis was found to be zinc deficient. The dermatitis improved with oral zinc therapy [83].

## Eosinophilic Pustular Folliculitis

Eosinophilic pustular folliculitis (Ofusi's disease) is a rare dermatosis that is characterized by a pruritic eruption, typically affecting the face, trunk, and proximal extremities [84]. The lesions are follicular pustules or erythematous papules which become confluent to form indurated plaques with occasional central healing and pustular margins.

Eosinophilic pustular folliculitis has been described in AIDS and ARC patients [84]. Two patients had *Demodex folliculorum* mite on skin biopsy and a third patient had a dermatophyte. Soeprono and Schinella [84] believe that this skin disease may represent a form of hypersensitivity of the skin to *D. folliculorum* and dermatophytes. One AIDS patient with Kaposi's sarcoma developed eosinophilic folliculitis that improved with trimethoprim-sulfamethoxazole treatment [85].

## Acute Exanthemata

An exanthem associated with acute HIV disease often may occur 1 to several weeks after viral exposure [86]. This exanthem is extremely important to recognize because it may allow diagnosis of possible HIV infection several weeks prior to seroconversion. The rash presents as an asymptomatic, fine, symmetrical, erythematous morbilliform eruption involving mainly the trunk and arms. The exanthem is transient, lasting from 3 days to several weeks. It may be associated with exanthemata in the oral cavity. Besides the exanthem, the patient may present with an acute febrile illness, malaise, sore throat, lymphadenopathy, abdominal pain, splenomegaly, and diarrhea [86,87]. The clinical syndrome may mimic infectious mononucleosis. Associated abnormalities include a transient decrease in T helper to T suppressor cell ratio, leukopenia, and thrombocytopenia [86].

When rhesus monkeys were infected with an HIV-like virus (STLV-III, simian T lymphotropic virus type III), between 1 and 3 weeks after inoculation 83% of the monkeys developed a transient cutaneous macular eruption of the face, groin, and trunk [88]. Histologically the affected skin was characterized by a superficial perivascular infiltrate of mononuclear cells with associated endothelial cell hypertrophy and degeneration. The histologic picture was remarkably similar to that found in AIDS or ARC patients with exanthematous rash or papular eruptions [89]. Interestingly, the rash was most severe and persistent in animals given the highest viral dose, which is suggestive of a dose-dependent phenomenon [88].

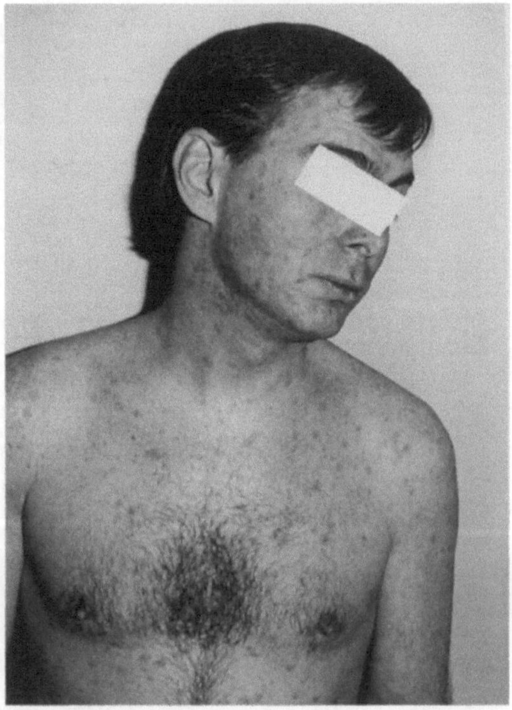

FIGURE 22.12. Exanthemata seen in early HIV infection. Lesions are discrete red macules and small patches which greatly resemble those of secondary syphilis or pityriasis rosea. This rash, which usually precedes seroconversion, disappears on its own within 1 to 3 weeks.

Because of the very strong similarity of the exanthemata in acute HIV infection and that seen in ARC and AIDS, as well as the similar histologic picture, we believe that these rashes are essentially the same. Patients with an acute HIV rash have blood abnormalities (leukopenia, thrombocytopenia, decreased T cell helper-to-suppressor ratio) similar to that seen in more advanced HIV infection. These initial blood abnormalities correct themselves as the exanthem disappears. When the immunosuppression becomes permanent, the exanthem may similarly become long lasting.

Another exanthem that occurs in acute HIV infection is associated with severe dysphagia and esophageal and oral ulcerations [87]. The eruption consists of fairly discrete erythematous and hemorrhagic lesions 2 to 3 cm in diameter resembling lesions of pityriasis rosea or secondary syphilis (Figs. 22.12 and 22.13). There may be a background of fine erythema. The eruption lasts a few days to 3 weeks and the esophageal ulcers and dysphagia may persist for up to 2 weeks. The oral ulcers are sharply demarcated and are found on the tongue or buccal mucosa [87].

## Papular Eruption

A clinically characteristic, chronic papular eruption has been described in patients with HIV disease. The lesions, which are often pruritic, appear as a few to hundreds of 2- to 5-mm skin-colored or reddish noncoalescing papules on the head, neck, upper trunk, and extremities.

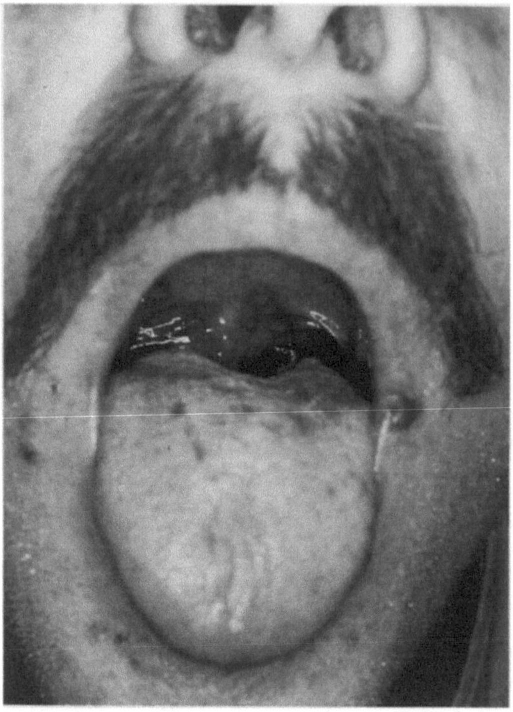

FIGURE 22.13. Another example of exanthema seen in early HIV infection. In addition to having discrete macular lesions on face and chin, this patient has small ulcers on the palate and has left angular stomatitis.

Histology shows a chronic, perivascular infiltrate of mononuclear cells with hyperchromatic nuclei in a lymphoeosinophilic perivascular infiltrate. Bizarre multinucleated cells in the dermis have also been described in these lesions [1,90].

We have recently seen lesions of various morphology (plaque, scab, vesicle) in a patient with AIDS. The histology in all lesions showed a pseudolymphomatous picture [2].

Patients with HIV disease have a deficiency in T helper cells as well as a decrease in Ia-positive Langerhans cells in the skin [91]. It has been postulated that the described papular eruption represents an abnormal host response to an infective process, which requires an intact cellular immunity for resolution [89]. This type of papular eruption may be seen in other viral infections such as the Gianotti-Crosti syndrome or hepatitis B.

## Atopic Dermatitis

Atopic dermatitis has been described in 50% of children with AIDS [87]. These eruptions tend to wax and wane. Interestingly, in both Wiskott-Aldrich syndrome and the ataxia-telangiectasia syndrome, as well as in other immunodeficiency syndromes of childhood, atopic dermatitis commonly occurs.

We recently saw two adult patients with atopic dermatitis. One was a 53-year-old man who had never had this disease until he developed AIDS. The other was a 23-year-old man who had mild atopic dermatitis in childhood that recurred in a severe form when he developed AIDS [2].

## Granuloma Annulare

Granuloma annulare has been described in AIDS patients [32,92,93]. One patient with a pathologic diagnosis of perforating granuloma annulare had an inflammatory infiltrate in his skin which was found to be predominantly composed of T suppressor cytotoxic cells [93].

## Pyoderma Gangrenosum

There is a report of a patient with a 6-year history of recurrent episodes of bilateral ulcers of the lower extremities [94]. Skin biopsy was consistent with pyoderma gangrenosum. The patient tested positive for the HIV antibody. He did not suffer from any other disease known to be associated with pyoderma gangrenosum. Several investigators have found a deficiency in cell-mediated immunity in patients with pyoderma gangrenosum [95].

## Premature Aging of Skin

The skin ages prematurely. Loss of facial fat and hollowing of the facial contour occur commonly, particularly in the late stages of AIDS [8].

## Bullous Pemphigoid

A patient with ARC presented with widespread excoriated erythematous papules measuring 3 to 10 mm in diameter with many scars as a result of scratching due to intense pruritus [96]. Direct immunofluorescence revealed linear deposits of IgG at the dermoepidermal junction. The patient was diagnosed as having bullous pemphigoid in its early papular prebullous form. He responded well to ritodrine, a beta-agonist.

## Erythema Elevatum Diutinum

Erythema elevatum diutinum is a chronic inflammatory dermatosis characterized by symmetrical persistent erythematous nodules and plaques primarily in an acral distribution. It is often associated with streptococcal infection. A patient with HIV-positive lymphadenopathy syndrome (persistent generalized lymphadenopathy) has been described with this skin disease [97].

### Transient Acantholytic Dermatosis (Grover's Disease)

Transient acantholytic dermatosis (Grover's disease) has been described in asymptomatic HIV-positive individuals [35].

## Drug Reactions

Hypersensitivity rashes have been reported in at least 40 to 60% of patients with *P. carinii* pneumonia treated with therapeutic doses of trimethoprim-sulfamethoxazole [8]. The rash is characteristically a widespread blanchable maculopapular eruption accompanied by fever [98]. We have seen similar rashes in patients treated with azidothymidine (AZT). Erythematous fixed drug reaction and generalized toxic erythemas with mucositis may occur as well [87].

Pentamidine is often used to treat *P. carinii* pneumonia in patients who are allergic to trimethoprim-sulfamethoxazole. Sterile abscesses often occur at injection sites because of the local irritating effects of pentamidine [82]. Ulceration of the skin with secondary bacterial infection may occur at the site of injection. The ulcers are managed with oral antibiotics, topical wound care, cavity opening, and in selected cases, wound closure by skin grafting [99].

Pyrimethamine-sulfadoxine has been used as prophylaxis against *P. carinii* pneumonia. The development of Steven-Johnson syndrome has been reported in AIDS patients receiving this drug [100]. Some of these patients had previously developed a maculopapular reaction when treated with trimethoprim-sulfamethoxazole. Therefore, pyrimethamine-sulfadoxine should be used with caution, especially in patients with hypersensitivity to trimethoprim-sulfamethoxazole [100].

*Cryptosporidium muris* is a protozoan that can cause gastroenteritis in AIDS patients [82]. It is treated with spiramycin, which can occasionally cause a rash [82]. Sulfadiazine, which is used to treat toxoplasmosis, can cause severe rashes as well [82].

Clofazimine is used to treat *M. avium*-intracellulare [91]. It produces a characteristic purplish discoloration of the skin and eyes [82].

Severe aphthosis has been described in a patient receiving interferon therapy [32].

Electron beam therapy, which is sometimes used to treat multiple small lesions of Kaposi's sarcoma, may cause hyperpigmentation [8].

Systemic chemotherapy with etoposide (VP-16), used to treat Kaposi's sarcoma, may cause alopecia and phototoxic hyperpigmentation [8].

## Urticaria and Pruritus

Recurrent urticaria has been reported as an early manifestation of HIV infection [22].

Patients frequently complain of intractable generalized pruritus with no identifiable cause [2]. This may or may not be associated with HIV exanthema. Scabies

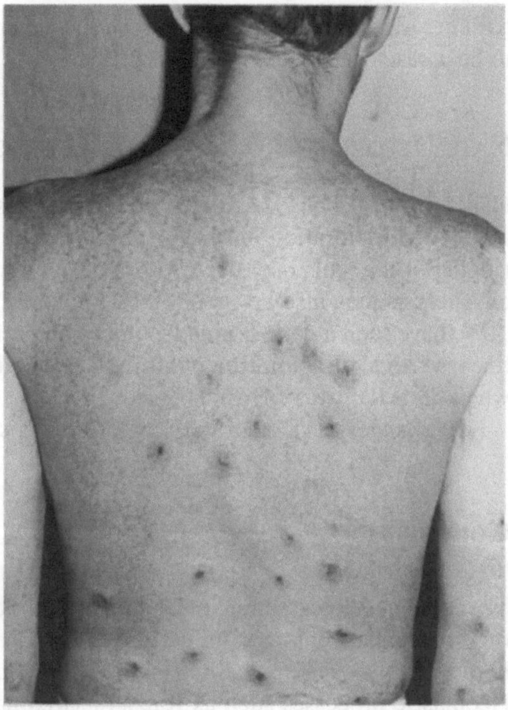

FIGURE 22.14. Multiple deep excoriations in an AIDS patient with severe pruritus. The itching was not helped by any therapeutic means. The patient was hospitalized for this problem without real benefit.

and lymphoma must be ruled out in such cases. Severe scratching may be manifested by excoriation and prurigo lesions (Fig. 22.14). This pruritus may be very difficult to control [2], although dapsone helps at times.

## Hair and Nail Changes

### ALOPECIA AREATA

Alopecia areata has been described in a patient with ARC [101]. In general, patients with alopecia areata have changes in T lymphocytes [102,103]. Since similar immunologic defects have been described in patients infected with HIV, Schonwetter and Nelson [101] suggested that the immunologic aberrations caused by the AIDS virus could cause alopecia areata.

### THINNING AND GRAYING OF HAIR

Hair changes associated with premature aging occur in AIDS [8]. The hair grays prematurely. Frontal recession, thinning of the hair, and diffuse alopecia may develop as well [8]. We have recently seen a case of sudden hair loss in an AIDS patient. Although clinically it looked like severe alopecia areata, biopsy showed it to be a case of telogen effluvium [2].

### Nail Deformities and Color Changes

Nail deformities have been reported in patients with AIDS. Some patients develop a yellow discoloration of the distal portion of the nail. Transverse or longitudinal ridging of the nails may occur. Loss of the lunula and opaqueness with or without onycholysis may also be seen [104]. Leukonychia has been described as well [8].

We have seen a dark-skinned Colombian patient who developed hyperpigmented linear vertical discoloration of his nails 6 months previously, apparently at the time when his AIDS was first diagnosed.

Nail changes associated with infection or psoriasis have been described earlier.

## Conclusion

There are numerous cutaneous manifestations of AIDS and related diseases. To further complicate matters, infections such as histoplasmosis, cryptococcosis, and herpes simplex may present as skin lesions that clinically mimic another disease. Neoplastic processes such as Kaposi's sarcoma and lymphoma may appear on the skin as small, benign-looking, and inconspicuous lesions. A lesion that looks like molluscum contagiosum could be molluscum contagiosum, Kaposi's sarcoma [1], histoplasmosis [44], cryptococcosis [40], or a mixed infection [68].

Biopsy, acid-fast and fungal staining, and appropriate culture of all skin lesions in AIDS patients are mandatory, even if the clinical diagnosis seems certain. When a patient at high risk for AIDS presents with any of the cutaneous manifestations discussed, the clinician should be alert to the possibility of this disease. Once HIV disease has been diagnosed, careful and thorough cutaneous follow-up is warranted. Such follow-up might allow early diagnosis and treatment of a potentially life-threatening complication, which could prolong the life of the HIV-infected victim.

### References

1. Warner LC, Fisher BK: Cutaneous manifestations of the acquired immunodeficiency syndrome. *Int J Dermatol* **25**:337–350, 1986.
2. Fisher BK, Warner LC: Cutaneous manifestations of the acquired immunodeficiency syndrome, update 1987. *Int J Dermatol* **26**:615–630, 1987.
3. Martin J: Acquired immunodeficiency syndrome (AIDS) and Kaposi's sarcoma. *Int J Dermatol* **23**:483–486, 1984.
4. Kramer RH, Fuh G, Hwang CBC, et al: Basement membrane and connective tissue proteins in early lesions of Kaposi's sarcoma associated with AIDS. *J Invest Dermatol* **84**:516–520, 1985.
5. McLeod WA: Kaposi's sarcoma in AIDS. *Contemp Dermatol*; charter issue:5–11, 1987.

6. Eversole LR, Leider AS, Jacobsen PI, et al: Oral Kaposi's sarcoma associated with acquired immunodeficiency syndrome among homosexual males. *J Am Dent Assoc* **107**:248–253, 1983.
7. Farthing CF, Staughton RCD, Rowland Payne CME: Skin disease in homosexual patients with acquired immune deficiency syndrome (AIDS) and lesser forms of human T-cell leukemia virus (HTLV-II) disease. *Clin Exp Dermatol* **10**:3–12, 1985.
8. Farthing CF, Brown SE, Staughton RCD: *A Colour Atlas of AIDS*. London: Wolfe Medical Publications, 1986.
9. Keith JE, Shaw Wilgis EF: Kaposi's sarcoma in the hands of an AIDS patient. *J Hand Surg* **11A**:410–413, 1986.
10. Lemlich G, Schwam L, Lebwohl M: Kaposi's sarcoma and acquired immunodeficiency syndrome. *J Am Acad Dermatol* **16**:319–325, 1987.
11. Volberding P: Therapy of Kaposi's sarcoma in AIDS. *Semin Oncol* **11**:60–67, 1984.
12. Schoeppel SL, Hoppe RT, Dorfman RF, et al: Hodgkin's disease in homosexual men with generalized lymphadenopathy. *Ann Intern Med* **102**:68–70, 1985.
13. Ziegler JL, Drew WL, Miner RC, et al: Outbreak of Burkitt's like lymphoma in homosexual men. *Lancet* **2**:631–633, 1982.
14. Lind SE, Gross PL, Andiman WA, et al: Malignant lymphoma presenting as Kaposi's sarcoma in a homosexual man with acquired immunodeficiency syndrome. *Ann Intern Med* **102**:338–340, 1985.
15. Conant MA, Wolberding P, Fletcher V, et al: Squamous cell carcinoma in sexual partner of Kaposi's patient. *Lancet* **1**:286, 1986.
16. Li FP, Osborn D, Cronin CM: Anorectal squamous cell carcinoma in two homosexual men. *Lancet* **2**:391, 1982.
17. Slazinski L, Stall JR, Mathew C: Basal cell carcinoma in a man with acquired immunodeficiency syndrome. (Letter) *J Am Acad Dermatol* **11**:140–141, 1984.
18. Ruocco V, Satriano RA: Basal cell cancer and classic Kaposi's sarcoma in a locally immunocompromised patient. *Int J Dermatol* **25**:594–596, 1986.
19. Safai B, Good RA: Basal cell carcinoma with metastasis: Review of literature. *Arch Pathol Lab Med* **101**:327–331, 1977.
20. Sitz KV, Koppen M, Johnson DF: Metastatic basal cell carcinoma in acquired immunodeficiency syndrome-related complex. *JAMA* **257**:340–343, 1987.
21. Moore GE, Cook DD: AIDS in association with malignant melanoma and Hodgkin's disease. *J Clin Oncol* **3**:1437, 1985.
22. Kaplan MH, Sadick N, McNutt NS, et al: Dermatologic findings and manifestations of acquired immunodeficiency syndrome (AIDS). *J Am Acad Dermatol* **16**:485–506, 1987.
23. Barlow RJ, Schulz EJ: Necrotizing folliculitis in AIDS-related complex. *Br J Dermatol* **116**:581–584, 1987.
24. Richard M, Mathieu-Serra A: Staphylococcal scalded skin syndrome in a homosexual adult. *J Am Acad Dermatol* **15**:385–389, 1986.
25. Yeager BA, Hoxie J, Weisman R, et al: Actinomycosis in the acquired immunodeficiency syndrome-related complex. *Arch Otolaryngol Head Neck Surg* **112**:1293–1295, 1986.
26. Johns RJ, Tierney M, Felsenstein D: Alteration in the natural history of neurosyphilis by concurrent infection with the human immunodeficiency virus. *N Engl J Med* **316**:1569–1572, 1987.
27. Berry CD, Hooton TA, Collier AC, et al: Neurologic relapse after benzathine penicillin therapy for secondary syphilis in a patient with HIV infection. *N Engl J Med* **316**:1587–1589, 1987.

28. Tramont EC: Syphilis in the AIDS era. (Editorial) *N Engl J Med* **316**:1600–1601, 1987.
29. Zakowski P, Fligiel S, Berlin OGW, et al: Disseminated *Mycobacterium avium*-intracellulare in homosexual men dying of acquired immunodeficiency. *JAMA* **248**:2980–2982, 1982.
30. de la Loma A, Manrique A, Rubrio R, et al: Generalized tuberculosis in a patient with acquired immunodeficiency syndrome. *J Infect* **10**:57–59, 1985.
31. Marchiando A: Scrofula followed by AIDS. (Letter) *Ear Nose Throat J* **63**:197–198, 1984.
32. Penneys NS, Hick B: Unusual cutaneous lesions associated with acquired immunodeficiency syndrome. *J Am Acad Dermatol* **13**:845–852, 1985.
33. Klein RS, Harris CA, Smal CB, et al: Oral candidiasis in high-risk patients as the initial manifestation of the acquired immunodeficiency syndrome. *N Engl J Med* **311**:354–358, 1984.
34. Bush DF: Overview of infectious diseases and other non-malignant conditions in the acquired immune deficiency syndrome. *Front Radiat Ther Oncol* **19**:52–58, 1985.
35. Muhlemann MF, Anderson MG, Paradinas FJ, et al: Early warning skin signs in AIDS and persistent generalized lymphadenopathy. *Br J Dermatol* **114**:419–424, 1986.
36. Perniciaro C, Peters MS: Tinea faciale mimicking seborrheic dermatitis in a patient with AIDS. *N Engl J Med* **314**:315–316, 1986.
37. Noppakun N, Head ES: Proximal white subungual onychomycosis in a patient with acquired immune deficiency syndrome. *Int J Dermatol* **25**:586–587, 1986.
38. Borton LK, Wintroub BV: Disseminated cryptococcosis presenting as herpetiform lesions in homosexual man with acquired immunodeficiency syndrome. *J Am Acad Dermatol* **10**:387–390, 1984.
39. Feldman SR, Kuttner BJ: Forehead ulcer in a homosexual man. *Arch Dermatol* **122**:821, 1986.
40. Rico MJ, Penneys NS: Cutaneous cryptococcosis resembling molluscum contagiosum in a patient with AIDS. *Arch Dermatol* **121**:901–902, 1985.
41. Taylor MN, Baddour LM, Alexander JR: Disseminated histoplasmosis associated with the acquired immune deficiency syndrome. *Am J Med* **77**:579–580, 1984.
42. Wheat LJ, Slama TG, Zeckel ML: Histoplasmosis in the acquired immune deficiency syndrome. *Arch Intern Med* **78**:203–210, 1985.
43. Bonner JR, Alexander WJ, Dismukes WE, et al: Disseminated histoplasmosis in patients with the acquired immune deficiency syndrome. *Arch Intern Med* **144**:2178–2181, 1984.
44. DeChavin MF, Revuz J, Deniau M: Histoplasmose a *Histoplasma duboisii* lesions cutanees simulant des molluscum contagiosum. *Ann Dermatol Venereol* **113**:715–716, 1983.
45. Mayorla F, Penneys NS: Disseminated histoplasmosis presenting as a transepidermal elimination disorder in an AIDS victim. (Letter) *J Am Acad Dermatol* **13**:842–844, 1985.
46. Hazelhurst JA, Vismer HF: Histoplasmosis presenting with unusual skin lesions in acquired immunodeficiency syndrome (AIDS). *Br J Dermatol* **113**:345–348, 1985.
47. Lipstein-Kresch E, Isenberg HD, Singer C, et al: Disseminated *sporothrix schenckii* infection with arthritis in a patient with acquired immunodeficiency syndrome. *J Rheumatol* **12**:805–809, 1985.
48. Bibler MR, Luber HJ, Glueck HI, et al: Disseminated sporotrichosis after treatment for acquired factor VIII inhibitor. *JAMA* **256**:3125–3126, 1986.

49. Sarma DP, Weilbacher TG: Molluscum contagiosum in the acquired immunodeficiency syndrome. *J Am Acad Dermatol* **13**:682–683, 1985.
50. Douglass MC, Mathes B, Thomas L: Molluscum contagiosum in the acquired immunodeficiency syndrome (Reply). *J Am Acad Dermatol* **13**:683, 1985.
51. Katzman M, Elmats CA, Lederman MM: Molluscum contagiosum in the acquired immunodeficiency syndrome. (Letter) *Ann Intern Med* **102**:413–414, 1985.
52. Lombardo PC: Molluscum contagiosum in the acquired immunodeficiency syndrome. *Arch Dermatol* **121**:824–825, 1985.
53. Siegal FP, Lopez C, Hammer GS, et al: Severe acquired immunodeficiency in male homosexuals, manifested by chronic perianal ulcerative herpes simplex lesions *N Engl J Med* **305**:1439–1444, 1981.
54. De Maubeuge J, Mascart-Lemone F, Clumeck N, et al: Acquired immunodeficiency manifested as severe genital herpes: Two cases. (Abstract) *Dermatologica* **168**:105–111, 1984.
55. Dotz WI, Berman B: Kaposi's sarcoma, chronic ulcerative herpes simplex and acquired immunodeficiency. *Arch Dermatol* **119**:93–94, 1983.
56. Macher AM: Infection in the acquired immunodeficiency syndrome: Epidemiologic, clinical, immunologic and therapeutic considerations. *Ann Intern Med* **100**:92–106, 1984.
57. Cone LA, Schiffman MA: Herpes zoster and the acquired immunodeficiency syndrome. (Letter) *Ann Intern Med* **100**:462, 1984.
58. Quinnan GV Jr, Maur H, Rook A, et al: Herpesvirus infections in the acquired immune deficiency syndrome. *JAMA* **252**:72–77, 1984.
59. Greenspan D, Greenspan JS, Conant M, et al: Oral "hairy" leukoplakia, in male homosexuals: Evidence of association with both papillomavirus and a herpes-group virus. *Lancet* **2**:831–834, 1984.
60. Greenspan D: Oral viral leukoplakia (hairy leukoplakia): A new oral lesion in association with AIDS. *Compend Contin Educ Dent* **6**:204–206,208, 1985.
61. Lupton GP, James WD, Redfield RR, et al: Oral hairy leukoplakia: A distinctive marker of human T-cell lymphotropic virus type III (HTLV-III) infection. *Arch Dermatol* **123**:624–628, 1987.
62. Conant MA: Hairy leukoplakia: A new disease of the oral mucosa. *Arch Dermatol* **123**:585–587, 1987.
63. Greenspan D: Acyclovir relative slows growth of oral hairy leukoplakia. Quoted in *The Medical Post* (Canada), MacLean Hunter, **23**(13):30, 1987.
64. Muggia FM, Lonberg M: Kaposi's sarcoma and AIDS. In *Cutaneous Oncology Med Clin North Am*, **70**(1):139–154, 1986.
65. Sadick N, Kaplan MH, Pahwa SG, et al: Unusual features of scabies complicating human T-lymphotropic virus type III infection. *J Am Acad Dermatol* **15**:482–486, 1986.
66. Glover R, Young L, Goltz RW: Norwegian scabies in acquired immunodeficiency syndrome: Report of a case resulting in death from associated sepsis. (Letter) *J Am Acad Dermatol* **16**:396–398, 1987.
67. Klotz-Levy B, Badillet G, Cavelier-Balley B, et al: Alternariose cutanée au cours d'un SIDA. *Ann Dermatol Venereol* **112**:739–740, 1985.
68. Boudreau S, Hines HC, Hood AF: Dermal abscesses with *Staphylococcus aureus*, cytomegalovirus and acid-fast bacilli. *J Cutan Pathol* **15**:53–57, 1988.
69. Gretzula JC, Penneys NS: Complex viral and fungal skin lesions of patients with acquired immunodeficiency syndrome. *J Am Acad Dermatol* **16**:1151–1154, 1987.

70. Karpatkin S: Idiopathic thrombocytopenic purpura in homosexual men. *Ann NY Acad Sci* **437**:58–64, 1984.
71. Fallon T, Abell E, Kingsley L, et al: Telangiectasias of the anterior chest in homosexual men. *Ann Intern Med* **105**:679–682, 1986.
72. Abramson SB, Odajynk CM, Weissman G, et al: Hyperalgesic pseudothrombophlebitis: New syndrome in male homosexuals. *Am J Med* **78**:317–320, 1985.
73. Torre D, Sampietro C, Fiori G, et al: Skin manifestations in infants with AIDS. *Int J Dermatol* **26**:459–460, 1987.
74. Eisenstat B, Wormser GP: Seborrheic dermatitis and butterfly rash in AIDS. (Letter) *N Engl J Med* **311**:358–364, 1984.
75. Soeprono FF, Schinella RA, Cockerell CJ, et al: Seborrheic-like dermatitis of acquired immunodeficiency syndrome; A clinicopathologic study. *J Am Acad Dermatol* **14**: 242–248, 1986.
76. Mathes BM, Douglass MC: Seborrheic dermatitis in patients with acquired immunodeficiency syndrome. *J Am Acad Dermatol* **13**:947–951, 1985.
77. McGinley KJ, Leyden JJ, Marples RR, et al: Quantitative microbiology of the scalp in non-dandruff, dandruff and seborrhoeic dermatitis. *J Invest Dermatol* **64**:401–405, 1975.
78. Ford GP, Farr PM, Ive FA, et al: The response of seborrhoeic dermatitis to ketoconazole. *Br J Dermatol* **26** (Supp 3):25, 1984.
79. Skinner RB Jr, Zanolli MD, Noah PW, et al: Seborrheic dermatitis and acquired immunodeficiency syndrome. (Letter) *J Am Acad Dermatol* **14**:147–148, 1986.
80. Johnson TM, Duvic M, Rapini RP, et al: AIDS exacerbates psoriasis. *N Engl J Med* **313**:1415, 1985.
81. Duvic M, Johnson TM, Rapini RP, et al: AIDS associated psoriasis and Reiter's syndrome. *Arch Dermatol* **123**:1622–1632, 1987.
82. Selwyn PA: AIDS! What is now known. III. Clinical aspects. *Hosp Pract* Sept. 15, 1986.
83. Tong TK, Andrew LR, Abey A, et al: Childhood acquired immune deficiency syndrome manifesting as acrodermatitis enteropathica, *J Paediatr* March, 426–428, 1986.
84. Soeprono FF, Schinella RA: Eosinophilic pustular folliculitis in patients with acquired immunodeficiency syndrome: Report of three cases. *J Am Acad Dermatol* **14**:1020–1022, 1986.
85. Jankins D Jr, Fisher BK, Chalvardjian A, et al: Eosinophilic pustular folliculitis in a patient with the acquired immunodeficiency syndrome. *Int J Dermatol* **27**:34–35, 1988.
86. Wantzin GRL, Lindhardt BO, Weismann K, et al: Acute HTLV-III infection associated with exanthema, diagnosed by seroconversion. *Br J Dermatol* **115**:601–606, 1986.
87. McLeod AW: Dermatologic manifestations of AIDS. *Medicine Nor Am* (2nd series) **32**:4448–4454, 1986.
88. Ringler DJ, Murphy GF, King W: An erythematous maculopapular eruption in macaques infected with an HTLV-III like virus (STLV-III). *J Invest Dermatol* **87**: 674–677, 1986.
89. James WD, Redfield RR, Lupton GP, et al: A papular eruption associated with human T-cell lymphotropic virus type III disease. *J Am Acad Dermatol* **13**:563–566, 1985.
90. Breadon J, Halder R, Minus H: Lichenoid eruption with atypical infiltrate in an AIDS patient. (Personal communication) presented at meeting of the American Society of Dermatopathology, 1986 New Orleans, LA.
91. Belsito DV, Sanchez NR, Baer RL, et al: Reduced Langerhans cell Ia antigen and ATPase activity with the acquired immunodeficiency syndrome. *N Engl J Med* **310**: 1279–1282, 1984.

92. Smith NP: AIDS, Kaposi's sarcoma and the dermatologist. *J Roy Soc Med* **78**:97–99, 1985.
93. Huerter CJ, Bass J, Bergfeld WF, et al: Perforating granuloma annulare in a patient with acquired immunodeficiency syndrome. *Arch Dermatol* **123**:1217–1220, 1987.
94. Schwartz BK, Clendenning WE, Blaski LG: Pyoderma gangrenosum in a patient with HTLV-III antibody. *Arch Dermatol* **122**:508–509, 1986.
95. Greenberg SJ, Jegasothy BV, Johnson RB, et al: Pyoderma gangrenosum: Occurrence with altered cellular immunity and a circulating serum factor. *Arch Dermatol* **118**:498–502, 1982.
96. Levy PM, Balavoine JF, Salomon D, et al: Ritodrine responsive bullous pemphigoid in patients with AIDS-related complex. *Br J Dermatol* **114**:635–636, 1986.
97. Da Cunha Bang F, Weismann K, Ralfkier E, et al: Erythema elevatum diutinum and pre-AIDS. *Acta Dermatol Venereol* (Stockh) **66**:272–274, 1986.
98. Kalter DC, Tschen JA, Klima M: Maculopapular rash in a patient with acquired immunodeficiency syndrome. *Arch Dermatol* **121**:1455, 1985.
99. Gottlieb JR, Lewis VL, Bashioum RW: Care of pentamidine ulcers in AIDS patients. *Plast Reconstr Surg* Oct:630–632, 1985.
100. Navin TR, Miller KD, Satriale RF, et al: Adverse reactions associated with pyrimethamine-sulfadoxine prophylaxis for *Pneumocystis carinii* infections in AIDS. *Lancet* June **8**:1332, 1985.
101. Schonwetter RS, Nelson EB: Alopecia areata and the acquired-immunodeficiency-related complex. (Letter) *Ann Intern Med* **104**:287, 1986.
102. Hordinsky MK, Hallgren H, Nelson D, et al: Suppressor cell number and function in alopecia areata. *Arch Dermatol* **120**:188–194, 1984.
103. Galbraith G, Thiers B, Vasely D, et al: Immunological profiles in alopecia areata. *Br J Dermatol* **110**:163–170, 1984.
104. Chernosky ME, Finely VK: Yellow nail syndrome in patient with acquired immunodeficiency disease. *J Am Acad Dermatol* **13**:731–736, 1985.

CHAPTER 23

# Balanitis and Vulvitis

Mohamed Amer

## Part 1. Balanitis

### Definition

Balanitis is defined as an acute or chronic inflammation of the glans penis and prepuce. Phimosis is commonly associated with it. It is rare in circumcised men.

### Predisposing Factors

Irritation by smegma, urine, or alkalies; external contact with clothing; friction; and trauma are the most common predisposing factors to balanitis. Exposure to venereal and vaginal pathogens plays a major role in its pathogenesis.

### Clinical Findings

The presentation differs according to the underlying cause.

#### Traumatic Balanitis

Accidental or coital trauma may cause inflammation of the glans penis. Itching and the resultant scratching of the penile skin (especially the glans), for example because of scabies, may cause moderate to severe balanitis.

#### Iatrogenic Balanitis

Contact Dermatitis

Although affecting the shaft rather than the glans, contact dermatis may cause balanitis. Local antiseptics and local anesthetic creams are the common offending agents.

### Fixed Drug Eruptions

These cause apprehension in the patient and confusion in medical attendants about their possible origin as being sexually transmitted. A fixed drug eruption can be diagnosed by its characteristic morphologic features, namely single, well-defined, superficial, erosive lesions with no regional lymphadenopathy. The lesion is preceded and accompanied by itching and burning. A history of drug taking is the mainstay of diagnosis. Provocation tests with gradual doses of the suspected drug(s) may be undertaken. Tetracycline is the most common causative drug, followed by exphenbutazone and acetylsalicylic acid [1]. Elimination of the offending drug(s) is the first and essential measure. This is usually followed by involution of the lesions in a short time. Symptomatic treatment is given in the form of antihistamines, orally or by injection, and corticosteroids are given in severe cases.

## Infective Balanitis

This is the usual cause of balanitis. It can be classified into types, as follows.

### Candidal Balanitis

In recent years, the importance of genital candidosis in men has been stressed. Four clinical types have been described:

1. Asymptomatic: *Candida* was isolated from 18% of asymptomatic men with a diligent search [2].
2. Hypersensitivity. The patient complains of burning and itching of the penis, which develops within hours of sexual intercourse. A generalized erythema of the glans and prepuce may be noted [3].
3. Typical. This type is mild with a dry, glazed, erythematous surface of the glans penis and the undersurface of the prepuce. There may be very small, irregular, eroded papules and a dispersed vesicular eruption, often with plaques of white cheesy matter. The fossa navicularis may be involved and there may be transient urethritis. Itching and scaly erythematous lesions may also be present on the penile and scrotal skin. In the obese, the groins may be involved.
4. Acute. An edematous fulminating type of balanoposthitis may occur with ulceration of the penis and a swollen fissured prepuce. This is often associated with diabetes mellitus.

### Trichomonal Balanitis

*Trichomonas vaginalis* is frequently recovered from the subpreputial sac [4] and has been associated with ulcerative lesions of the penis. It is not clear whether *T. vaginalis* causes ulcers or whether it merely colonizes ulcers caused by other agents.

### Genital Herpes

Genital herpes is caused by herpes simplex virus (HSV or *Herpesvirus hominis*). Genital herpes is mainly transmitted sexually. Most cases are caused by herpesvirus type 2, as opposed to type 1, which is usually associated with lesions elsewhere on the body, such as the mouth and eyes; however, occasional cases of genital herpes may be due to type 1 as a result of orogenital contact. There are biologic antigenic differences between the two types.

The primary disease is associated with constitutional symptoms, including fever, malaise, and muscular pain. The initial lesions are grouped vesicles that often only irritate or give a pricking pain. The vesicles soon rupture, resulting in polycyclic, shallow, mostly nonindurated, sometimes tender ulcers on the glans penis. Secondary infection, however, is common.

## Genital Warts

Condylomata acuminata, or genital warts, are caused by a papillomavirus that may be sexually transmitted. The incubation period may be as long as 9 months. The sites commonly affected are the glans penis; the prepuce, including the mucosal surface; the penile shaft; and the external meatus.

The warts are flesh colored. They may be sessile or pedunculated. Their number and size may vary from a few pinhead-sized ones to several small and large warts covering the whole of the glans penis, looking almost like a cauliflower.

Spontaneous regression may occur in some and relapse in others.

## Parasitic Balanitis

### *Amebiasis*

This type is caused by *Entamoeba histolytica*. Penile lesions may occur after intercourse. The ulcer has irregular and undermined edges with a granulomatous base. Diagnosis is made by identification of the parasite in stools and in exudate from the infected sites or histologic examination of the biopsy material.

### *Scabies*

Burrows on the genitals have a rather different appearance from the classic lesions on the hand and wrist. They are raised, slightly elongated, nodular lesions with the burrow track seen as a thin black, irregular line.

### *Schistosomiasis*

This type is caused by *Schistosoma haematobium*. Lesions may develop in any part of the male genital tract. Diagnosis is made by finding the terminal spined eggs in the urine and from histologic examination of the biopsy material.

## Syphilitic Balanitis

This follows the primary chancre. The glans shows a whitish coalescent surface on the edematous background.

### Mycoplasma Balanitis

This may accompany mycoplasma urethritis. It responds to tetracycline, 2 g per day for 2 weeks.

### Chlamydial Infection

This may be associated with the penile lesions of Reiter's disease. It can be treated with tetracyclines or erythromycin, 2 g daily for 3 weeks.

### Balanitis Associated with *Gardnerella vaginalis* Infection

About 7% *G. vaginalis* can be isolated in specimens from unselected men. Much heavier growth of the organism is obtained from preputial swabs than from concomitant urethral swab [4]. Typically the condition is mild with preputial irritation and an offensive fishy odor. It is associated with signs of increased subpreputial mucoid discharge and mild inflammation of the glans penis and prepuce. It is treated with oral metronidazol in a dosage of 400 to 500 mg twice daily for 5 days.

### Erosive Balanitis

This is an infection due to Vincent's organisms and it occurs only in patients with some degree of phimosis. Subpreputial foul-smelling discharge is noticed by the patient. When the prepuce is retracted and the pus removed with saline swab, the mucous surfaces of the prepuce and glans penis are seen to be reddened with a number of small, round, superficial erosions over the surface. Treatment is with daily saline washes. Circumcision may be indicated if balanitis is recurrent.

## Balanitis Due to Other Causes

### Balanitis Circinate

Balanitis circinate is almost diagnostic of Reiter's disease; it occurs in up to 69% of men with this disease.

Spongiform pustules of the skin are the most distinctive histopathologic finding of Reiter's disease detected by a light microscope. Hyperkeratosis, parakeratosis, and acanthosis may also be present in cutaneous lesions, which resemble those of psoriasis. Ultrahistopathology [5] shows small to medium-sized pustules in the upper epidermis. The thin flattened keratinocytes form a spongelike trabecular network. Neutrophils are not found inside the keratinocytes. The fine structure of balanitis circinate resembles that of pustular psoriasis.

### Plasma Cell Balanitis

Synonyms for this condition are pseudoerythroplastic balanitis and balanitis circumscripta plasmacellularis (Zoon's balanitis). The clinical appearance is similar to that of erythroplasia of Queyrat or Bowen's disease of the glans penis. In some instances erosions with a tendency to bleed are present. Like erythroplasia, this disorder is seen almost exclusively in uncircumcised men.

## Histopathology

The histologic findings of balanitis are those of inflammation with spongiosis and moderate to severe inflammatory infiltrate. In the infective variety, the offending organism can be demonstrated by the application of specific strains. In Zoon's balanitis, the histopathologic findings are specific. They include epidermal atrophy and erosion, absence of epidermal dysplasia, and a bandlike upper dermal inflammatory infiltrate composed primarily of plasma cells. Occasional lymphocytes, histiocytes, and mast cells may be found within the infiltrate, as may hemosiderin deposits.

## Management

Gentle but thorough washing of the affected area with an emollient nondetergent soap should precede any other measure. Successful treatment of balanitis depends on eradication of the offending causes, if possible.

Antifungal therapeutic agents used for candidal balanitis are imidazoles (e.g., clotrimazole and miconazole) or polyenes (e.g., nystatin and candicidin). Twice daily application for 2 weeks suffices for clinical cure. Eradication of candidal vaginitis in female patients is an important step to preventing recurrence in the male.

In primary genital herpes, intravenously administered acyclovir (5 mg/kg every 8 hours) has reduced the duration of viral shedding by 80%, shortened the signs and symptoms of the disease by a mean of 5 days, and quickened the time to healing of lesions by a mean of 12 days over placebo-treated patients [6].

Plasma cell balanitis is notably resistant to treatment. Topical corticosteroids provide a measure of symptomatic relief and clinical improvement, but rarely result in permanent cure. Irradiation and superficial electrodessication have been reported efficacious.

# Part 2. Vulvitis

## Definition

Vulvitis is inflammation of the vulva. The vulva is a region in which three specialties are interested, namely, dermatologists, venereologists, and gynecologists. This has led, in the past, to multiplication of disease nomenclature, with resulting confusion.

The boundaries of the vulva consist of the lower part of the mons veneris superiorly, the perineum inferiorly, and the labia majora laterally. The inner limit of the vulva is the introitus of the vagina bounded by the hymen, beyond which the vagina proper begins. The clitoris, urethral orifice, and Bartholin's gland contained within these boundaries are conveniently considered part of the vulva. The labia minora are naturally contained in this area and form an important part of the vulva.

## Clinical Findings

The lax tissues of the vulva encourage edema rather than vesiculation. Bullous lesions become erosive or vegetating. Intertriginous lesions spread from the inguinal or abdominal folds, and secondary infection is common in obese middle-aged or elderly patients. Lichenification frequently complicates the situation and may mask any pruritic inflammatory vulval lesions.

In vulvitis the vulva is swollen, reddened, and covered with slight or profuse exudation. In severe cases the inflammation involves the skin of the adjacent areas of the thighs. The patient complains of burning, itching, and tenderness. As the result of scratching and laceration of the skin, extensive excoriation develops.

The clinical findings may be classified according to the underlying etiology. The following working classification may help in clinical practice.

### Inflammatory Lesions Principally Affecting the Vulva Itself

#### Infection of Hair Follicles

Staphylococcal and streptococcal infections of the hair follicles of the mons and labia majora may lead to folliculitis, furunculosis, and/or intertrigo. The latter is due to irritation and infection of retained secretions in the skin folds, usually in the obese patient, and to friction of unhygienic underclothes or sanitary napkins.

#### Infection of Sebaceous Cysts

Infection of sebaceous cysts with production of boggy swellings may lead to pain and tenderness in the vulval region.

#### Inflammation

Inflammation of the vulva may occur after accidental, coital, obstetric, or operative trauma. The most important cause of traumatic vulval infection is scratching secondary to itchy vulval dermatoses.

#### Sexually Transmitted Infection

Seven sexually transmitted infections have been considered, as follows:

The primary chancre of syphilis.
Eroded papules or condylomata lata of secondary syphilis.
Gummatous ulcers of tertiary syphilis.
Chancroid ulcer.

Lymphogranuloma venereum (primary lesion and ulceration associated with elephantiasis).
Granuloma inguinal.
Herpes genitalis.

The clinical pictures of these diseases are mentioned elsewhere in this book.

*Vulvovaginitis in Children*

Vulvovaginitis in children due to organisms other than the gonococcus or *Candida* is generally regarded as uncommon. Gonococcal vulvovaginitis presents variable signs and symptoms. There may be no complaint at all, or only an observation of discharge on the underwear by the child's mother. Some girls complain of malaise, soreness, itching, discomfort in walking, or sometimes dysuria and frequency.

Local examination reveals a reddened, edematous vulva with a purulent discharge. Examination of the rectum may reveal redness and mucuslike discharge due to associated gonococcal proctitis [7].

*Erysipelas of the Vulva*

This is now a very rare disease and readily amenable to antibiotic therapy.

*Seminal Vulvitis*

Most patients with this condition are atopic and have developed reaginic antibodies to all human seminal plasma.

*Salivary Vulvitis*

A relatively common cause of vulval itching is the increasingly common practice of oral-genital contact.

## Inflammatory Lesions Primarily Affecting Structures in the Vulva

### Infection of Bartholin's Gland

An abscess of Bartholin's gland due to distal blocking of the duct may be due to pyogenic organisms or may complicate gonococcal infection. *Chlamydia trachomatis* can also infect Bartholin's gland.

There will be swelling of the vulva on the affected side. The abscess can be felt between the fingers with the thumb on the outer surface of the labium majus and the index finger in the vagina. Attacks often follow intercourse, and recurrent mild attacks may occur until fibrosis supervenes. Persistent lymphoedema usually follows repeated attacks.

### Infection of the Paraurethral and Suburethral Glands

This is usually the result of chronic urethritis, often of gonococcal origin. The glands open beside or just inside the urethral meatus. The opening appears red and edematous, and when pressed by the gloved finger against the anterior vaginal wall may yield a small bead of pus.

## Secondary Inflammatory Lesions of the Vulva

In these infections the primary site of infection is elsewhere.

### Trichomonas Infection of the Vagina

Infection with *T. vaginalis* is a frequent cause of vaginitis and vulvitis. *T. vaginalis* is a common inhabitant of the female genital tract, and the problem of pathogenicity is similar to that of *Candida* and depends on a favorable environment for growth. Infection is rare in children and after the menopause. *T. vaginitis* causes a frothy, malodorous, grayish-green watery discharge and a bright red or petechiae-studded vaginal mucosa.

### Candidal Vulvovaginitis

In one study, *C. albicans* was isolated from the vagina of 22% of 226 women college students at the University of Washington [8]. Changes in host factors are probably responsible for transition to pathogenicity and are generally not directly associated with sexual contact. Pregnancy; diabetes; use of systemic antibiotics, contraceptive pills, or immunosuppressive drugs; and factors related to cell-mediated immunity may all favor precipitation and persistence of infection.

### Vulvitis Secondary to Chronic Infected Lesions of Cervix

Infection of the cervix represents a reservoir for perinatal transmission of pathogenic microorganisms.

### Vulvitis Secondary to Urinary or Bowel Fistula.

## Rare Inflammatory Lesions of the Vulva

### Malakoplakia of the Vulva

This is an unusual granulomatous response to infection, usually *Escherchia coli* but sometimes *Pseudomonas* or *Staphylococcus aureus*. Diagnosis is made by searching for and finding Michaelis-Guttman bodies in the close-packed histocytes of the infiltrate.

### Mycobacterial Infection

Tuberculosis of the genital tract is rare. Unilateral Bartholin's gland infection has been reported. On the other hand, vulval lesions are not common in *M. lepra* infection.

### Erosive Vulvitis

This condition of the vulva clinically resembles that seen in the mouth, with which it may be associated. The diagnosis is made bacteriologically by isolating the *Spirella*. This is sensitive to large doses of penicillin.

### Actinomycosis

Vulval infection with *Actinomyces* is extremely rare. It presents the usual characteristics such as branny lesion with typical sulfur granules in the discharge. Multiple sinuses may be present with fistulae formation.

### Parasitic Infestation

*Enterobius vermicularis* (threadworm), scabies, filariasis, schistosomiasis, and amebic dysentery, among other organisms, all may cause vulvovaginitis.

### Circinate Vulvitis

Like circinate balanitis, this may occur in Reiter's syndrome. The vulvitis consists of shallow circinate erosion. Although circinate vulvitis has been reported in four cases, Reiter's syndrome is uncommon in women [9].

### Vulvodynia and the Burning Vulva Syndrome

These terms have been used synonymously. Both are characterized by the complaint of chronic vulval soreness or burning. Vulvodynia has several etiologies; it can be produced, for example, by a chronic *Candida* infection. Patients with burning vulva syndrome are usually, but not always, young. Their past experience is often of multiple sexually transmitted infections, and they tend to be emotionally labile.

### Vulvitis Circumscripta Plasmacellularis

In this condition a lesion analogous to balanitis circumscripta plasmacellularis is observed on the vulva.

## References


1. Sehgal VH, Gangwani OP: Genital fixed drug eruptions. *Genitourin Med* **62**:56–58, 1986.
2. Radin P, Kolator B: Carriage of yeast on the penis. *Br Med J* **1**:1123–1124, 1976.
3. Oates JK: Sexually transmitted skin diseases. *Br J Sex Med* **3**:8–10, 1976.
4. Kinghorn GR, Jones BM, Chowdhury FH, et al: Balanoposthitis associated with *Gardnerella vaginalis* infection in men. *Br J Vener Dis* **58**:127–129, 1982.
5. Kanerva L, Kousa M, Niemi KM, et al: Ultrahistopathology of balanitis circinate. *Br J Vener Dis* **58**:188–195, 1982.
6. Covey L, Benedetti JA, Fife KH, et al: Intravenous acyclovir for the treatment of primary genital herpes. *Ann Intern Med* **98**:914–921, 1983.

7. Farid M: *Sexually Transmitted Diseases*. Cairo: Ain-Shams University Press, 1981, pp. 97–98.
8. Holmes KK, Hardh PA, Sparling PF, et al: *Sexually Transmitted Diseases*. New York: McGraw-Hill, 1984, p. 1570.
9. Daunt SO, Kotowski KD, Orelly AP, et al: Ulcerative vulvitis in Reiter's syndrome: A case report. *Br J Vener Dis* **58**:405–407, 1982.

CHAPTER 24

# Sexually Transmitted Diseases in the Tropics

Peter Piot and Marie Laga

## Introduction

As is the case for most other infectious diseases, sexually transmitted diseases (STD) are common in many parts of the developing world. This may have multiple causes, such as a larger pool of infected individuals, lack of control programs, antimicrobial resistance of causative organisms, poor health care facilities in general, poor health-seeking behavior, and socioeconomic factors [1]. Table 24.1 shows infection rates of various sexually transmitted agents in pregnant women.

The burden of STD in the tropics is particularly severe because of a high frequency of complications and sequelae, including urethral stricture, epididymitis, and AIDS in men; endometritis, pelvic inflammatory disease (PID), ectopic pregnancy, infertility, and AIDS in women; and congenital syphilis, neonatal conjunctivitis and pneumonia, and congenital infection with human immunodeficiency virus (HIV) in the newborn.

The disease spectrum may also be different from that seen in Europe and North America. Genital ulcer disease is much more common, with chancroid often being the leading cause. Gonorrhea occurs relatively more commonly, with sometimes high prevalence rates in the sexually active population. Syphilis is a major public health problem in some countries, resulting in high rates of congenital syphilis. AIDS and HIV-related disease are not only common in some areas, but also not confined to specific high-risk groups such as homosexual men or intravenous drug abusers [2,3].

In addition, antimicrobial resistance is a major problem in infections with *Neisseria gonorrhoeae* and *Haemophilus ducreyi*, making some cheap treatment regimens ineffective, and thereby favoring the spread of these infections.

Epidemiologic studies suggest that, at least in some parts of the developing world, prostitutes play a major role in the spread of STD. They may exhibit very high infection rates for all STD agents, as shown in Table 24.2. Because developing countries face many other severe health problems, STDs are rarely considered a priority by the health authorities. Consequently, funds for STD control programs are usually minimal or nonexisting, despite high direct and indirect costs due to complications and sequelae of STD.

TABLE 24.1. Prevalence of selected sexually transmitted agents in some developing countries.

| | | | Percent positive | | | |
|---|---|---|---|---|---|---|
| City/country | Year | Number tested | Gonorrhea | *Chlamydia trachomatis* | VDRL/ RPR | Human immunodeficiency virus (HIV) |
| Bangui, Central African Republic | 1980 | | 9 | | 9 | |
| Ethiopia | 1977 | | | | 13 | |
| Gambia | 1982 | | 7 | 7 | | |
| Abidjan, Ivory Coast | 1986 | | | | | 3 |
| Nairobi, Kenya | 1986 | | 7 | 29 | 4 | 2 |
| Kampala, Uganda | 1986 | | | | | 14 |
| Kinshasa, Zaire | 1986 | | | | | 8 |

Data from Piot and Meheus [1], Quinn et al. [3], Piot et al. [36], Denis et al. [37], and Carswell [39].

In this chapter we will briefly review some common problems of STD in the tropics. The reader is referred to two recently published textbooks for a more in-depth discussion of STD in the developing world [4,5].

## Sexually Transmitted Diseases in the Perinatal and Puerperal Periods

As a result of high STD rates in general, pregnant women in many developing countries may have high prevalence rates for agents such as *N. gonorrhoeae*, *Chlamydia trachomatis*, *Treponema pallidum*, and human immunodeficiency virus (HIV) (Table 24.1). These microorganisms may have a negative impact on pregnancy outcome, as discussed in other chapters. One complication that is particularly common in some populations is postpartum endometritis/salpingitis. For example, in one study in Nairobi, Kenya, over 20% of women developed endometritis or salpingitis during the puerperal period, with gonococcal and chlamydial infections during labor as the major risk factors [6]. Similarly, 18% of mothers of infants with neonatal conjunctivitis suffered from pelvic inflammatory disease; 65% of them were infected with *N. gonorrhoeae* [7]. Further studies are needed to elucidate the etiology of puerperal infections and to define their role in secondary infertility. It is noteworthy that the majority of cases (85%) of involuntary infertility in sub-Saharan Africa are due to bilateral tubal occlusion—a sequel of pelvic inflammatory disease [8]. This is another illustration of the impact of STD on maternal health.

Congenital syphilis is still an important problem in many parts of the world. Its incidence may be as high as 14 to 700 per 100,000 births [1]. In addition, endemic treponematoses, which are still occurring in some parts of Africa, Latin America, and the Middle East, may be another reason for positive serologic tests for syphilis

TABLE 24.2. Infection rate of some sexually transmitted agents among female prostitutes in developing countries

| | | | Percent positive | | |
|---|---|---|---|---|---|
| City/area | Year | Number tested | Gonorrhea | Human immunodeficiency deficiency virus | Serologic test for syphilis |
| Abidjan, Ivory Coast | 1986 | 101 | | 20 | |
| Nairobi, Kenya | 1985– | 71 | 46 | 53 | |
| | 1986 | 286 | | 61 | |
| Butare, Rwanda | 1984 | 33 | | 88 | |
| Kinshasa, Zaire | 1985 | 377 | | 27 | |

Data from D'Costa et al. [16], Piot et al. [36], Denis et al. [37], Mann et al. [40], and Van de Perre et al. [41].

in an adult or child. In the absence of typical clinical lesions, a differential diagnosis of venereally acquired syphilis may be very difficult.

The incidence of neonatal conjunctivitis is high in populations with high prevalence rates of STD, particularly when eye prophylaxis at birth is not applied [9]. Sexually transmitted bacterial agents are the major causes of ophthalmia neonatorum in Africa, where 15 to 50% of cases are due to *N. gonorrhoeae* and *C. trachomatis*. Corneal lesions with keratitis develop in approximately 15% of cases of gonococcal ophthalmia, and may result in blindness [10]. Because of the high prevalence of penicillinase-producing strains of *N. gonorrhoeae* (PPNG) in most parts of the developing world, penicillin is no longer the drug of choice for the treatment of gonococcal ophthalmia neonatorum. Systemic single-dose therapy with ceftriaxone or kanamycin is recommended [11,12].

Neonatal infection with *C. trachomatis* results also in considerable infant morbidity in the tropics. In a prospective cohort study in Nairobi, exposed infants suffered more conjunctivitis, pneumonia, and diarrhea than did controls [13]. The clinical spectrum of chlamydial infection following perinatal exposure was similar to that observed in developed countries.

## Genital Ulcer-Lymphadenopathy Syndrome

Genital ulcerations are among the more complex clinical problems in patients with STD, and occur commonly in the developing world, where adequate facilities for proper diagnosis and therapy are scarce.

### FREQUENCY

Genital ulcerations are present in 10 to 70% of patients seen in STD clinics in Asia and Africa [14]. For instance, in Swaziland, up to half of all male patients with STD had a genital ulceration [15]. Studies in Nairobi have documented the relatively high

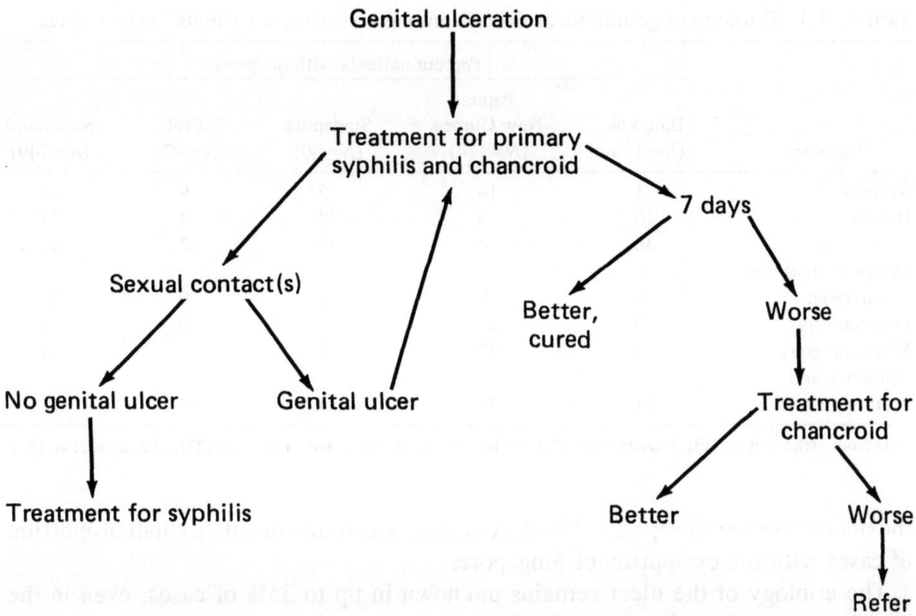


FIGURE 24.1. Management of genital ulceration in the absence of diagnostic facilities. From Meheus and Piot [32].

frequency of genital ulcerations among low-class prostitutes, who are important transmitters of genital ulcer disease, particularly chancroid [16,17].

Several surveys suggest that syphilis has become an important problem in many tropical areas, where previously the endemic treponematoses were often controlled [1,18]. Prevalence rates for positive serologic tests for syphilis are shown in Tables 24.1 and 24.2; however, because foci of endemic treponematoses still exist, interpretation of a positive serologic test for syphilis may be difficult in asymptomatic patients from such areas.

Genital herpes, the major cause of genital ulcer disease in the industrialized world, is much less commonly seen in the tropics, but well-documented data are lacking. Lymphogranuloma venereum is a relatively rare cause of genital ulcer disease in most countries, and presents usually as an inguinal lymphadenopathy syndrome.

## ETIOLOGY

The etiology of genital ulcerations in different areas in the tropics is shown in Table 24.3. There is clearly regional variation in the etiology of genital ulcer disease. Chancroid is apparently the leading cause of genital ulceration in Africa and Southeast Asia (Fig. 24-2) [15,19–22]. However, syphilis and donovanosis – a rare disease in most places – were the main diagnoses in Papua New Guinea [23]. Genital herpes,

TABLE 24.3. Etiology of genital ulcer disease among consecutive patients in the tropics.

| Diagnosis | Percent patients with diagnosis | | | | |
|---|---|---|---|---|---|
| | Bangkok (*N*=120) | Papua New Guinea (*N*=174) | Singapore (*N*=60) | Nairobi (*N*=97) | Swaziland (*N*=149) |
| Syphilis | 1 | 14 | 5 | 9 | 17 |
| Herpes | 10 | 0 | 28 | 4 | 11 |
| Chancroid | 36 | 0 | 48 | 62 | 42 |
| Lymphogranuloma venereum | 0 | 9 | 0 | 0 | 12 |
| Donovanosis | 0 | 22 | 0 | 0 | 1 |
| Mixed etiology | 2 | 37 | 5 | 2 | 4 |
| Unknown and other causes | 51 | 18 | 14 | 13 | 13 |

Data from Meheus et al. [15], Nsanze et al. [20], Taylor et al. [22], Vacca and MacMillan [23], and Rajan et al. [42].

the major cause in Europe and North America, was found in only a small proportion of cases with the exemption of Singapore.

The etiology of the ulcer remains unknown in up to 35% of cases, even in the best documented studies. Occasional cases may be due to *Pthirus pubis*, *Entamoeba histolytica*, *Sarcoptes scabiei*, and *Trichomonas vaginalis*. *Neisseria gonorrhoeae* is occasionally isolated from genital ulcers, but it is not clear whether this is due to contamination from urethral or cervical secretions. Erosive balanoposthitis and superficial ulcers may be caused by an association of nonsyphilitic spirochetes and anaerobic bacteria [24]. Serologic tests for syphilis remain negative in such cases; however, in general, the epidemiologic and clinical features and the response to antimicrobial therapy of ulcers of unknown etiology in Africa are similar to those that are culture positive for *H. ducreyi*, suggesting that they are caused by undetected *H. ducreyi* [25,26]. In addition, serum antibodies to *H. ducreyi* can be detected in most such cases [27].

## Clinical Findings and Differential Diagnosis

The clinical presentation of genital ulcer disease is frequently atypical, particularly in developing countries where mixed infections are common and patients often present late in the course of their disease. The reader is referred to the respective chapters in this book for a discussion of the different causes of lymphadenopathy-genital ulcer syndrome.

In the tropics there is often little correlation between the clinical presentation and the classic description of primary syphilis. The aspect of the chancre is frequently nonspecific, with a purulent base due to other infections. In a series of male patients in Johannesburg, the only reasonably sensitive clinical marker of syphilis was the finding of discrete, bilateral, rubbery inguinal lymph nodes associated with genital ulcers [19]. Because of high rates of positive reactions for syphilis serology among

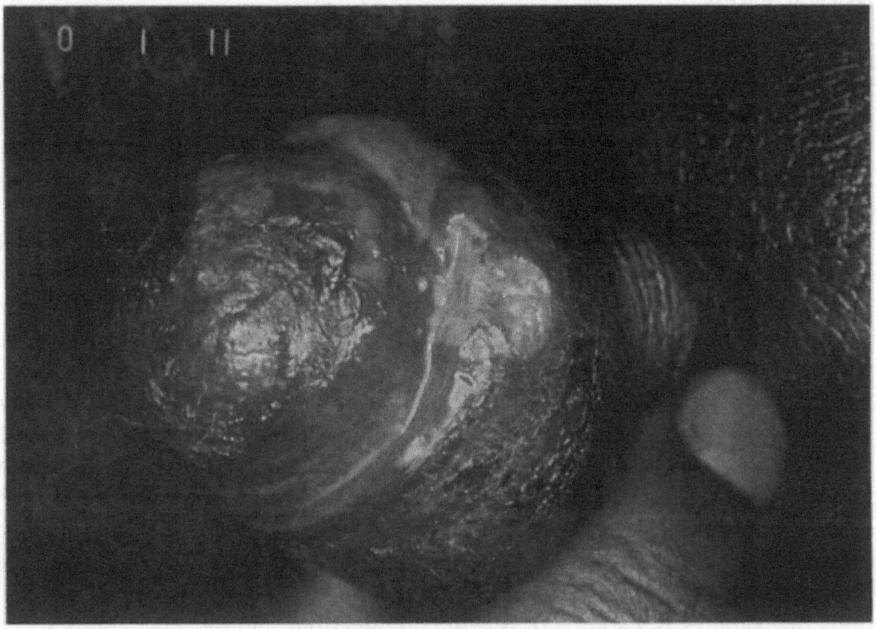



FIGURE 24.2. Chancroid can be devastating in many tropical areas.

patients with other causes of genital ulceration and among controls, the performance of serologic tests for syphilis is poor for the differential diagnosis of genital ulcers in some areas such as southern Africa; however, because of the higher incidence of syphilis in many parts of the developing world, patients with any sexually transmitted disease should be evaluated for syphilitic infection.

In Africa, the overall accuracy of a clinical diagnosis of genital ulceration was 40 to 70% in centers with extensive experience with this syndrome [19,28]. Genital ulcers in women may be even less typical than in men [29,21]. Women in Johannesburg tended to have more mixed infections than men, and inguinal lymphadenopathy was less common in women with chancroid than in men [29]. Even extensive laboratory investigations fail to determine the cause of genital ulcers in 20 to 35% of cases (Fig. 24.2).

Patients with lymphogranuloma venereum usually present with unilateral or bilateral lymphadenopathy, and only a minority have an ulcer, which is rather discrete; however, they may also present with more extensive genital ulcerations from which the L serovars of *C. trachomatis* can be isolated [18].

Extensive, persistent, and necrotic genital ulcerations are mostly due to herpes simplex virus and should prompt investigations for infection with human immunodeficiency virus (HIV), since this may be an opportunistic infection associated with AIDS [30,31].

### Management

As the accuracy of a clinical diagnosis is often poor, genital ulcers should be thoroughly investigated using all laboratory tests available, including tests for *T. pallidum*, herpes simplex virus, and *H. ducreyi* in patients who presumably acquired their infection in the tropics. The laboratory diagnosis of chancroid has been drastically improved in recent years (see chap. 6), but experience and appropriate isolation media are rarely available.

Specific treatment regimens are discussed elsewhere in this book. Well-evaluated simple and fairly inexpensive treatment regimens are now available for syphilis and chancroid; however, diagnostic facilities are often very limited or not available, the clinical presentation is frequently atypical, mixed infections are common, and patients have often already taken some form of therapy before presentation at a health care facility. Therefore, standard management of genital ulcerations is now recommended in developing countries [32,33]. Standard management regimens should be based on the local etiology of genital ulcerations and on the local effectiveness of antibiotics against different causes of genital ulcer disease. In the absence of laboratory facilities, all genital ulcerations in the tropics may be treated with benzathine penicillin, 2.4 million units intramuscularly, combined with single-dose therapy for chancroid (see chap. 6). This recommendation is based on the considerations that syphilis is a source of severe complications and sequelae and that chancroid is the most common cause. Ulcers of undetermined etiology are usually cured by the latter part of this treatment regimen. Figure 24.1 shows an example of standard management of genital ulcerations at basic health services level.

## Problems of Antimicrobial Resistance

Bacterial strains are generally less susceptible to antimicrobial agents in the tropics. At least 50% of gonococcal strains in Africa and Asia are now resistant to penicillin, either because of beta-lactamase production or because of chromosomally mediated resistance (Table 24.4). The majority of these isolates are also resistant to tetracycline. Therefore, patients with a gonococcal infection acquired in the tropics should be treated with a drug that is effective against PPNG (see Chap. 5). Though spectinomycin-resistant strains have occasionally been seen in the Far East, such strains are rare.

Similarly, *H. ducreyi* isolates are usually resistant to ampicillin, tetracycline, and, often, to sulfonamides. Effective single-dose treatment regimens for chancroid have recently been developed (see chap. 6).

## AIDS in the Tropics

Infection with human immunodeficiency virus (HIV) and the acquired immunodeficiency syndrome (AIDS) often follow a different epidemiologic pattern in the

TABLE 24.4. In vitro antimicrobial susceptibility of *Neisseria gonorrhoeae* isoates in Africa.

| | | Percent of strains resistant to | | |
|---|---|---|---|---|
| Geographic origin | Year | Penicillin | Tetracycline | Spectinomycin |
| Central African Republic | 1983 | 44 | 7 | 0 |
| Kenya | 1985 | 77 | 0 | 0 |
| Rwanda | 1986 | 56 | 18 | 0 |
| Zaire | 1986 | 52 | 24 | 0 |

Data from Laga et al. [12], Bogaerts et al. [43], and Meheus et al. [44].

tropics, and may have different clinical features, compared with the disease in Europe and North America. However, the biology and modes of transmission of HIV infection are basically the same in all parts of the world.

## EPIDEMIOLOGY

The geographic distribution and the incidence of AIDS and HIV infection are difficult to assess in most developing countries. This is mainly due to poor surveillance activities in general, and limited diagnostic facilities for HIV infection and associated opportunistic diseases. In many parts of Africa, major foci of HIV infection are now occurring [3]. In one city in central Africa, the annual incidence of AIDS was estimated at 550 to 1,000 cases per 1 million population in 1984–1985, with a current female/male ratio of 1.1:1 [34]. In Haiti, the proportion of women with AIDS has been increasing to a female/male ratio of 1:1.8, suggesting that heterosexual transmission is becoming increasingly important [35]. Whereas AIDS is predominantly an urban problem in most countries, large rural outbreaks are occurring in others.

Seroprevalence rates for HIV antibody in health populations in Africa vary widely (Table 24.1). In random surveys of the general population, of blood donors, and of pregnant women, HIV seropositivity rates between 0.5 and 18% have been reported from Africa and the Caribbean, which is much higher than those observed in the industrialized world [3]. Among high-risk groups, such as patients with STD and female prostitutes, seroprevalence rates of up to 88% have been found (Table 24.2). Longitudinal data on East African prostitutes demonstrate that HIV infection can disseminate as fulminantly in a population of very promiscuous heterosexuals as in promiscuous homosexual men [36].

The recent isolation of the HIV-related human retrovirus from West Africans may further complicate the epidemiology of HIV infection in Africa. Seroprevalence rates for HIV-2 antibody of less than 1% in the general population, but as high as 14% among prostitutes, were found in West Africa [37].

In contrast to AIDS in North America and Europe, an overwhelming majority of AIDS cases in Africa are heterosexual men and women, and transmission is mostly by heterosexual contact, both from male to female and from female to male [3]. Characteristics of AIDS patients are those of other patients with a STD.

TABLE 24.5. Clinical manifestations among AIDS patients in Africa.

| Signs or symptoms | Percent of 196 consecutive patients with symptoms |
|---|---|
| Weight loss 10% of body weight | 99 |
| Asthenia | 91 |
| Fever >1 month | 54 |
| Diarrhea >1 month | 41 |
| Cough | 37 |
| Dyspnea | 23 |
| Headache >1 month | 33 |
| Pruritus | 30 |
| Amenorrhea (women) | 42 |
| Dysphagea | 35 |
| Oral thrush | 47 |
| Pruritic papular eruption | 20 |
| Generalized lymphadenopathy | 11 |
| Varicella zoster lesions | 9 |
| Convulsions or other focal neurologic manifestations | 6 |

Data from Colebunders et al. [30].

Other modes of transmission of HIV infection in Africa include blood transfusions and perinatal acquisition, and probably also contaminated injection sites and scarifications.

AIDS is becoming a public health problem in Africa on the same scale as malaria, malnutrition, and respiratory and diarrheal diseases. The impact of this pandemic on demography, economic development, and health care programs remains to be assessed, but is likely to be significant.

## Clinical Aspects

The clinical expression of HIV infection may vary among different populations, depending on the occurrence of endemic opportunistic infections. Table 24.5 lists the most common clinical manifestations of AIDS in Africa, based on a series in Zaire [5]. The most common manifestations include weight loss, asthenia, fever, persistent diarrhea, oral thrush, and cough. Persistent generalized lymphadenopathy is less frequently observed in African patients, but chronic diarrhea and a distinct pruritic papular skin eruption are common [30,31].

A chronic diarrhea-wasting syndrome ("slim disease") is found in approximately half of the African AIDS cases, but others may present predominantly with fever of unknown origin. Skin and mucosal abnormalities are very common in patients with HIV infection. A generalized, pruritic, maculopapular eruption was found in 20 to 60% of patients with AIDS in Kishasa [38]. It occurs often during the initial phase of the disease, but is generally intermittent during the course of the illness. Its etiology is unknown. Histologic examination shows nonspecific perivascular infiltration of the skin and subcutaneous tissues with mononuclear cells and eosinophils. Varicella zoster is also observed as an initial manifestation of HIV disease in approximately 10% of cases, and is recurrent in one fourth of such cases [30].

The most frequent opportunistic diseases in African patients with AIDS include candidal esophagitis, tuberculosis, cryptococcal meningitis, cerebral toxoplasmosis, and generalized infection with cytomegalovirus. *Pneumocystis carinii* pneumonia, which is found in over half of the European and North American AIDS cases, occurs less often in Africans, whereas tuberculosis, cryptococcosis, and toxoplasmosis are more frequent.

In general, one should consider HIV infection in any patient coming from an HIV-endemic area who presents with one or more of the signs and symptoms mentioned above.

## Control

Control of AIDS and HIV infection has become an immediate public health priority in many African countries. Programs focus on changing sexual behavior through health education, since the overwhelming majority of infections are acquired by heterosexual contact. At the same time, these programs should reduce the incidence of other sexually transmitted diseases, which are also associated with considerable morbidity. This is also the major approach to control of perinatal transmission of HIV. Such programs aimed at changing sexual behavior are a formidable undertaking without precedent. Encouraging results have been obtained in a group of prostitutes in East Africa, who were actively counseled and given free condoms. This program resulted in a dramatic increase in the use of condoms by the prostitutes' clients.

Screening programs for blood donors have been initiated in most countries, but cost and logistic problems are major drawbacks when setting up a blood bank screening infrastructure. The recent development of rapid, simple, and cheap diagnostic assays for HIV antibody should be extremely helpful. The identification of high-risk donors on epidemiologic and clinical grounds has not been successful in Africa [3]. Finally, campaigns against unnecessary and contaminated injections may not only limit the further spread of HIV infection, but also reduce transmission of other injection-transmitted infections such as hepatitis B.

## References


1. Piot P, Meheus A: Epidémiologie des maladies sexuellement transmissibles dans les pays en développement. *Ann Soc Belge Méd Trop* **63**:87–110, 1983.
2. Piot P, Caraël M: Epidemiological and sociological aspects of HIV infection in developing countries. *Br Med Bull* **44**:68–88, 1988.
3. Quinn TC, Mann JM, Curran JW, et al: AIDS in Africa: An epidemiologic paradigm. *Science* **234**:995–963, 1986.
4. Arya, Osoba AO, Benett D: *Tropical Venereology.* London: Churchill Livingston, 1987.

5. Osoba AO (Ed): *Sexually Transmitted Diseases in the Tropics. Clinical Tropical Medicine and Communicable Diseases*. Eastbourne, England: Bailliere, Tindal, 1987.
6. Plummer FA, Laga M, Brunham RC, et al: Postpartum upper genital tract infections in Nairobi: Epidemiology, etiology and risk factors. *J Infect Dis* **156**:92–98, 1987.
7. Fransen L, Nsanze H, D'Costa LJ, et al: Parents of infants with ophthalmia neonatorum: A high risk group for sexually transmitted diseases. *Sex Trans Dis* **12**:150–155, 1985.
8. Cates W, Farley TMM, Rowe PJ: Worldwide patterns of infertility: Is Africa different? *Lancet* **2**:596–598, 1985.
9. Laga M, Plummer FA, Nsanze H, et al: Epidemiology of ophthalmia neonatorum in Kenya. *Lancet* **2**:1145–1149, 1986.
10. Fransen L, Nsanze H, Klauss V, et al: Ophthalmia neonatorum in Kenya: Role of *Neisseria gonorrhoeae* and *Chlamydia trachomatis*. *J Infect Dis* **153**:862–869, 1986.
11. Fransen L, D'Costa L, Nsanze H, et al: Single dose kanamycin therapy of gonococcal ophthalmia neonatorum. *Lancet* **2**:1234–1236, 1984.
12. Laga M, Namaara W, Brunham RC, et al: Single-dose therapy of gonococcal ophthalmia neonatorum with ceftriaxone. *N Engl J Med* **315**:1382–1385, 1986.
13. Datta P, Laga M, Plummer FA, et al: Longitudinal study of perinatal exposure to *Chlamydia trachomatis* in Nairobi, Kenya *J Infect Dis* (in press).
14. World Health Organization: *Non-Gonococcal Urethritis and Other Selected Sexually Transmitted Diseases of Public Health Importance. Technical Report Series 660*, Geneva: World Health Organization,
15. Meheus A, Van Dyck E, Ursi JP, et al: Etiology of genital ulcerations in Swaziland. *Sex Trans Dis* **10**:33–35, 1983.
16. D'Costa LJ, Plummer FA, Bowmer I, et al: Prostitutes are a major reservoir of sexually transmitted diseases in Nairobi, Kenya. *Sex Trans Dis* **12**:64–67, 1985.
17. Plummer FA, D'Costa LJ, Nsanze H, et al: Epidemiology of chancroid and of *Haemophilus ducreyi* in Nairobi, Kenya. *Lancet* **2**:1293–1295, 1983.
18. Piot P, Meheus A: Genital ulcerations in the troipcs. In JD Oriel and JRW Harris (Eds): *Recent Advances in Sexually Transmitted Diseases*. Churchill Livingston, Edinburgh, 1986, pp. 261–272.
19. Duncan MO, Bilgeri YR, Fehler HG, et al: The diagnosis of sexually acquired genital ulcerations in black patients in Johannesburg. *S Afr J Sex Trans Dis* **1**:20–23, 1981.
20. Nsanze H, Fast M, D'Costa LJ, et al: Genital ulcers in Kenya: A clinical and laboratory study. *Br J Vener Dis* **57**:378–381, 1981.
21. Plummer FA, D'Costa LJ, Nsanze H, et al: Clinical and microbiological studies of genital ulcers in Kenyan women. *Sex Trans Dis* **12**:193–197, 1985.
22. Taylor DN, Duangmani C, Suvongse C, et al: The role of *Haemophilus ducreyi* in penile ulcers in Bangkok, Thailand. *Sex Trans Dis* **11**:148–151, 1984.
23. Vacca A, MacMillan LL: Anogenital lesions in Papua New Guinea. *Papua New Guinea Med J* **23**:70–73, 1980.
24. Piot P, Duncan M, Van Dyck E, et al: Ulcerative balanoposthitis associated with non-syphilitic spirochaetal infection. *Genitourin Med* **62**:44–46, 1986.
25. Plummer FA, D'Costa LJ, Nsanze H, et al: Antimicrobial therapy of chancroid: Effectiveness of erythromycin. *J Infect Dis* **148**:726–731, 1983.
26. Plummer FA, Nsanze H, D'Costa LJ, et al: Single-dose therapy of chancroid with trimethoprim-sulfametrole. *N Engl J Med* **309**:67–71, 1983.
27. Museyi K, Van Dyck E, Vervoort T, et al: Detection of serum IgG antibodies to *Haemophilus ducreyi* in an enzyme immune assay *J Infect Dis* **157**:1039–1043, 1988.

28. Fast MV, D'Costa LJ, Nsanze H, et al: The clinical diagnosis of genital ulcer disease in men in the tropics. *Sex Trans Dis* **11**:72–76, 1984.
29. Duncan MO, Ballard RC, Bilgeri YR, et al: Sexually acquired genital ulcers in Kenyan women. *Sex Trans Dis* **12**:193–197, 1985.
30. Colebunders R, Mann J, Francis H, et al: La clinique du SIDA en Afrique. *Méd Mal Infect* **15**:350–355, 1986.
31. Piot P, Kapita B, Colebunders R, et al:*A Handbook on AIDS in Africa*. Geneva: World Health Organization, 1988.
32. Meheus A, Piot P: Lutte contre les maladies sexuellement transmissibles dans les pays en développement. *Ann Soc Belge Méd Trop* **63**:281–312, 1983.
33. Meheus AZ: Practical approaches in developing countries. In KK Holmes, P A Márdh, PF Sparling, et al (Eds): *Sexually Transmitted Diseases*. New York: McGraw-Hill, 1984, pp. 998–1008.
34. Mann JM, Francis H, Quinn T, et al: Surveillance for AIDS in a central African city, Kinshasa, Zaire. *JAMA* **255**:3255–3259, 1986.
35. Johnson WD, Liautaud B, Thomas F, et al: Changing patterns of AIDS epidemiology. (Abstract) 2nd Sexually Transmitted Disease World Congress, Paris, 25–28 June, 1986.
36. Piot P, Plummer FA, Rey MA, et al: Retrospective seroepidemiology of HIV infection in Nairobi populations. *J Infect Dis* **155**:1108–1112, 1987.
37. Denis F, Barin F, Gershy-Damet G, et al: Prevalence of human T-lymphotropic retroviruses type III (HIV) and type IV in Ivory Coast. *Lancet* **1**:408–411, 1987.
38. Colebunders R, Mann JM, Francis H, et al: Generalised papular pruritic eruption: A manifestation of human immunodeficiency virus infection in African patients. *AIDS* **1**:117–121, 1987.
39. Carswell JW, Sewankambo N, Lloyd G, et al: How long has the AIDS virus been in Uganda? *Lancet* **1**:1217, 1986.
40. Mann JM, Quinn TC, Piot P, et al: HIV seroprevalence among prostitutes in Kinshasa: Sexual practices associated with seropositivity. *AIDS* (in press).
41. Van de Perre P, Clumeck N, Caraël M, et al: Female prostitutes: A risk group for infection with human T-cell lymphotropic virus type III. *Lancet* **2**:525–526, 1985.
42. Rajan VS, Doraisingham M, Sng EH, et al: Polymicrobial aetiology of genital ulcers. *Sing Med J* **23**:207–214, 1982.
43. Bogaerts J, Vandepitte J, Van Dyck E, et al: In vitro antimicrobial sensitivity of *Neisseria gonorrhoeae* from Rwanda. *Genitourin Med* **62**:217–220, 1986.
44. Meheus AZ, Widy-Wirski R, D'Costa J, et al: Treatment of gonorrhoea in males in the Central African Republic with spectinomycin and procaine penicillin. *Bull WHO* **62**:89–94, 1984.

CHAPTER 25

# Sexually Transmitted Disease in Children

Hilary A. Lavery

In 1916, venereal disease in the United Kingdom was defined as syphilis, gonorrhea, and chancroid, but 26 pathogens resulting in sexually transmitted diseases (STDs) are now recognized (Table 25.1). Carcinoma of the cervix is associated with herpes simplex virus (HSV) and the human papillomavirus (HPV), and is considered by some to be a STD. The increasing number of infections now known to be sexually transmitted, and also transmitted by other routes, for example, intestinal infections, reflects the widening variety of sexual activity being increasingly recognized.

Children may be infected by transplacental, intrapartum, or postpartum transmission or as a result of voluntary or involuntary sexual activity (sexual abuse) or of artificial insemination. The latter is performed 30,000 to 60,000 times annually in the United States, with the rate of infection ranging from 6.7 to 9.4 per 1,000 inseminations. It is difficult to assess the risk of STD in victims of sexual assault, as many surveys are unable to give information about preexisting infection or about voluntary sexual activity that took place after the assault, especially in adolescents; however, one STD is identified in 26% of cases. Some refute that all the pathogens in Table 25.1 are sexually transmitted in children, but as Herman-Giddens [1] stated, STDs in adults are also sexually transmitted in children, and to fail to make this diagnosis leaves children open to further abuse.

Full evaluation for all STDs is mandatory, because many are asymptomatic. Since 20 to 35% of abused children have had anal or oral penetration [2–5] (58% of boys and 13.4% of girls in one series had been sodomized [6]), systematic genital and extragenital cultures are required. When the assailant is a homosexual, particular attention must be paid to the infections prevalent in the community, for example, hepatitis B virus, human T cell lymphotropic virus type III, and intestinal infections (giardiasis, amebiasis, and shigellosis). Pharyngeal cultures are essential, as their routine use has revealed a disturbingly high incidence of pediatric STD, especially gonorrhea [7]. Such cultures are also needed in the asymptomatic contacts of children with gonococcal infection [8]. The siblings of an assaulted child also have a high incidence of sexual assault [9] and must be interviewed, examined, and assessed for STD.

STD may be the first indicator of sexual abuse and should be considered such until proven otherwise. The true incidence of sexual abuse is unknown because it is largely a concealed problem; 83% of men and 58% of women had dept it a secret until the time of one survey [10]. Over80% of victims under age 18 are assaulted by a person

TABLE 25.1. Sexually transmitted pathogens.

| | |
|---|---|
| *Treponema pallidum* | Hepatitis A |
| *Neisseria gonorrhoeae* | Hepatitis B |
| *Chlamydia trachomatis* | Human T lymphotropic retrovirus type III |
| *Mycoplasma hominis* | Human T lymphotropic retrovirus type I |
| *Ureaplasma urealyticum* | Cytomegalovirus (CMV) |
| *Candida albicans* | *Calymmatobacterium granulomatis* |
| *Trichomonas vaginalis* | *Haemophilus ducreyi* |
| *Gardnerella vaginalis* | *Campylobacter* |
| *Sarcoptes scabiei* | *Shigella* |
| *Pthirus pubis* | *Entamoeba histolytica* |
| Herpes simplex virus | *Giardia lamblia* |
| Condylomata acuminata | *Salmonella* |
| Molluscum contagiosum | *Streptococcus* |

they know, with more than half of these assailants being relatives, usually the fathers. Approximately 25 to 30% of these children are assaulted more than once by the same person [6,11]. At the age of 16 years, 5 to 9% of boys and 15 to 20% of girls have experienced unwanted sexual touching or assault. One in two men and one in three women are victims of a sexual offence at some time during their lives [12]. In the United States, over 336,000 children are sexually abused each year, a figure that includes one in every four preadolescent and adolescent girls. This represents 9% of all reported cases of sexual abuse. The vast majority of cases are girls (only 17.3% boys), while white and hispanic races become victims less frequently than black.

Each infection will now be considered, first as voluntarily or involuntarily acquired, and then due to vertical transmission.

## Syphilis

Syphilis is systemic from the onset, chronic, and infectious, with the arbitrary division between early and late being 2 years. Early lesions are considered infectious; late are not (Table 25.2). Syphilis is found in up to 6% of sexually abused children [13].

### ACQUIRED SYPHILIS

#### Primary

After an incubation period of 9 to 90 days, a macule that evolves into a papule and then into an ulcer develops at the site of sexual activity. The primary chancre is classically painless and associated with nonsuppurative regional lymphadenopathy. Without treatment it heals in 3 to 8 weeks.

#### Secondary

This usually occurs 6 to 8 weeks after the appearance of the chancre and is associated with constitutional symptoms, a generalized symmetrical nonitchy rash typically affecting the palms and soles, mucosal ulcers, and enlarged lymph nodes.

TABLE 25.2. Classification of syphilis.

| | | | |
|---|---|---|---|
| Acquired | Early | Primary<br>Secondary<br>Early latent | |
| | Late | Late latent<br>Tertiary<br>Cardiovascular<br>Neurosyphilis | |
| Congenital | Early | | |
| | Late | | |
| | Stigmata or scars | (1) of early lesions in CS<br>Saddle nose<br>Bulldog face<br>Rhagades<br>Hutchinson's teeth<br>Moon's molars | (2) of late lesions in CS<br>Corneal opacities<br>Choroidoretinitis<br>Optic atrophy<br>Nerve deafness<br>Frontal and parietal bossing of skull<br>Gummatous scars |

CS, congenital syphilis.

### Latent

Latent syphilis may be suspected from the history and is established by serology. Sixty percent of untreated patients will not suffer further.

### Tertiary

This occurs 3 or more years after the primary stage. It usually affects the skin, mucous membranes, and subcutaneous and submucous tissues and bones. The characteristic lesion is the gumma.

### Quaternary

This phase encompasses cardiovascular syphilis and neurosyphilis, which includes meningovascular syphilis, tabes dorsalis, and general paralysis of the insane.

## Congenital Syphilis

The number of cases of congenital syphilis in the United States increased from 104 in 1978 to 244 in 1984, in parallel with the increase in primary and secondary syphilis, which accounted for 9.4 cases per 100,000 in 1977 and 14.1 cases per 100,000 in 1983. The increased incidence of early infectious syphilis in Singapore, which rose from 8.7 per 100,000 in 1980 to 25 per 100,000 in 1984, may also be followed by an increased incidence of congenital syphilis [14]. Two thirds of patients with congenital syphilis are asymptomatic at birth and develop signs in 3 to 8 weeks. Nearly all have signs by 3 months. The major clinical criteria for the diagnosis of acute congenital syphilis are snuffles, maculopapular or vesiculobullous eruption, condylomata, osteochondritis, and periostitis. Minor criteria include perioral fissures, mucous patches, hepatosplenomegaly, lymphadenopathy, pseudoparalysis, and CNS involvement, which has been reported in 60% of patients. Late congenital syphilis may present as frontal bossing, flattened maxilla, protruding mandible, saddle nose, high arched palate, Hutchinson's teeth, Moon's molars, interstitial keratitis, eighth-nerve deafness, sternoclavicular thickening, Clutton's joints, and sabre tibia. Patients may develop tertiary and quaternary syphilis. Methods of diagnosis and treatment are summarized in Table 25.3.

## Endemic Treponematosis

The causative agents of yaws (*T. pertenue*), endemic syphilis (*T. pallidum*), and pinta (*T. carateum*) are morphologically indistinguishable. Yaws is found in tropical Africa, Southeast Asia, and India; yaws and pinta in tropical America; and endemic syphilis in the Middle East. Yaws and pinta have primary lesions but these are uncommon in endemic syphilis. All have secondary stages and long periods of latency, and there is probably no congenital disease. Treatment is benzathine penicillin, 2.4 megaunits intramuscularly.

## Gonorrhea

One million cases of gonorrhea were reported in the United States in 1983. This figure was thought to represent half the actual number of cases. In children aged 0 to 9 years there were 1,169 cases reported in 1956 and 2,708 cases in 1974. In Nigeria, 36.5% of cases are girls aged 1 to 11 [15]. Gonorrhea is found in 3 to 26% of sexually abused children [13]. Even handicapped children are at risk [16]. The penicillinase-producing stains (PPNG) account for 0.5% of all reported U.S. cases; the first case report in a child was in 1986 [17]. In Malaysia, 41% of gonococcal cases are due to PPNG; correspondingly, 31% of girls younger than 12 years with gonococcal vulvovaginitis are infected with PPNG strains. The nonpenicillinase-producing (chromosomal) resistance strain (CMRNG) has now been reported in 17 states in the United States. Adolescents may be asymptomatic, or boys may have dysuria and discharge following an incubation period of less than 2 weeks and girls may have vaginal discharge (40%) or dysuria (12%). Pharyngeal gonorrhea is usually asymptomatic but may cause a sore throat, and rectal gonorrhea is either asymptomatic or associated with discharge and tenesmus. Complications include disseminated gonococcal infection and pelvic inflammatory disease (PID). PID is usually asymptomatic, but lower, often colicky, abdominal pain; menstrual irregularity; fever; pelvic tenderness; and a pelvic mass may occur. Gonococcal infection has been found in 40% of women with PID, and tubal occlusion occurs in 24% after one episode of gonococcal salpingitis.

TABLE 25.3. Diagnosis and treatment of sexually transmitted diseases in children.

| Organism | Presentation | Congenital transmission | Diagnosis | Treatment |
|---|---|---|---|---|
| *Treponema pallidum* (syphilis) | Chancre; regional lymphadenopathy | Antepartum | Dark-field microscopy; serology: specific FTA ABS TPHA, nonspecific VDRL | Primary, secondary, tertiary: APPG 600,000 units* IM × 14 d<br>Quarternary or late congenital: prednisone 5 mg qid × 2 d, followed by 900–1200 units APPG × 21 d*<br>Penicillin allergy: erythromycin, tetracycline □ 500 mg po qid × 21 d*<br>For congenital < 2 y 250,000 units APPG/kg, total dose over 10 d<br>If penicillin allergy: erythromycin 50 mg/kg in divided doses × 15 d<br>Age 2–10: half adult dose |
| *Neisseria gonorrhoea* | Asymptomatic; vulval or abdominal pain; purulent urethral discharge; vulvovaginal discharge 5–10 days following coitus | Intrapartum | Gram-negative intracellular diplococci; modified New York City culture medium | >45 kg, APPG 4.8 million units IM plus probenecid po 1 g (followed by tetracycline □ or erythromycin 500 mg qid × 14 d<br><45 kg, APPG 100,000 units/kg IM plus probenecid 25 mg/kg po if >2 y, plus tetracycline □ or erythromycin 40 mg/kg/d in 4–5 doses for 14 d<br>If penicillin sensitivity and >45 mg or <45 mg, tetracycline □ or erythromycin as above<br>Ophthalmia neonatorum prophylaxis: 1% silver nitrate solution within 2 h of delivery; erythromycin 0.5% ophthalmic ointment in each eye within 2 h of delivery<br>Hospitalization and isolation for 24 h, ACPG 25,000 units/kg IV qid × 7 d; irrigate eyes with saline; examine and treat mother as well |

TABLE 25.3. *Continued.*

| Organism | Presentation | Congenital transmission | Diagnosis | Treatment |
|---|---|---|---|---|
| *Neisseria gonorrhoea* (cont.) | | | | If PPNG or CMRNG: Cefotaxime 1.0 g IM in appropriate dose |
| *Chlamydia trachomatis* | Asymptomatic; dysuria, mucoid or mucopurulent discharge 8–21 d after coitus | Intrapartum | Giemsa-stained conjunctival swab. Genital swab: (a) tissue culture with cyclohexamide-treated McCoy cells, (b) immunofluorescent slide test | >45 kg, tetracycline hydrochloride □ 500 mg po qid × 14 d<br><45 kg, tetracycline □ 50 mg/kg/d po in 4 divided doses to maximum of 500 mg for 7 d<br><8 years, erythromycin ethylsuccinate 50 mg/kg/d po in 4 divided doses for 7 d<br>Conjunctivitis prevention: erythromycin 0.5% ophthalmic ointment<br>Treatment: irrigate eyes with saline, erythromycin syrup 10 mg/kg po qid × 14 d<br>*Pneumonia*: Erythromycin syrup 10 mg/kg qid × 21 d |
| *Candidosis* | Asymptomatic; malodorous white discharge pH 4–5; severe pruritus, dyspareunia, dysuria, white cottage cheese plaques | Intrapartum | | Miconazole, clotrimazole, butoconazole, topically bd × 7 d; oral nystatin, if required (side effects of oral ketoconazole have not yet been evaluated in pediatric therapy) |
| *Gardnerella vaginalis* | Asymptomatic; pruritus; homogenous thin gray or white malodorous discharge; vaginal flour-paste discharge pH 5–5.5 | ? | Clue cells; gram-negative rods; fishy odor with KOH<br>Casmann's agar culture medium | Metronidazole 15 mg/kg/d po in 3 divided doses × 7 d, maximum dose 250 mg<br>Older adolescents: 500 mg po bd × 7 d<br>Treat sexual partners |

TABLE 25.3. *Continued.*

| Organism | Presentation | Congenital transmission | Diagnosis | Treatment |
|---|---|---|---|---|
| *Trichomonas vaginalis* | Asymptomatic; severe pruritus, dysuria, dyspareunia, green frothy malodorous discharge, vulval erythema and excoriations, punctate vaginal hemorrhage and strawberry cervix; pH 5–6.5 | Rarely intrapartum | Wet mount–motile flagellated organisms; Papanicolaou smear; oxoid culture medium. | Metronidazole 15 mg/kg/d in 3–5 doses × 7 d to maximum dose of 250 mg bd × 7 d<br>Treat sexual partners |
| *Haemophilus ducreyi* (chancroid) | Fever, malaise, painful vesicle pustule/ulcer with painful inguinal lymphadenopathy | – | Gram-negative bacillus on chocolate agar of 1% isovitalex and vincromysin | Erythromycin 500 mg po qid × 10 d*<br>Tetracycline 500 mg po qid × 10 d*<br>Bubo aspiration |
| *Calymmatobacterium granulomatis* | Papulonodular lesion with pseudobubo formation | – | Donovan bodies in tissue smears and biopsies | Tetracycline 500 mg po qid × 14 d*<br>Surgical treatment of complications |
| Lymphogranuloma venereum | Fever, conjunctivitis, iiritis, arthralgia, proctitis, tenesmus, rectal stricture | – | Tissue culture; group antibody: LGV CFT; RIP; Type-specific antibody: MIF | Sulfadiazine 1 g po tid × 21 d*<br>Tetracycline 500 mg po qid × 10 d*<br>Minocycline 100 mg po bd × 20 d*<br>Bubo aspiration<br>Surgical treatment of complications |
| *Sarcoptes scabiei* | Nocturnal pruritus, burrows | – | Presence of mites, biopsy | Lindane 1%, lotion washed off after 12 h |
| *Pthirus pubis* | Pruritus, excoriation, sky-blue macules | – | Nits on hair shafts; lice on skin | Lindane 1%, shampoo for 5 minutes |

TABLE 25.3. *Continued.*

| Organism | Presentation | Congenital transmission | Diagnosis | Treatment |
|---|---|---|---|---|
| Molluscum | Flesh-colored nodules with umbilication | – | Isolation of pox virus | Surgical removal<br>Topical phenol trichloroacetic acid and podophyllin or systemic inisoplex |
| Herpes genitalis | Fever, malaise, anorexia, genital pain, paresthesia, dysuria, grouped vesicles, painful inguinal lymphadenopathy | Antepartum, intrapartum, and postpartum | Tzanck test (shows multinuclear cells and inclusion bodies), electron microscopy; tissue culture | 5% idoxuridine in dimethyl sulfoxide qid $\times$ 4 d; 5% acyclovir ointment 5 times daily $\times$ 5 d |
| Cytomegalovirus | Jaundice, hepatosplenomegaly, purpura, thrombocytopenia, intrauterine infection | Antepartum, intrapartum, postpartum | Positive cell culture; serology | No specific treatment |
| *Staphylococcus*, *Streptococcus* | Vaginal discharge | Group B hemolytic streptococci<br>Intrapartum: 75% of infants colonized, 1% develop disease<br>Postpartum: Late onset<br>Group B streptoccal sepsis | Positive culture for appropriate organism | Penicillin, cephalosporin |

TABLE 25.3. *Continued.*

| Organism | Presentation | Congenital transmission | Diagnosis | Treatment |
|---|---|---|---|---|
| Enterobiasis | Nocturnal perineal pruritus; gastrointestinal symptoms; vulvovaginal contamination from feces | – | Adult worms in stool | Pyrantel pamoate 10 mg/kg po, repeated in 2 and 4 wks to a maximum of 1 g<br>Avoid $<$ 2 years and during pregnancy |
| *Entamoeba histolytica* | Diarrhea; mucoid stool; vulvovaginal contamination from feces | – | Amebas in stool; serology | Metronidazole 15 mg/kg/d in 3 divided doses to a maximum of 250 mg $\times$ 7 d<br>Adolescents 500 mg bd $\times$ 7 d |
| *Giardia lamblia* | Asymptomatic; fecal contamination; diarrhea; malabsorption syndrome; vaginal discharge | – | Protozoal flagellate in feces | Metronidazole 15 mg/kg/d in 3 divided doses to a maxinum of 250 mg $\times$ 7 d<br>Older adolescents 500 mg bd $\times$ 7 d |
| *Shigella* species | Fever; malaise; fecal contamination; diarrhea; blood, mucus, pus in stool | – | Stools–WBC and RBC, positive for *Shigella* | Tetracycline 50 mg/kg/d in 4 divided doses to a maximum of 500 mg $\times$ 7 d<br>Older adolescents 500 mg qid $\times$ 7 d |

ACPG, aqueous crystalline penicillin G; APPG, aqueous procaine penicillin G; d, day; y, years; IM, intramuscular; po, oral; PPNG, penicillinase-producing *Neisseria gonorrhoea*; CMRNG, chromosomal resistant strain *Neisseria gonorrhoea*.

* Dose stated is for adolescents; if younger, age-related dose.

☐ Tetracycline should be avoided if $<$ 8 years.

TABLE 25.4. Causes of nonspecific urethritis (NSU).

| | |
|---|---|
| *Chlamydia trachomatis* | Urethral stricture |
| Candidosis | Warts |
| *Ureaplasma urealyticum* | Herpes simplex virus |
| *Gardnerella vaginalis* | Syphilis |
| Trichomoniasis | Neoplasms |
| Upper urinary tract infection | Crystelluria |
| Trauma | Hypersensitivity |
| Foreign body | |

### MATERNAL-NEONATAL TRANSMISSION

The incidence of gonorrhea in pregnant women is 1 to 7.5% [17a-17f]. It is usually asymptomatic. All mothers should thus be screened at the first prenatal visit. Follow-up smears and cultures should be done in any infected woman after therapy is completed. A rectal culture is especially important. Gonorrhea in this site accounts for 30% of treatment failures, even when the initial test was negative.

Coexistent STD occurs in 30 to 50% of patients. The high-risk populations of young adults and adolescents, those from a low socioeconomic background, those with a history of STD including PID, and those from areas where there is a high incidence of gonorrhea must have third-trimester screening and peripartum cultures. Disseminated gonococcal infection frequently occurs late in pregnancy or at delivery, but PID may occur in the first trimester.

Untreated infection may result in abortion, chorioamnionitis, endometritis, intrauterine growth retardation, premature rupture of the membranes, prematurity, maternal peripartum fever, and neonatal sepsis. The risk of vertical transmission is 30%, resulting in ophthalmia neonatorum (Fig. 25.1) and less commonly gonococcal arthritis, sepsis, and meningitis. Infants born to infected mothers should have cultures done on material from all sites exposed during delivery—mouth, conjunctivae, pharynx, umbilical cord, vagina, and anorectum, with blood cultures if there was prolonged rupture of the membranes. Eighty-one cases of ophthalmia neonatorum were reported in 1984 in the United States. The incubation period is 36 to 48 hours, and characteristically there is bilateral conjunctivitis with orbital edema. Gonococcal vulvovaginitis, which accounts for 37% of vulvovaginitis cases presenting to the pediatric gynecologist, may be asymptomatic or the child may have an erythematous edematous excoriated vulva with a thick creamy-yellow discharge. Methods of diagnosis and treatment are given in Table 25.3.

## Nonspecific Genital Infection

Nonspecific genital infection encompasses also nonspecific urethritis and proctitis. *C. trachomatis* accounts for 50 to 60% of cases; 5 to 10% are due to the other causes listed in Table 25.4 and the etiology of the remainder are unknown. Four to six percent of sexually abused adolescents have nonspecific genital infection [18].

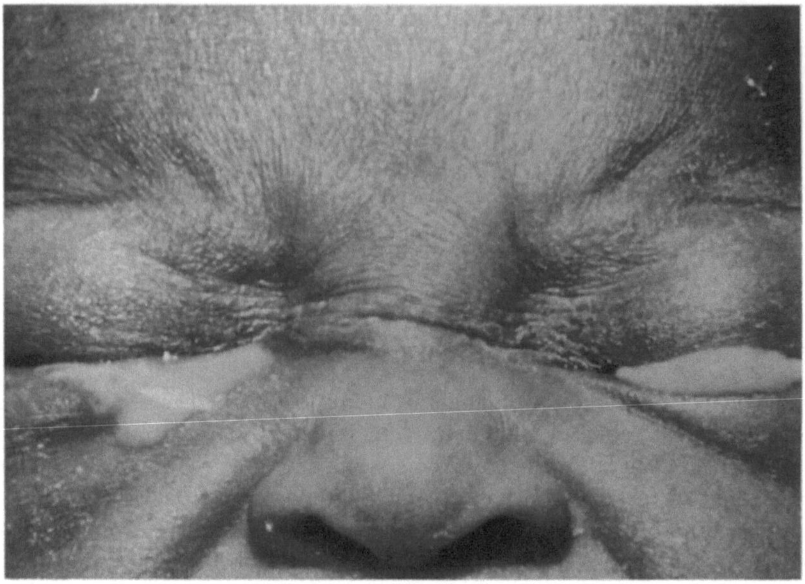

FIGURE 25.1. Gonococcal ophthalmia in a child. Reproduced by permission of Dr. David Oriel, University College Hospital, London, England.

## Chlamydial Infection

### In Adolescents

Chlamydial cervicitis has been reported in 8 to 24.7% of adolescents, with 30 to 60% of those infected being asymptomatic. This infection is more prevalent in pregnant than in nonpregnant teenagers. Ten to thirty percent of cervical chlamydial infections ascend to involve the fallopian tubes; a sexually active 15-year-old in Scandinavia has a 1 in 8 risk of salpingitis, compared with a 1 in 80 risk for a 24-year-old. Physical findings include vaginal discharge, cervical inflammation, and mucopurulent endocervical discharge. In adolescent boys, chlamydia is more common than gonococcal infection. In one series, 46% of boys had significant pyuria and of these, 23% had chlamydia infection [19]. Complications include epididymitis.

### In Neonates

Infection in neonates is a direct reflection of the rate of maternal colonization during pregnancy. Fifteen to twenty percent of exposed infants have upper nasopharyngeal infection, 33% develop pneumonia, and 18 to 50% have conjunctivitis. *C. trachomatis* infection in the mother may also be associated with spontaneous abortion, intrauterine growth retardation, prematurity, and perinatal death; a relationship to the sudden infant death syndrome has been postulated.

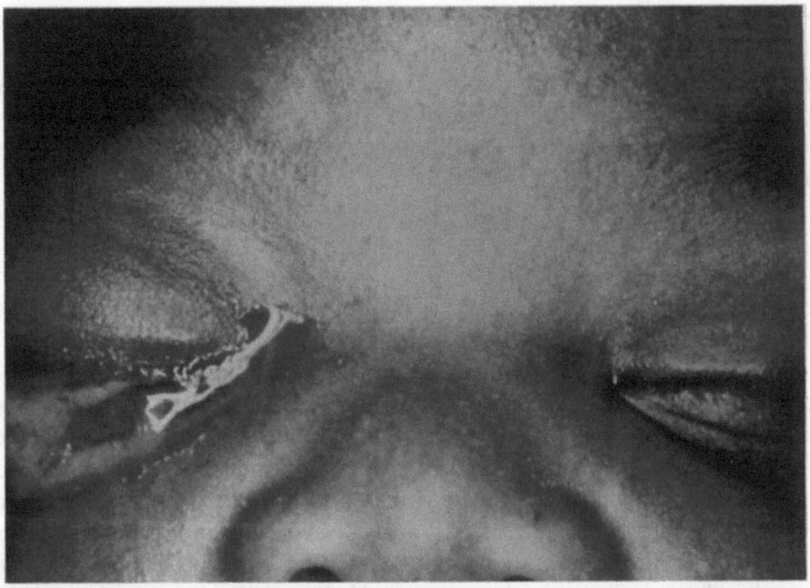

FIGURE 25.2. Chlamydial ophthalmia in a child. Reproduced by permission of Dr. David Oriel, University College Hospital, London, England.

### *Chlamydial Conjunctivitis*

This condition is more common than gonococcal infection as a cause of ophthalmia neonatorum. The onset is usually 5 to 12 days postnatally with a mucoid discharge from one eye. This becomes purulent over several days, with subsequent chemosis, bulbar erythema, and bilateral involvement developing within the first week (Fig. 25.2). From 19 to 83% of infants have nasopharyngeal carriage of chlamydia when first seen. Untreated, the conjunctivitis will clear after several weeks or months, but ocular carriage may persist for over 2 years. Visual acuity is usually unimpaired, but microscopic corneal sequelae are likely to occur if initial treatment is delayed for more than 12 days.

### *Chlamydial Pneumonia*

This condition, first described in 1975, is now one of the most common forms of pneumonia during the first 3 months of life, accounting for 15% of cases of afebrile pneumonia in Dallas, Texas, 25% in Birmingham, Alabama, and 73% in Chicago [19a,b,c]. The diagnosis is based on the clinical syndrome and documentation of nasopharyngeal carriage of *C. trachomatis*. It usually presents between 3 and 11 weeks of age with 1 to 2 weeks of mucoid rhinorrhea. This is followed by a characteristic cough, which is short and repetitive but does not build up to a crescendo and is not followed by emesis. Ninety-five percent of affected infants are afebrile, 50%

have concurrent or previous conjunctivitis, and chest radiology shows hyperexpansion with diffuse interstitial or alveolar infiltrates.

Untreated infants gradually improve after 5 to 7 weeks, but abnormalities in pulmonary function have been described 7 to 8 years after hospitalization for chlamydial pneumonia of infancy [20]. Methods of diagnosis and treatment are summarized in Table 25.3.

## Reiter's Syndrome (RS)

RS is a multisystem disease characterized by urethritis, nonsuppurative arthritis, and conjunctivitis. It occurs in genetically predisposed individuals. The HLA-B27 antigen is present in 76% of affected adults and 86% of children. In Britain and North America RS is associated with nonspecific urethritis, but in other parts of the world it frequently follows diarrheal illness, with nonspecific urethritis occurring in the dysenteric illness. One to three percent of men with nonspecific urethritis subsequently develop RS, but of the 37 pediatric cases reported [20a,b], 70% had diarrhea. Whether intestinal mucosal alteration is an early event causing pathogen multiplication, or whether RS is an immunologic expression following exposure to enteric antigen, is unknown. Two cases have occurred in boys following sexual activity; with the earlier onset and increased frequency of sexual adolescent activity more cases may be reported. In children the course of disease is milder and there are fewer recurrences than in adults. Diagnosis and treatment are the same as in adults (see chap. 9).

## Candidosis

Twenty-eight percent of girls between 2 months and 15 years of age have yeasts as normal vaginal flora [21]. Yeasts are isolated less commonly in 3- to 10-year-olds than in girls younger or olders, as *Candida* tends to flourish in the estrogenic vagina. Its presence should therefore indicate the possibility of sexual abuse [22]. If sexual abuse is excluded, the other predisposing factors are diabetes mellitus; use of broad-spectrum antibiotics, antimitotic agents, or corticosteroid drugs; and in the adolescent, pregnancy or use of contraceptives. The cardinal symptom is pruritus with a curdlike, non-foul-smelling, white discharge, and external dysuria. On examination the vulva may be erythematous and edematous, with white plaques adherent to the vaginal mucosa. The neonate may be affected due to intrapartum infection, presenting with oral candidiasis and skin infections, for example, diaper rash. Methods of diagnosis and treatment are summarized in Table 25.3.

## Gardnerella Vaginitis

*Gardnerella vaginalis* infrequently affects children, since it prefers the estrogenic vagina. When found it should raise suspicion of sexual abuse [22]. The infection may be asymptomatic or there may be a thin copious discharge that has a characteristic pungent amine or fishy odor when 10% potassium hydroxide (KOH) is added to it. Methods of diagnosis and treatment are given in Table 25.3.

## Trichomoniasis

This is uncommon in prepubertal girls, as this organism also prefers an estrogenic environment. Again, if infection is found in this age group, sexual abuse must be considered. Infection may be asymptomatic (3.6% of asymptomatic girls aged 1–9 years had infestation) [22a], or there may be offensive yellow vaginal discharge associated with vulval irritation and pain, external dysuria, and dyspareunia. Infection may be acquired intrapartum with the female infant developing vaginal colonization (as high as 5% of cases). Complications include infection of the urethra and of Bartholin's and Skene's glands. The organism may spread to the fallopian tubes. Methods of diagnosis and treatment are summarized in Table 25.3.

## Chancroid

*H. ducreyi* occurs most commonly in tropical Africa, South America, and the Far East. Following an incubation period of 1 to 8 days (rarely 60 days) a genital ulcer appears, usually on the labium minora in the girl and the prepuce in the boy. Complications include phimosis, paraphimosis, phagedena, and extragenital lesions. Methods of diagnosis and treatment are given in Table 25.3.

## Granuloma Inguinale

*C. granulomatis* has a worldwide distribution but is more prevalent in tropical and subtropical regions. Although sexually transmitted, it is not considered very contagious. The presenting feature is usually a genital ulcer which, if untreated, may enlarge. Complications include fibrosis, neoplastic change, and extragenital lesions. Methods of diagnosis and treatment are given in Table 25.3.

## Lymphogranuloma Venereum

This disease is caused by L1, L2, and L3 immunotypes of *C. trachomatis*. It has three stages: (a) a primary genital lesion, usually a small painless ulcer, 3 to 30 days after exposure, occurring on the glans penis or vaginal wall, followed by (b) lymphadenitis 2 to 6 weeks later, associated with constitutional symptoms and (c) the bubo stage, during which the chronic inflammatory process may progress to fibrosis and lymphatic obstruction, with vaginal and rectal stricture. Methods of diagnosis and treatment are shown in Table 25.3.

## Scabies

*Sarcoptes scabiei* var *hominis*, first identified 300 years ago, occurs in cyclical epidemics at approximately 30-year intervals. Characteristically there is nocturnal itch 4 weeks after infestation, associated with a symmetrical polymorphous eruption of red papules, vesicles, pustules, nodules, and eczematous areas. The burrow is best observed in older children in the finger webs and flexor aspects of the wrists, but in infants and children under 5 years of age they are on the palms and soles and less commonly the legs and buttocks. The differential diagnosis includes atopic dermatitis, contact dermatitis, papular urticaria, prurigo nodularis, lichen planus, dermatitis hepatiformis, herpes gestationis, reticulosis, syphilis, Darier's disease, pityriasis rosea, and vasculitis. Methods of diagnosis and treatment are given in Table 25.3.

## Pediculosis

One third to one half of patients with pediculosis have coexistent STD. Although *Pthirus pubis* prefers the pubic area, the louse is found in various short-haired regions, for example, the perianal area, trunk, legs, beard, and moustache. In children lice in the eyelids are usually *P. pubis*, and this organism may also affect the edges of the scalp in children. Fifty percent of cases may be asymptomatic, but severe pruritus usually occurs about 30 days after infestation. On examination there may be characteristic maculae cerulae. Methods of diagnosis and treatment are summarized in Table 25.3.

## Condyloma Acuminatum

Over 30 or more types of the etiological agent, human papillomavirus (HPV), have been identified. Types 1, 2, 3, 4, and 10 are associated with common skin warts and types 6, 11, 16, and 18 with genital lesions. Condyloma acuminatum was first classified as a venereal disease in 1954. The incidence has increased 459% in the last 15 years in the United States, with most patients being in the 15 to 29-year-old age group. Only 69 cases of genital disease in children have been reported. Transmission to children may occur during delivery, in close nonsexual contact, or from sexual contact, but sexual abuse must always be suspected and carefully excluded before environmental contamination or innocent family contact is assumed. When cases have been reviewed retrospectively, at least 50% had a sexual etiology [22b]. HPV typing may in future be beneficial in this respect. Children with condyloma acuminatum must have close review not only in relation to sexual abuse but also to contagiousness. The child may have been infected with an oncogenic type of HPV—HPV-16 or HPV-18. As the child may symptomatically shed the virus at some point in time, the future sexual partner may be at risk. The incubation period is 3 to 20 months. Then flesh-colored, focal, and verrucous tumors occur on the genital and anorectal area (Fig. 25.3), with cervical lesions being flat and wartlike. These may not be detectable macroscopically, and colposcopy is thus advised in all cases of vulval condyloma acuminatum. The diagnosis is confirmed by histology.

Treatment involves ensuring that the infected parts are kept cool and dry; prompt administration of topical agents, for example, 10 to 20% podophyllin (which should be washed away by the patient after 2–4 hours) and trichloracetic acid; electrocautery; and/or cryotherapy. Use of human lymphoblastoid interferon has been successful in two children [22c] who had been sexually abused; it had the advantage of minimizing further physical and psychologic trauma to these children. Long-term effects have not been evaluated.

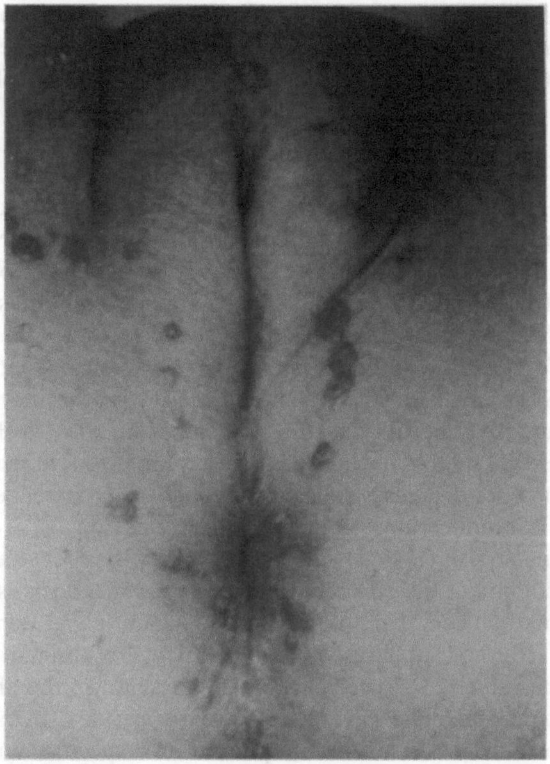

FIGURE 25.3. Perianal warts in a child. Reproduced by permission of Dr. David Oriel, University College Hospital, London, England.

There is a 60% positive history of juvenile laryngeal papillomatosis in children of women who had perineal warts at delivery. Most children present within 1 year with hoarseness (range birth [rare] to 5 years) but any child with hoarseness should be evaluated for juvenile laryngeal papillomatosis. The warty red growths, often multiple, predominantly affect the true cord but also involve the false cord, arytenoid, epiglottis, and frequently the trachea. The lesion is rarely more than 1 cm in diameter. Secondary infection may cause further respiratory distress, and asphyxia may occur. Removal of the lesion is often followed by obstinate recurrences. Although in practically all cases there is spontaneous cure around the time of puberty, due to the high incidence of the condition in children born to mothers with condyloma acuminatum, and the associated morbidity and even mortality, all such mothers should be delivered by cesarean section.

## Molluscum Contagiosum

In the period 1966 to 1983 there has been an 11-fold increase in patient visits to private physicians in the United States because of molluscum contagiosum [22d]. There is some dispute that this condition is sexually acquired in children, but if it is found, and especially if it is confined to the genital area, evidence of sexual abuse should be sought. Flesh-colored papules with central umbilication, which often becomes secondarily infected, occur after an incubation period of 1 week to 6 months. Methods of diagnosis and treatment are shown in Table 25.3.

## Herpes Genitalis

Herpes genitalis is usually caused by herpes simplex virus type II and less commonly by HSV-I. Physician patient consultations for this condition increased 15-fold from 1966 to 1984 in the United States [22e], from 29,560 to 450,570. Although the incidence in children is unknown, in affected children sexual abuse is frequently found. After an incubation period of 4 to 5 days there is a prodromal phase of malaise and fever, followed 2 days later by genital vesicles that readily burst, leaving erosions. Systemic features are common and the lesions may take 6 weeks to heal. Recurrent attacks affect at least 60% of people infected with HSV-II but are less common with HSV-I infection. Most patients have four to five recurrences in the first year but the number decreases subsequently and the recurrences are milder.

Complications include urinary retention or severe constipation (first attack), meningitis (HSV-I), encephalitis (HSV-II; first attack), neonatal infection, and carcinoma of the cervix. The differential diagnosis is herpes zoster, chancroid, traumatic ulcers, carcinoma, erosive balanitis and Behcet's syndrome.

Methods of diagnosis and treatment are summarized in Table 25.3. Serology is of no value [23]. Affected women must inform the obstetrician if they become pregnant and must have at least yearly cervical cytology. Sexual contact should be avoided when lesions are present or suspected, but as fewer than 25% of patients with genital herpes are symptomatic and transmission can frequently be traced to persons with asymptomatic or unrecognized disease, the prospect of increased reporting of infection in adults and neonates unfortunately exists.

Neonatal herpes is estimated as affecting 400 to 1,000 infants annually in the United States [22f]. In the period 1966 to 1969 the incidence was 2.6 cases per 100,000 in King County, Washington; in 1982 it was 28.2 per 100,000 live births [22e]. Primary genital herpes infections in the mother are thought more likely to result in neonatal transmission than recurrent episodes, but most mothers of infants with neonatal herpes in the United States are young, primigravid, white, and asymptomatic at delivery or with no history of genital herpes. Intravenous acyclovir is the drug of first choice in neonatal herpes, but there is still considerable morbidity, even in those infants who survive.

## Acquired Immune Deficiency Syndrome (AIDS)

AIDS is the diagnosis in those who have a reliably diagnosed disease at least moderately indicative of underlying cellular immune deficiency and no known underlying cause of such deficiency, nor any other cause of reduced resistance that might predispose to the diagnosed disease. The AIDS-related complex (ARC) is diagnosed in those with two or more symptoms or signs, or a specific chronic unexplained condition for 3 months or longer, together with two or more abnormal laboratory values and persistent generalized lymphadenopathy (PGL) with nodes present in at least two extrainguinal sites for more than 3 months. The etiological agent is the lymphadenopathy-associated-virus/human T cell lymphotropic virus type III (LAV/HTLV-III) known now as the human immunodeficiency virus (HIV). Nonvertical transmission results in the clinical spectrum of acute HIV disease with a glandular feverlike syndrome; PGL; diffuse pneumonitis, usually due to *Pneumocystis carinii* pneumonia; gastrointestinal manifestations, diarrhea being the common presenting symptom of AIDS; CNS involvement, which includes opportunistic infection by cytomegalovirus, *Cryptococcus neoformans*, and herpes simplex virus causing meningoencephalitis, mass lesions due to toxoplasmosis or CNS lymphomas, progressive multifocal leukoencephalopathy caused by papovavirus, diffuse subacute brain disease, and progressive dementia; skin manifestations; and malignant disease. Approximately 5% of AIDS patients develop non-Hodgkin's lymphoma; Kaposi's sarcoma is particularly prevalent in homosexual men. AIDS in children accounts for approximately 1% of the U.S. cases, typical findings being failure to thrive, persistent candidiasis (resistant oral candidiasis is characteristic), recurrent opportunistic infections, hepatosplenomegaly, lymphadenopathy, interstitial pneumonia, recurrent or protracted diarrhea, and altered immune function. Gram-negative sepsis is a particular feature in children, being reported in 20%. In a life table analysis of 64 affected children younger than age 13 [24], there were two distinct courses: development of *P. carinii* pneumonia, usually at a mean age of onset of 5.5 months, and development of opportunistic infections, occurring at a mean age of 14.3 months. However, length of survival from the time of diagnosis in each group was similar, being slightly less than 3 months, with 75% being dead within 1 year.

Pahwa et al. [25] reviewed 36 children and emphasized the neurologic manifestations of pediatric AIDS infection (five children had microcephaly). Psychomotor retardation is being increasingly recognized in affected children. All 36 children in Pahwa's study had a marked deficit of thymulin; the onset of thymic damage may play a crucial role in determining the evolution of immunodeficiency and disease severity in infected children. One child in this series developed renal tubular acidosis, and this may emerge as a feature of HIV infection. Of note, two children had evidence of HIV in the peripheral blood lymphocytes but were negative for antibody, providing evidence of a seronegative virus-infected state in children. Although horizontal transmission has not been confirmed, an 11-year-old apparently healthy male sibling of a 2-year-old affected child was found to be seropositive. Sexual abuse will have to be excluded before this can be considered as transmission of virus via body secretion.

At present vertical transmission and transmission by breast feeding appear to be the predominant sources of infection to the newborn. Sixty-seven cases of AIDS have been diagnosed in 12,000 to 17,000 hemophilia patients in the United States [25a], a frequency of 0.5%. This suggests a less severe infection in hemophilia patients than in homosexual men exposed to HIV. It may be that chronic activation of the immune system by factor VIII concentrate may prepare it for more vigorous response after HIV infection. Chapter 21 in this volume discusses methods of diagnosis and treatment. Table 25.5 summarizes treatment.

TABLE 25.5. Treatment of AIDS.

| | |
|---|---|
| Immune reconstruction | Alpha-interferon<br>Gamma-interferon<br>Interleukin-2<br>Isoprinosine |
| Antiviral action | Suramine<br>HPA-23 (antimoniotungstate)<br>Foscarnate<br>Azidodeoxythymidine |
| Specific therapy | |
| Kaposi's sarcoma | Vinblastin, 4–8 mg* in weekly doses |
| *P. carinii* pneumonia | Cotrimoxazole, 15–20 mg/kg/day × 21 days<br>Pentamadine, 4 mg/kg/day × 21 days |
| Cytomegalovirus | DHPG BW 795 U — Gancyclovir 5 mg/kg IV every 12 hours for 2 weeks; maintenance 5 mg/kg IV daily |
| *T. gondii* infection | Pyrimethamine 25 mg/day* + sulfadoxine 100 mg/kg/day to maximum of 8 g + 1-2 tablets folinic acid* for 6 weeks; maintenance pyrimethamine 50 mg + sulfadoxine 1 g weekly |
| Cryptococcus neoformans | Amphotericin B 0.3 mg/kg/day for 6 weeks; maintenance flucytosine 100 mg/kg/day |

*Weight-related dose for pediatric patients.

## Hepatitis

Although this may be due to a number of conditions, viral hepatitis is traditionally restricted as being due to hepatitis A (HAV), hepatitis B (HBV), and hepatitis non-A non-B (HNANB). These have incubation periods respectively of 3 to 5 weeks, 5 to 28 weeks, and 2 to 26 weeks. HAV is transmitted via the intestinal-oral route and is an important pathogen for homosexuals, with the annual incidence in susceptible homosexuals being 22%. The risk of infection depends on the number and frequency of partners involved in oral-anal sex.

If an adolescent has indulged in homosexual activity or a child has been abused, human normal immunoglobulin (HNIG) provides effective protection if given within 2 weeks of exposure. The dose is 250 mg IM in children and 500 mg IM in adolescents. HBV can be recognized by several antigens, including HBsAg, which is an indicator of carrier infection. Such carriers occur in 0.1 to 0.2% of the population in the United Kingdom, 5% in Mediterranean areas, and up to 20% in tropical countries. HBeAg indicates high levels of HBsAG viral activity and infectivity. HBV is transmitted by sexual contact, particularly in homosexuals and especially if there has been rectal intercourse. HBV transmission also occurs in 20 to 50% of infected mothers. The infected infants have a 60 to 90% chance of being chronic carriers of HBV with risk of chronic liver disease. Those exposed, for example, infants or children who have been abused, may be given the specific hepatitis B immunoglobulin (HBIG), 500 mg in 5 ml if over 10 years of age, 250 mg in 2.5 ml if less than 10 years old. This must be given within 48 hours of exposure and the dose repeated if there is recurrent or ongoing infection after 1 month. HNANB is the most common cause of posttransfusion hepatitis in the Western world, but there is no real evidence of sexual transmission.

## Cytomegalovirus

Cytomegalovirus is present in 90% of homosexual men and is found in 65% of patients with AIDS or PGL. Most young adults are asymptomatic but occasionally have headache, backache, abdominal pain, or sore throat. On examination there may be pharyngitis, hepatosplenomegaly, and occasionally jaundice and polyneuritis. Methods of diagnosis and treatment are summarized in Table 25.3. Sixty to seventy percent of pregnant women have serum antibodies on initial attendance at the antenatal clinic, and 1 to 4% develop primary infection during pregnancy. Congenital cytomegalovirus infection is symptom- and sign-free in 95% of infants, with those who develop features having jaundice, hepatosplenomegaly, microcephaly, encephalitis, chorioretinitis, pneumonia, and rash. Complications include sensorineural deafness and mental retardation.

## Balanitis

Poor hygiene and a tight prepuce predispose to balanitis. The condition is frequently caused by yeast, streptococci and certain anaerobic bacteria, and occasionally by *T. vaginalis*. Diabetes and broad-spectrum antibiotics may exacerbate candidal balanitis. On examination there may be patchy erythema or superficial erosions, while thin purulent secretions suggest trichomoniasis. The diagnosis is made clinically, with confirmation by microscopy and culture. Treatment includes scrupulous hygiene; topical nystatin cream twice a day for candidisis; oral metronidazole, 15 mg/kg/day in three divided doses for 7 days to a maximum daily dose of 250 mg if less than 10 years, and 400 mg twice a day for 5 days if over age 10 for trichomonal or anaerobic infection; and cotrimoxazole, two twice a day for 7 days with subsequent reduction if under age 10 for streptococcus infection.

Complications include phimosis, paraphimosis, and phagedena. Specific forms of balanitis are circinate balanitis, Stevens-Johnson syndrome, Behçet's syndrome, balanitis xerotica obliterans (lichen sclerosus), and erythroplasia of Queyrat. The last requires histology for differentiation.

## Vulvitis

Vulvitis is the most frequent gynecologic problem among prepubertal girls. The prepubertal vulva and vagina lack the protection of the labial fat pads and pubic hair, thick estrogenised vaginal mucosa, and acidic pH of the adult. In addition, the close anatomic vicinity of the rectum promotes fecal material contamination. Poor perineal hygiene may also contribute. Although vulvitis is usually nonspecific, the cause must always be sought and treated. In all cases good hygiene practice should be taught to patients and parents.

## Behçet's Syndrome

Behçet's syndrome is a chronic multisystem disease of unknown etiology causing oral and genital ulceration and eye inflammation. It is more common in certain countries, for example, Turkey and Japan. It is not considered sexually transmitted, but may occur in families, and a genetic predisposition may be responsible. The differential diagnosis is Stevens-Johnson syndrome, syphilis, and hand-foot-and-mouth disease. Although there is no one specific therapy, levamisole has been helpful [26].

## Proctitis

Proctitis can affect both boys and girls and may be asymptomatic or manifest as discharge or bleeding. On examination there may be no abnormality, erythema, or mucopus. It is due to *N. gonorrhoea*, *N. meningitidis*, *C. trachomatis*, *T. pallidum*, other spirochetal infections, human papillomavirus, herpes simplex virus, and non-specific causes, for example, trauma, allergy, idiopathic bowel disease (Crohn's and solitary ulcer syndrome), shigellosis, salmonellosis, *Campylobacter*, amebiasis, and *Giardiasis*. Gonococcal and chlamydial proctitis was once thought to be due to contamination. It is now thought that all gonococcal proctitis in girls is due to direct penile anal penetration, and 55% of asymptomatic and 75% of symptomatic women with chlamydial proctitis admit to anal intercourse [25b].

The other infections have already been discussed. Shigellosis is due to fecal contamination of food. About 30 to 60% of those infected in the major cities in the United States are male homosexuals. *Salmonella* requires a high dose, $10^{-5}$ to $10^{-7}$, of organisms to produce enterocolitis. It can rarely be transmitted sexually, due to oroanal intercourse.

*Campylobacter jejuni* may also be transmitted in this way. Amebiasis caused by *Entamoeba histolytica* is rare in temperate climates unless there has been overseas travel. It has now been described in homosexuals in the United States, and is thought to be transmitted by oroanal or penorectal intercourse followed by orogenital contact. Giardiasis has also been reported in homosexual men; the route again is thought to be oroanal transmission. Methods for diagnosis and treatment of these various conditions are described in Table 25.3.

Of note, anal cancer, a rare condition, has a higher incidence in homosexual men. With the reported high incidence of sodomy in sexually abused children and the increasing rate of anal intercourse reportedly occurring in voluntary activity, it is essential that proctitis be sought for in any child suspected of having an STD.

## Cervical Carcinoma

Invasive cervical cancer is the third most common genital cancer in the United States, with 45,000 new cases of carcinoma-in-situ being detected annually. It is thought to be related to early marriage, two or more marriages, voluntary intercourse before the age of 20, and two or more sexual partners. Many regard it as a venereal disease. Although there is no direct evidence for a transmissible agent, there is a strong association between herpes simplex virus type II and human papillomavirus. Preinvasive or invasive lesions develop in the transformation zone, which is the area originally covered by columnar epithelium that has now been replaced by squamous epithelium through metaplasia. Three phases have been associated with the most active metaplastic changes: late fetal life, adolescence, and first pregnancy. It is the immature metaplastic cell of the ectocervix which is believed to be susceptible to genetic alteration by some sexually transmitted agent. This explains why the sexually active teenager, especially one with multiple partners, is at greater risk for development of preinvasive cervical lesions.

## Sexual Abuse

The increase in incidence of sexual abuse—one in every four preadolescent and adolescent girls in the United States is abused each year—means that every physician must be aware of this problem. Indications may be behavioral, for example, insomnia, fearful dreams, night terrors, generalized withdrawal, clinging behavior, separation anxiety, enuresis, encopresis, excessive masturbation, and sexually explicit acts. The detailed physical examination must include specific attention to erythema, bruising, lacerations, discharge, and relaxation of the pubococcygeal muscles. The normal dimensions for the hymenal opening are 4 mm for a child under age 5 and 5 mm for a child between 5 and 10 years of age. Synechiae or adhesions between the hymen and labia minora may also indicate sexual abuse. Separation of the buttocks usually causes anal sphincter contraction, but a sodomized victim shows a paradoxical relaxation. Gentle stroking of the perineal skin usually causes sphincter contraction, but this reflex is lost following sodomy. Anorectal skin tags may be missing, and there may be hyperpigmentation and a thickening of the skin around the anus. Colposcopic assessment of the vulva, with photographic documentation, may be helpful. There must be detailed clinical and laboratory investigation of all STDs, with a review appropriate to the long incubation periods these diseases may have. Not only must any infection be treated, but the possibility of pregnancy must be considered. Two thirds of abused children are emotionally disturbed, not only by the offence but by its consequences, and long-term support is necessary.

## Conclusion

The decrease in effectiveness of the church and subsequent lowering of moral values and codes may have contributed to the increasing incidence of sexual abuse. Whatever the cause, the net result of mounting pressure on young adolescents to indulge in early sexual activity and with more frequent partners and increasing incidence of homosexual activity has been a marked increase in the incidence of sexually transmitted diseases in children. Physicians must not only be aware of the problem, searching for it in all suspicious cases, but must remember that such a disease is an indication of sexual abuse until proven otherwise. Not only do abused children have the problem of the actual abuse, with resulting possible infection and pregnancy, but some sexually transmitted diseases have oncogenic potential. Such children require close review and supportive therapy.

## References


1. Herman-Giddens M: Condylomata acuminata in children and sexual abuse. *Genitourin Med* **6**:68, 1985.
2. Hayman CR, Lanza C: Sexual assault on women and girls. *Am J Obstet Gynecol* **109**:480–486, 1971.
3. Edward JR, Gold EM: Epidemiology and management of sexual assault victims. *Obstet Gynecol* **53**:381–387, 1979.
4. Kaufman A, Vandermeer J, DiVasto P, et al: Follow-up of rape victims in a family practice setting. *South Med J* **69**:1569–1571, 1976.
5. Holmstrom LL, Burgess AW: Sexual behavior of assailants during reported rapes. *Arch Sex Behav* **9**:427–439, 1980.
6. Rimsza ME, Niggemann EH: Medical evaluation of sexually abused children: A review of 311 cases. *Pediatrics* **69**:8–14, 1982.
7. McClure EM, Stack MR, Tanner T, et al: Pharyngeal culturing and reporting of pediatric gonorrhea in Connecticut. *Pediatrics* **78**:509–510, 1986.
8. Nair P, Glazer-Semmel E, Gould C, et al: *Neisseria gonorrhoeae* in asymptomatic prepubertal household contacts of children with gonococcal infection. *Clin Pediat* **25**:160–163, 1986.
9. Tilelli JA, Turek D, Jaffe AC: Sexual abuse of children: Clinical findings and implications for management. *N Engl J Med* **302**:319–323, 1980.
10. Finkel KC: Sexual abuse of children in Canada. *Can Med Assoc J* **130**:345,348, 1984.
11. Miller J, Moeller D, Kaufman A, et al: Recidivism among sex assault victims. *Am J Psychiat* **135**:1103–1104, 1978.
12. Badgley RF (Chmn): *Sexual Offenses Against Children*. Report of the Committee on Sexual Offenses Against Children and Youths (Cat No. J2-50/1984E). Ottawa: Departments of Justice and of National Health and Welfare, 1984.
13. Frau LM, Alexander ER: Public health implications of sexually transmitted diseases in pediatric practice. *Pediatr Infect Dis* **4**:453–467, 1985.
14. Thirumoorthy T, Lee CT, Lim KB: Epidemiology of infectious syphilis in Singapore. *Genitourin Med* **62**:75–77, 1986.
15. Alausa KO, Osoba AO: Epidemiology of gonococcal vulvovaginitis among children in the tropics. *Br J Vener Dis* **56**:239–242, 1980.
16. Demmler GJ, Wells D, Heitkamp JW, et al: *Neisseria gonorrhoeae* ventriculoperitoneal shunt infection in a child. *Pediatr Infect Dis* **4**:419–420, 1985.
17. Hammerschlag MR: Infection due to penicillinase-producing *Neisseria gonorrhoeae* in a sexually abused girl. *Pediatr Infect Dis* **5**:603, 1986.

17a. Kraus YW, Yen SSC: Gonorrhea during pregnancy. *Obstet Gynecol* **31**:258–260, 1968.
17b. Cave VY, Bloomfield RD, Hurdle ES, et al: Gonorrhea in the obstetric and gynecology clinic: Incidence in a voluntary hospital in an urban community. *JAMA* **210**:309, 1969.
17c. Spence MR: Gonorrhea in a military prenatal population. *Obstet Gynecol* **42**:223, 1973.
17d. Corman LB, Levison ME, Knight R, et al: The high frequency of pharyngeal gonococcal infection in a prenatal clinic population. *JAMA* **230**:568, 1974.
17e. Jones DED, Brame RY, Jones BP: Gonorrhea in obstetric patients. *Am Vener Dis Assoc* **2**:30–32, 1976.
17f. Edwards LE, Barrada MI, Hamann AA, et al: Gonorrhea in pregnancy. *Am J Obstet Gynecol* **132**:637–641, 1978.

18. Hammerschlag MR, Doraiswamy B, Alexander ER, et al: Are rectogenital chlamydial infections a marker of sexual abuse in children? *Pediatr Infect Dis* **3**:100–104, 1984.
19. Adger H, Shafer M-A, Sweet RL, et al: Screening for *Chlamydia trachomatis* and *Neisseria gonorrhoeae* in adolescent males: Value of first-catch urine examination. *Lancet* **2**:944–945, 1984.
19a. Rettig PJ: Infections due to Chlamydia trachomatis from infancy to adolescence. *Pediatr Infect Dis* **5**:449–457, 1986.
19b. Stagno S, Braskield DM, Brown MB, et al: Infant pneumonitis associated with cytomegalovirus, Chlamydia, Pneumocystis and Ureaplasma: A prospective study. *Pediatrics* **322**-329, 1981.
19c. Tipple MA, Beem MO, Saxon EM: Clinical characteristics of the afebrile pneumonia associated with Chlamydia trachomatis infection in infants less than 6 months of age. *Pediatrics* **63**:192–197, 1979.
20. Weiss SG, Newcomb RW, Beem MO: Pulmonary assessment of children after chlamydial pneumonia of infancy. *J Pediatr* **5**:659–664, 1986.
20a. Rosenberg AM, Petty RE: Reiter's disease in children. *Am J Dis Child* **133**:394–398, 1979.
20b. Sehgal VN, Koranne RV, Shyam Prasad AL: Unusual manifestations of Reiter's disease in a child. *Dermatologia* **170**:77–79, 1985.
21. Hammerschlag MR, Alpert S, Rosner I, et al: Microbiology of the vagina in children: Normal and potentially pathogenic organisms. *Pediatrics* **62**:57–62, 1978.
22. De Jong AR: Vaginitis due to *Gardnerella vaginalis* and to *Candida albicans* in sexual abuse. *Child Abuse Neglect* **9**:27–29, 1985.
22a. Jones JY, Vamauchi T, Lambert B: Trichomoniasis vaginalis infestation in sexually abused girls. *Am J Dis Child* **139**:840–847, 1985.
22b. Shelton TB, Jerkins YR, Noe HN: Condyloma acuminatum in the pediatric patient. *J Urol* **135**:548–549, 1986.
22c. Trofater KY Jr, English PB, Hughes BE, et al: Human lymphoblastoid interferon (Wellferon) in primary therapy of two children with condylomata acuminatum. *Obstet Gynecol* **67**137–140, 1986.
22d. Becker TM, Blount JH, Douglas J, et al: Trends in molluscum contagiosum in the United States. *Sexually Transmitted Dis* **13**:89–92, 1986.
22e. Becker TM, Stone KM, Cates WJ: Epidemiology of genital herpes infections in the United States: The current situation. *J Reprod Med* **31**:3[illegible]-364, 1986.
22f. Nahmias AJ, Keyserling HL, Kerrick GM: Herpes simplex. In: Infectious Diseases of the Fetus and Newborn Infant. Third edition. SJ Remington, JO Klein (Eds.). Philadelphia, W.B. Saunders, 1983, p. 636–678.
23. Lavery HA, Connolly JH, Russell JD: Incidence of herpes genitalis in Northern Ireland in 1973–83 and herpes simplex types 1 and 2 isolated in 1982–84. *Genitourin Med* **62**:24–27, 1986.
24. Lampert R, Milberg J, O'Donnell R, et al: Life table analysis of children with acquired immunodeficiency syndrome. *Pediatr Infect Dis* **5**:374–375, 1986.
25. Pahwa S, Kaplan M, Fikrig S, et al: Spectrum of human T-cell lymphotropic virus type III infection in children: Recognition of symptomatic, asymptomatic and seronegative patients. *JAMA* **265**:2299–2305, 1986.
25a. Changing patterns of acquired immunodeficiency syndrome in hemophilia patients: United States. *MMWR* **34**:241, 1985.
25b. Stamm WE, Quinn TB, Mkrtichian EE, Wang S-P, Schuffler MD, Holmes KK: Chlamydial pruritis. In: Chlamydial infections. PA Maroh, KK Holmes, JD Oriel, et al (Eds.). Elsevier Biomedical Press, Amsterdam, 1982, p. 111–114.
26. Lavery HA, Pinkerston JH: Successful treatment of Behçet's syndrome with levamisole. *Br J Dermatol* **113**:372–373, 1985.

CHAPTER 26

# Dermatologic Manifestations of Sexually Transmitted Diseases in the Canine

Kevin Shanley

## Introduction

Most sexually transmitted diseases (STDs) in veterinary medicine do not have dermatologic manifestations and therefore are inherently different from many STDs in human medicine. As such, this group of diseases is addressed by the specialty of theriogenology, which is defined in *Dorland's Illustrated Medical Dictionary* as "that branch of veterinary medicine which deals with reproduction, including the physiology and pathology of male and female reproductive systems and the clinical practice of veterinary obstetrics, gynecology and semenology." The American College of Theriogenologists was recognized by the American Veterinary Medical Association as a distinct specialty in 1974.

There are numerous STDs of large animals (bovine, equine, porcine, ovine, caprine) and very few in small animals (canine, feline). Contagious dermatologic diseases that may be transmitted by direct contact during copulation include

Sarcoptic mange: *Sarcoptes scabiei* (canine, porcine, ovine, bovine, equine)
notoedric mange: *Notoedres cati* (feline)
Psoroptic mange: *Psoroptes ovis* (ovine, bovine)
Pediculosis (canine, feline, ovine, caprine, bovine, equine, porcine)
Cheyletiellosis: *Cheyletiella blakei* and *C. yasquri* (canine, feline)
Chorioptic mange: *Chorioptes bovis* (bovine, ovine)
Dermatophytosis: *Microsporum canis*, *M. gypseum*, *Trichophyton mentagrophytes* (canine, feline); *T. equinum*, *T. mentagrophytes*, *M. canis*, *M. gypseum* (equine); *T. verrucosum*, *T. mentagrophytes* (bovine); *M. nanum* (porcine); *T. mentagrophytes* (caprine, ovine)
Psorgatic mange: *Psorgates ovis* (ovine, bovine)
Ticks and ked infestation: *Melophagus ovinus* (ovine)

I have chosen to discuss only those venereally transmitted diseases that frequently present with dermatologic signs. This small group of diseases includes transmissible venereal tumor and *Brucella canis*, both seen only in the dog.

# Transmissible Venereal Tumor

## Overview

Canine transmissible venereal tumor (TVT) is the first known transplantable tumor [1]. It is probably a naturally occurring allograft tumor [1–3] and may affect genital or extragenital locations. TVT is equally common in both sexes and is found most frequently in free-roaming, sexually active, young, large-breed dogs in a congested urban setting [4]. In one study, 83% of affected dogs weighed more than 20 kg, 30% were German Shepherds, and 87% were younger than 5 years old [4]. TVT is endemic in the southern United States, Puerto Rico, and parts of Africa, Europe, and South America [5]. Although spontaneously regressing TVT is common in the experimental setting, it is probably a rare phenomenon in nature [2,4]. Chemotherapy is effective in most cases.

## Synonyms

Synonyms are transmissible sarcoma, transmissible lymphosarcoma, contagious venereal tumor, TVT, venereal lymphosarcoma, infectious granuloma, Sticker tumor, venereal granuloma, and transmissible venereal sarcoma.

## Definition

Canine transmissible venereal tumor is an uncommon, usually benign round-cell tumor seen in young adult dogs. It usually is transmitted by coitus.

## Clinical Findings

TVT usually manifests in the genital area, although it may be found in extragenital sites. In the male dog, TVT is found most frequently on the penile shaft, on the preputial mucosa, or on the haired skin of the external prepuce (see Figs. 26.1 and 26.2). In females, the most common genital site is the vaginal vestibule, although the tumor can be seen externally at or near the mucocutaneous junction. Large TVTs near the female urethral orifice may cause dysuria. Extragenital sites of TVT in males and females include the dermis or panniculus of the neck, trunk, extremities, and head. They have also been found in the oral and nasal cavities.

Genital TVTs usually begin as pale-pink to intensely hyperemic masses varying in size from 0.1 to 15 cm in diameter (average 3–6 cm) [6,7]. They tend to grow rapidly at first, then slowly later on, which may suggest inhibition by the immune system [8]. As they grow they take on a more lobulated, papillomatous or cauliflowerlike appearance and usually are sessile, but may be pedunculated. Genital TVTs are often friable and easily traumatized, leading to ulceration, hemorrhage, and secondary bacterial infection. A common presenting complaint, particularly in males, is the presence of a serosanguinous to hemorrhagic genital exudate [1].

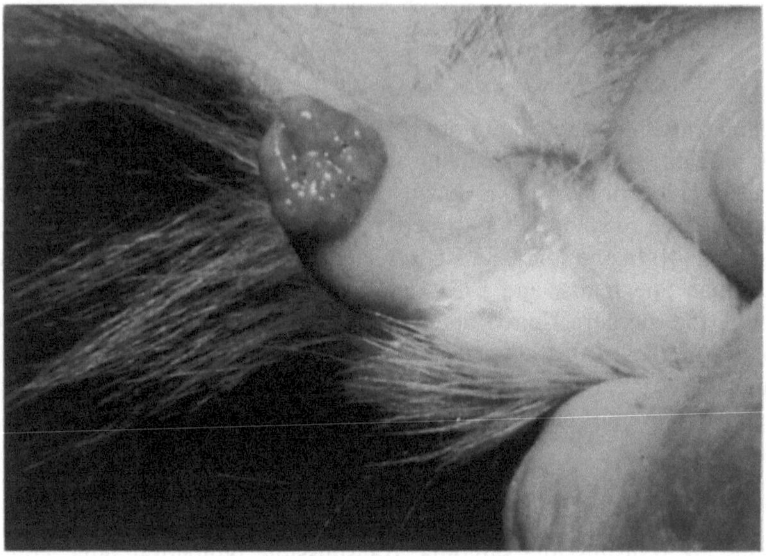

FIGURE 26.1. Well demarcated TVT of the exteriorized penis.

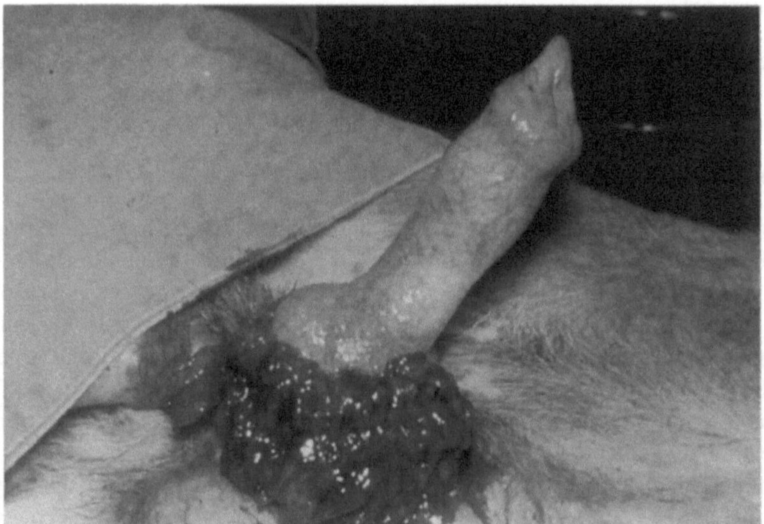

FIGURE 26.2. Transmissible venereal tumor with a hemorrhagic surface at the base of the penile shaft.

TVTs involving extragenital anatomic sites are considered to be naturally occurring allograft transplantations of tumor cells due to licking or biting [1,2]. Extragenital TVTs are usually well circumscribed and tend to be less friable, pedunculated, and lobulated than genital TVTs. True metastatic disease is considered rare [2,4], but has been reported to involve the internal iliac lymph nodes (female); the superficial inguinal and lumbar lymph nodes (male); and the brain, eye, thoracic and abdominal viscera, and panniculus. Dogs with poor nutrition and concurrent diseases may have a higher incidence of metastatic disease [2].

## Histopathology

The TVT is classified as a round-cell tumor of skin and genital mucosa. On routine hematoxylin and eosin sections, vascular stroma, which separates large sheets of cells, is minimal. The cells are round to polyhedral in shape with a large nucleus and variable amounts of cytoplasm (see Figs. 26.3 and 26.4). Average cell diameter is 17 μ [5]. The nuclei often contain one or two prominent nucleoli with marked chromatin clumping. Mitotic figures are common and there is a variable nucleocytoplasmic ratio [1]. The cytoplasm may have a vacuolated appearance due to the presence of lipid droplets [5]. Aggregates of lymphocytes are scattered diffusely throughout the tumor parenchyma, primarily in a perivascular location. Other cells involved with the local host reaction include plasma cells and macrophages.

## Natural History

TVT has worldwide distribution and has been recognized since 1876 [1]. It is the first known transmissible and transplantable tumor. The etiology of TVT is unknown. Although several inconsistent reports in the literature suggest the presence of a virus or of viruslike particles, most experimental evidence does not support a viral etiology. Transmission of the tumor by cell-free filtrates has occurred but is not consistently reproducible [3].

The most plausible explanation is that TVT is a naturally occurring allograft that is transplanted to a susceptible host at the site of damaged genital, nasal, ocular, or oral mucosa or via injection into the dermis or panniculus from a bite wound [1,3,4]. TVTs from different cell lines of widely varying geographic locations have almost identical histocompatibility antigens. Chromosome studies further support the TVT cell transplantation theory rather than a viral etiology. A negatively heteropyknotic marker chromosome is present in most TVT cells, regardless of geographic origin [9]. A unique feature of TVT is that its cells usually contain 59 chromosomes (range of 57–64) compared with the normal canine karyotype of 78 chromosomes. All except the sex chromosomes in normal canine cells are acrocentric. The presence of approximately 15 to 19 metacentric or submetacentric chromosomes in canine TVT cells suggests an end-to-end fusion of numerous pairs of acrocentric chromosomes, leading to a reduction in the normal chromosome number of 78 in TVT cells [9]. Autoradiographic studies also support the cellular mode of transmission [1].

FIGURE 26.3. Histopathology of a TVT. Note minimal stroma, monotonous sheets of cells with large nuclei and variable amounts of cytoplasm. (Hematoxylin & eosin, 10X).

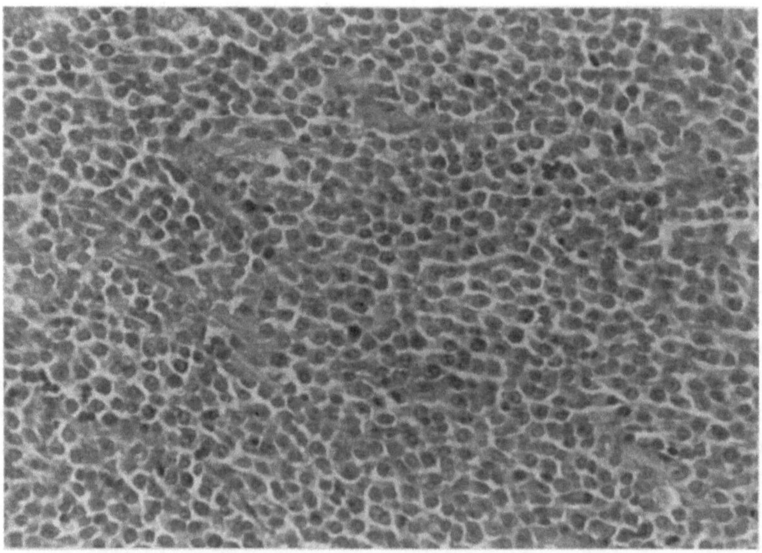

FIGURE 26.4. Close-up view of Fig. 25.3 (Hematoxylin and eosin, 25X).

The behavior of the TVT is probably linked to a modification of the host immune response to the major histocompatibility antigens, although the exact mechanism is unknown. Spontaneous regression of experimentally induced TVT has been reported frequently. Although this has not been documented in naturally occurring TVT, it probably can occur [2,4].

## Complications

Complications due to TVT are uncommon. Metastatic disease occurs in less than 5% of patients. The most common metastatic sites include the regional lymph nodes, eye, spleen, and brain. Intranasal TVTs can cause epistaxis and sneezing. Genital TVT in females may block the urethral orifice and cause dysuria, hematuria, and stanguria. TVTs frequently are located at easily traumatized sites, which may predispose them to secondary bacteria infection.

## Differential Diagnosis

Genital TVT should be differentiated from other genital tumors including leiomyoma, lipoma, leiomyosarcoma, and fibroma in the female and papilloma and squamous cell carcinoma in the male [5]. In females, leiomyomas are seen more frequently than TVTs, but the patient is older (average age 10.6 years), and the tumor is noninvasive, nonmetastatic, and grows slowly. Leiomyoma is usually found as an incidental lesion at necropsy or during an ovariohysterectomy [5]. Other tumors of the female genitalia are found less frequently than TVTs. In males, primary or metastatic tumor of the penis or prepuce other than TVT is rare.

Extragenital TVT should be differentiated from other round-cell tumors including canine histiocytoma, mast cell tumor, cutaneous lymphosarcoma, and neuroendocrine carcinoma (Merkel cell tumor). Cytologic examination of TVT shows numerous round to pleomorphic cells containing large basophilic nuclei with clumped chromatin and one or two nucleoli (Fig. 26.5). The pale, basophilic cytoplasm is variable in amount; may have several large vacuoles from lipid accumulation; and has distinct borders. Mast cell tumors are readily differentiated from TVTs due to the metachromatic staining of cytoplasmic granules, the presence of numerous eosinophils, and a low mitotic index. Cutaneous lymphosarcoma cells have minimal cytoplasm and deeply basophilic homogeneous nuclei. Canine cutaneous histiocytoma (CCH) is more difficult to differentiate from TVT, as it also has a high mitotic index and affects young dogs. CCH is commonly found on the head and limbs and is a firm, alopecic, button-shaped, well-circumscribed dermoepidermal tumor. The cells characteristically are pleomorphic with large amounts of cytoplasm. They do not contain the vacuoles that can be associated with TVT. Also, the cytoplasm is more eosinophilic on H and E staining, and nucleoli often are absent. Histiocytoma is frequently associated with a lymphocytic infiltrate at the base of the tumor, whereas TVT has numerous aggregates of lymphocytes dispersed throughout the tumor. CCH is much more common than TVT.

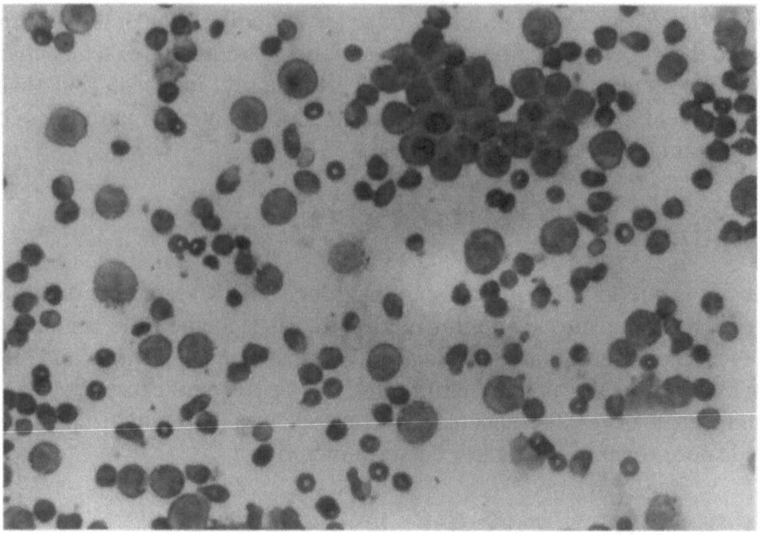

FIGURE 26.5. Cytology of a TVT from a fine needle aspirate. Note round cells with large basophilic nuclei and variable amounts of pale, basophilic cytoplasm. (Diff-Quick stain).

## MANAGEMENT

Numerous therapeutic modalities have been used to treat TVT, including surgical excision, radiation therapy, and chemotherapy. Immunotherapy using serum from dogs in remission from TVT has been successful in an experimental setting [1]. Surgical therapy has been associated with local recurrence of the TVT in approximately 20 to 25% of genital cases [2,6] and in 60% of cases of extragenital TVT [6]. TVT is quite radiosensitive, but this mode of therapy is available only at large referral hospitals. Radiation doses of 450 to 500 rads given once or twice usually are curative.

The therapy of choice in most instances is chemotherapy. TVT is most sensitive to vincristine sulfate or doxorubicin. Vincristine sulfate is less expensive and has fewer side effects than doxorubicin. The dosage for vincristine sulfate is 0.5 mg/m² of body surface area given IV once weekly for two to seven treatments. Doxorubicin is given in a dosage of 30 mg/m² of body surface area IV every 21 days for two to three treatments [1,3,5,6]. Combination chemotherapy using vincristine sulfate and methotrexate with either prednisone or cyclophosphamide also has been used successfully [1,3,5].

## PROGNOSIS

In most cases, the prognosis for TVT is good. Chemotherapy and radiation therapeutic regimens consistently provide complete cure in 80 to 95% of tumors.

# Brucellosis

## Overview

Canine brucellosis is a nonfatal, contagious bacterial disease of dogs. It is transmitted most frequently by contact with postabortion vaginal discharge, venereally, or by contact with other mucosal surfaces. It is difficult to diagnose due to its insidious nature and variety of clinical presentations. It is a zoonotic disease. Therapy in canines usually is unsuccessful.

## Synonyms

Synonyms for brucellosis are canine brucellosis and beagle fever.

## Definition

Canine brucellosis is caused by the intracellular bacteria *Brucella canis*, which is a small, nonmotile, gram-negative coccobacillus. It is a rough strain of *Brucella* and therefore has less endotoxin and causes less cellular damage or pyrexic reaction compared with smooth strains of *Brucella*.

# Clinical Findings

Canine brucellosis is most common in hunting breeds, but affects all breeds. Although there is no age or sex predilection [10], sexually mature, intact dogs that are free roaming or exposed to large numbers of other dogs are more likely to become infected. Exposure may occur at field trials, obedience schools, dog shows, or boarding and breeding kennels.

No specific signs are diagnostic for brucellosis. In fact, many infected dogs are asymptomatic. Dogs usually are afebrile, as *B. canis* lacks the lipopolysaccharide cell wall constituent of other brucella organisms that is associated with endotoxic properties [11]. When present, dermatologic signs usually are limited to a scrotal dermatitis or dull dry haircoat. The scrotal dermatitis occurs within 5 weeks postinfection and is characterized by alopecia, mild to moderate erythema primarily affecting the ventral aspect of the scrotum, a moist serous exudate, and occasionally multifocal yellow to brown crusting (Fig. 26.6). A superficial secondary bacterial infection with *Staphlococcus intermedius* often is present. These lesions are probably due to excessive licking by the dog because of an underlying epididymitis, rather than invasion of the skin by brucella organisms. *Brucella canis*, however, has been cultured from the sanguinopurulent discharge from the skin over the lateral hocks and right forepaw in a Beagle bitch with nodular pyogranulomatous dermatitis [12].

Another common finding associated with brucella infection in male dogs is an enlarged scrotum, due to serosanguinous exudate accumulation in the tunics and

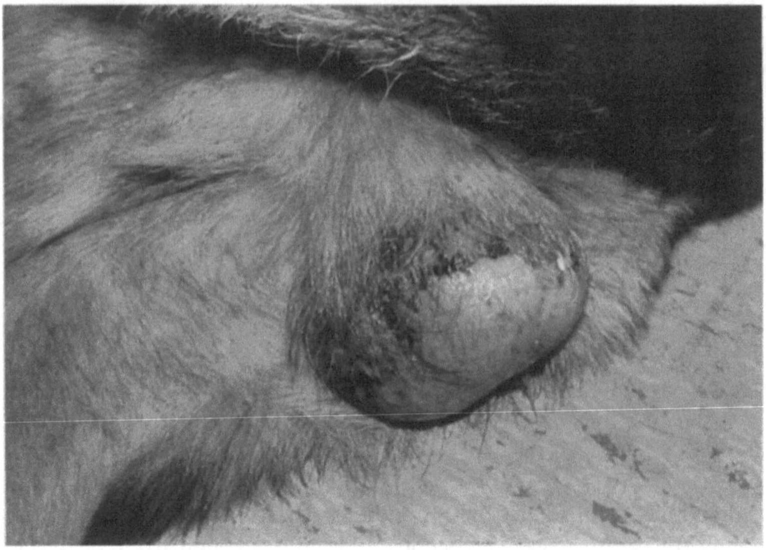

FIGURE 26.6. Erythema, erosion and serous exudation typical of scrotal dermatitis due to Brucellosis.

inflammation of the tail of the epididymis (Fig. 26.7). In bitches, the primary clinical finding is abortion. Brucella abortions are most common during days 45 to 55 of the 63-day canine gestation period [13]. Most aborted pups are dead or die within 48 hours and may be autolyzed. Surviving pups are bacteremic and hyperglobulinemic, usually have a generalized peripheral lymphadenopathy, and may be febrile with a leukocytosis [11]. A mucoid to serosanguinous vaginal discharge can persist for up to 6 weeks in affected bitches. The dogs subsequently may have normal litters, additional abortions, reduced litter sizes, or intermittent reproductive failures [11,13,14]. Brucellosis may cause undetected early embryonic death with abortion or fetal resorption during days 10 to 35 of gestation, and may be perceived as a lack of conception. Uncommon findings include lymphadenopathy, prostatitis, decreased libido, semen abnormalities, and decreased exercise tolerance. The lymphadenopathy usually is regional at the site of inoculation early in the course of disease, but can become generalized and include splenomegaly with chronic infection [11]. Prostatitis is characterized by lymphocytic infiltration, which leads to destruction of the lobules and to fibrosis [14]. Brucella localization in the prostate accounts for therapeutic failures, recurrent bacteremia, and the chronic nature of the disease. Bilateral testicular atrophy and associated aspermia and decreased libido develop as the disease becomes chronic. Semen abnormalities are detectable as early as 5 weeks postinfection, and over 90% of sperm are abnormal by 20 weeks postinfection. Abnormalities include immature sperm, bent tails, swollen midpieces, and deformed acrosomes [11].

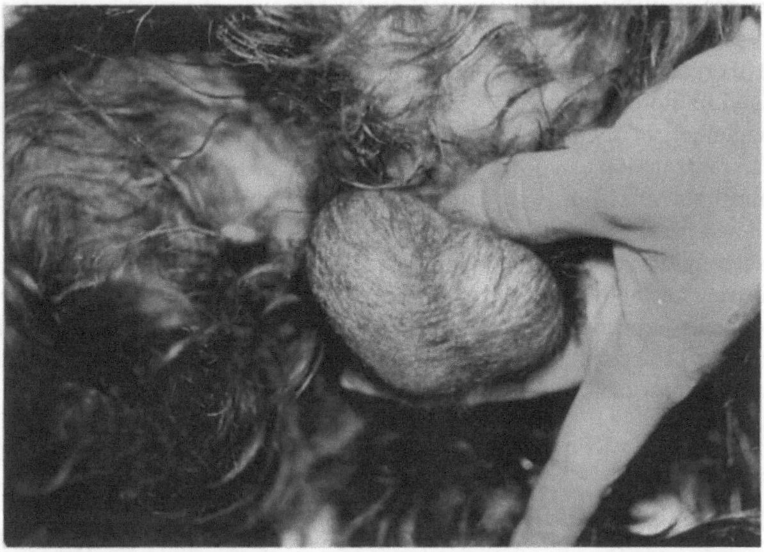

FIGURE 26.7. Scrotal edema and testicular asymmetry due to *Brucella canis*.

Infrequent clinical findings include discospondylitis, glomerulonephritis, and recurrent anterior uveitis (see section on complications).

## Histopathology

Since scrotal skin lesions are due to excessive licking rather than to invasion of the organism, histopathologic changes are nondiagnostic. They may include orthokeratotic hyperkeratosis of the epidermis, an eroded or ulcerated surface with dilation of the superficial dermal vasculature, and a perivascular mononuclear cell infiltrate.

Lymph nodes exhibit diffuse lymphoreticular hyperplasia and plasma cell infiltration. Phagocytized intracellular organisms may be seen in macrophages with the aid of special stains. The prostate, epididymis, scrotum, and penile sheath may show a necrotizing vasculitis. Uterine tissue often has a subacute to chronic endometritis with glandular hyperplasia [11].

## Natural History

Canine brucellosis was initially reported in 1966 in a New Jersey Beagle kennel and soon thereafter in numerous other states, although its origin is unknown. It cross-reacts antigenically with *B. ovis* but is similar morphologically to *B. suis* [11].

Natural transmission usually occurs by the venereal or oral routes. The minimum infectious dose by the oral route is approximately $2 \times 10^6$ organisms [11]. Accurate data are not available for the venereal route; however, it probably requires many fewer organisms [11,14]. Infection by the conjunctival route requires approximately $10^4$ to $10^5$ organisms. Transmission also occurs by the transmammary and intranasal routes and in utero [15,16].

High numbers of organisms are present in the semen for at least 8 weeks, although venereal transmission can occur for at least 2 years postinfection [10,14,15]. Urine concentrations vary from $10^3$ to $10^6$ organisms per milliliter. Casual contact between infected and noninfected dogs is unlikely to result in transmission [13].

A bacteremic state occurs within 3 weeks of transmission, at which time an agglutinating antibody response is detectable. The bacteremia is present for 1 to 3 years. Organisms proliferate in mononuclear phagocytic cells and remain intracellular throughout the course of infection. This results in generalized lymphoid hyperplasia and a polyclonal hyperglobulinemia.

## Complications

In addition to the previously mentioned reproductive tissue damage, nonreproductive tissues are affected as a result of the bacteremia or circulating immune complexes. Discospondylitis, anterior uveitis, meningoencephalitis, and glomerulonephritis have been reported secondary to brucellosis. Dogs with discospondylitis are reluctant to move, afebrile, have back pain, and have neurologic deficits [14]. The lumbar vertebrae are commonly affected, and paresis or ataxia may develop. Anterior uveitis and corneal edema may result from antibody formation.

Recurrences are associated with increased titers in the aqueous humor. Retinal detachment may occur in severe cases. Chronic nonsuppurative meningoencephalitis has been reported in experimentally infected dogs [17]. The glomerulopathy probably is immune complex induced.

*B. canis* has a mild zoonotic potential. The at-risk population includes laboratory personnel, animal caretakers, veterinarians, and owners of affected dogs [10,11,18]. Presenting signs include fatigue, fever, weight loss, lymphadenopathy, and malaise. Blood cultures and serologic examination should be used to diagnose human infections. Human brucellosis due to *B. canis* is much less severe compared with brucellosis contracted from other species. Most people respond well to tetracycline therapy. The most common means of transmission is contact with aborted fluid and tissues from affected bitches. Urine may also act as a vehicle for transmission.

## Differential Diagnosis

The list of conditions to be included in the differential diagnosis of scrotal dermatitis includes contact irritation, allergic contact dermatitis, flea allergy dermatitis, atopic dermatitis, food allergy, pemphigus foliaceus, pelodera dermatitis, hookworm dermatitis (ancylostomiasis and uncinariasis), and dermatophytosis. Contact irritation is the most common cause of scrotal dermatitis in my experience. Signalment, history, and physical examination usually make a simple task of differentiating the remaining list of diseases from brucellosis. No testicular or epididymal changes are expected with contact irritation as compared with brucellosis.

Several serologic assays are available to confirm the diagnosis of brucellosis. Most tests are invalid if taken within 4 weeks of infection or after recent antibiotic administration, as agglutinating titers may be low enough to cause a false-negative reaction. The standard rapid slide agglutination test (RSAT) has high sensitivity and is therefore a useful screening test. The high rate of false-positives requires additional diagnostics for confirmation. The addition of 2-mercaptoethanol to the RSAT has increased the specificity of commercially available test kits. True-positives are confirmed by the agar-gel immunodiffusion (AGID) test or the tube agglutination test (TAT), or by bacterial isolation from blood, lymph nodes, bone marrow, vaginal discharges, urine, or semen [10,11,14,15,18].

## Management

Recommendations for management of dogs infected with brucella vary depending on value and intended use of the dog and the willingness of the client to live with the public health risks. Options include therapy, observation, or euthanasia. Animals used for breeding purposes have little chance of becoming completely free of disease, and therefore usually do not return to breeding programs. Infected males are particularly difficult to clear due to localization of organisms in the prostate gland, where adequate antibiotic concentrations are difficult to achieve. Neutering pet animals is recommended to reduce zoonotic risk from genital fluids.

No single therapy has been routinely successful. Long-term antibiotic therapy using tetracycline, chloramphenicol, sulfonamides, and aminoglycosides has shown mixed results. Combination antibiotic therapy is more effective. Minocycline (25 mg/kg orally every 12 hours for 14 days) and streptomycin (10 mg/kg intramuscularly every 12 hours for 7 days) have been used successfully. Weekly repositol oxytetracycline injections (20 mg/kg IM) and streptomycin (15 mg/kg every 12 hours for 7 days) are also recommended. Long-term studies are necessary to assess efficacy, as animals may become bacteremic many months after cessation of therapy. Increased pup survival and decreased incidence of abortions in pregnant bitches occur with combination antibiotic therapy. No vaccine is currently available for prevention. Local disinfection using iodophors or quaternary ammonium compounds is effective for environmental control [11]. Problem kennels must undergo rigorous programs of serologic testing, isolation of new dogs, husbandry, and removal of affected dogs from the breeding pool in order to eliminate brucella.

## Prognosis

Although brucellosis in dogs is not fatal, it may result in the demise of the animal. The lack of an effective therapy and the zoonotic risk often lead clients to choose euthanasia, even though the affected dog may have few clinical signs. Breeders often choose euthanasia, because brucellosis essentially ends the reproductive career of the affected animal.

## References

1. Richardson RC: Canine transmissible venereal tumor. *Compend Cont Ed Pract Vet* **3**:951–959, 1981.
2. Calvert CA: Canine viral and transmissible neoplasias. In CA Greene (Ed): *Clinical Microbiology and Infectious Diseases of the Dog and Cat*. Philadelphia: WB Saunders, 1984, pp. 461–465.
3. Brown NO, MacEwen EG, Calvert C: Transmissible venereal tumor in the dog. *Calif Vet* **3**:6–9, 1981.
4. Calvert CA: Transmissible venereal tumor in the dog. In R Kirk (Ed): *Current Veterinary Therapy. VIII*. Philadelphia: WB Saunders, 1983, pp. 413–415.
5. Herron MA: Tumors of the canine genital system. *J Am Anim Hosp Assoc* **19**:981–994, 1983.
6. Withrow SJ, Susaneck SJ: Tumors of the canine female reproduction tract. In DA Morrow (Ed): *Current Therapy in Theriogenology. II*. Philadelphia: WB Saunders, 1986, pp. 526–527.
7. Strafuss AC: Clinical veterinary oncology. *Vet Clin North Am* **15**:485–486, 1985.
8. Cohen D, Steel GG: Thymidine labelling studies in a transmissible venereal tumor of the dog. *Br J Cancer* **26**:413, 1972.
9. Weber WT, Nowell PC, Hare WCD: Chromosome studies of a transplanted and a primary canine venereal sarcoma. *J Nat Cancer Inst* **35**:537–547, 1965.
10. Barton CL: Canine brucellosis. *Vet Clin North Am*, **7**:705–710, 1977.
11. Greene CE, George LW: Canine brucellosis. In CE Greene (Ed): *Clinical Microbiology and Infectious Diseases of the Dog and Cat*. Philadelphia: WB Saunders, 1984.
12. Dawkins BG, Machotka SV, Suchmann D, et al: Pyogranulomatous dermatitis associated with *Brucella canis* infection in a dog. *J Am Vet Med Assoc* **181**:1432–1433, 1982.
13. Carmichael LE, Kenney RM: Canine abortion caused by *Brucella canis*. *J Am Vet Med Assoc* **152**:605–616, 1968.
14. Pollock RVH: Canine brucellosis: Current status. *Compend Cont Educ Pract Vet* **1**:255–268, 1979.
15. Soderberg SF: Canine breeding management. *Vet Clin No Am*. **16**:419–433, 1986.
16. Krakowka S: Transplacentally acquired microbial and parasitic diseases of dogs. *J Am Vet Med Assoc* **171**:750–753, 1977.
17. Carmichael LE, George LW: Canine brucellosis: New knowledge. *Dev Biol Standard* **31**:237–250, 1976.
18. Swenson RM, Carmichael LE, Cundy KR: Human infection with *Brucella canis*. *Ann Intern Med* **76**:435–438, 1972.
19. Currier RW, Raithel WF, Martin RJ, et al: Canine brucellosis. *J Am Vet Med Assoc* **180**:132–133, 1982.

# Index

**T**

U

MIX
Papier aus verantwortungsvollen Quellen
Paper from responsible sources
FSC® C105338

If you have any concerns about our products,
you can contact us on
**ProductSafety@springernature.com**

In case Publisher is established outside the EU,
the EU authorized representative is:
**Springer Nature Customer Service Center GmbH**
**Europaplatz 3, 69115 Heidelberg, Germany**

Printed by Libri Plureos GmbH
in Hamburg, Germany